Introductory Statistical Inference
with the Likelihood Function

Charles A. Rohde

Introductory Statistical Inference with the Likelihood Function

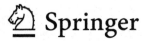 Springer

Charles A. Rohde
Bloomberg School of Health
Johns Hopkins University
Baltimore, MD, USA

ISBN 978-3-319-37481-9   ISBN 978-3-319-10461-4 (eBook)
DOI 10.1007/978-3-319-10461-4
Springer Cham Heidelberg New York Dordrecht London

Printed on acid-free paper

Springer is part of Springer Science+Business Media (www.springer.com)

To the memory of
Henry Laurence (Curly) Lucas
Advisor and Mentor
and my family
Savilla and RD
David Brooks Kitchel II
Denise Kitchel
David Brooks Kitchel III
Parker Kitchel

Preface

This book is a result of many years of teaching introductory statistical theory at the Johns Hopkins University Department of Biostatistics. It is designed for advanced undergraduates or master's level students.

The approach used is to introduce students to statistical theory without the use of too many advanced mathematical concepts which often inhibit the understanding of the basic philosophical foundations of statistics. In particular, attention is paid to the continuing debate on the foundations of statistics and the reasons why statistics "works" using any one of the major philosophical approaches to the subject. Most standard texts pay little or no attention to the contrasts between schools of statistical thought and how they related to each other. In particular I emphasize the Law of Likelihood as a way to connect various approaches.

Students must be made aware of the fact that there are no agreed upon methods for solving all of the problems to which modern statistics is asked to find solutions. I suspect that many of the current ad hoc procedures currently used will continue to be used for decades to come. A student can, however, be equipped at a modest level of mathematics with tools necessary to understand the myriad of statistical methods now available. The explosion of statistical packages in the last twenty years makes it possible for almost any one to perform analyses deemed intractable just a few years ago. This book is about some of the basic principles of statistics needed to criticize and understand the methods for analyzing complex data sets. I have included a short chapter on finite population sampling since I believe that every statistician should have some knowledge of the subject and since it forms the basis for much of what we know about contemporary society. It also clearly illustrates the need for some understanding of the foundations of statistics. I also included a section in the appendix on interpretations of probability, a subject which is often omitted in statistics texts. The remainder of the appendix consists of material on probability and some mathematical concepts which I find convenient to have in one place for reference.

A word on regularity conditions is in order. It often happens that a result is true provided some conditions are assumed. These are called **regularity conditions**.

In this book I am cavalier about these since being precise provides an additional layer of mathematics and often obscures the statistical concepts. In many cases it is easier to prove results from scratch rather than verify a list of regularity conditions.

I have tried to cite references for the many examples in the text. Unfortunately, as is often the case when lecture notes are developed into a book, some sources have been forgotten. I apologize in advance for these omissions and will correct them on the website as I become aware of them. The text is deliberately thin on exercises. Many more (with solutions) will appear on the website.

I thank the many students who have suffered through versions of these notes. I thank Richard Royall for many discussions and advice on statistics in general and likelihood in particular. Finally, I thank my wife, Savilla, for putting up with me.

Baltimore, Maryland
Charles A. Rohde
July 2014

Contents

Chapter 1
Introduction

1.1 Introductory Example

I have a list of 100 individuals, numbered 1–100. Associated with each is their disease status, diseased, d, or not diseased, $\bar{d}$.

I select a random sample (without replacement) of size 20 and record the disease status of each individual selected.

From basic probability theory the probability of obtaining x diseased in the sample of size 20 is given by the hypergeometric, i.e.,

$$\mathbb{P}(X = x) = \frac{\binom{D}{x}\binom{100-D}{20-x}}{\binom{100}{20}} \quad \text{for} \quad \max\{0, D-80\} \le x \le \min\{20, D\}$$

where D is the number of diseased individuals among the 100.

1. The problem is to use the observed value of x and the model, the hypergeometric, to learn about D. Equivalently, we want to learn about the proportion of diseased individuals $p = D/100$.
2. This is the fundamental problem of parametric statistical inference, reasoning from observed data to the parameters of the population which generated the data.
3. In fact, everything you need to know (well, almost everything) about parametric statistical inference is present in this example.

Suppose that the observed value in the sample was $x = 5$. What have we learned about D?

1. Clearly we have learned that D cannot be 0, 1, 2, 3, 4.
2. Nor can it be 100, 99, 98, 97, 96, 95, 94, 93, 92, 91, 90, 89, 88, 87, or 86.
3. What about 16 or 53 or 81?

© Springer International Publishing Switzerland 2014
C.A. Rohde, *Introductory Statistical Inference with the Likelihood Function*, DOI 10.1007/978-3-319-10461-4_1

The sample proportion is

$$\widehat{p} = \frac{5}{20}$$

and we might reason that the population proportion is about the same so that

$$\frac{\widehat{D}}{N} = \frac{5}{20} \text{ or } \widehat{D} = 25$$

is a good guess for the value of D.

1. But, how good?
2. What about values close to $\widehat{D}$, etc.?

1.1.1 Likelihood Approach

For any value of D we can calculate the probability of observing 5 in our sample. Thus

$$\mathbb{P}_D(5) = \frac{\binom{D}{5}\binom{100-D}{15}}{\binom{100}{20}} \text{ for } D = 0, 1, 2, \ldots, 100 \qquad (1.1)$$

It seems axiomatic that D_2 does better than D_1 at explaining the observed data if

$$\mathbb{P}_{D_2}(5) > \mathbb{P}_{D_1}(5)$$

which is a simple statement of the **Law of Likelihood** to be formalized later.

Comparisons between values of D can be facilitated by dividing each of the probabilities in (1.1) by their maximum. We call this the **likelihood** of D:

$$\mathscr{L}(D; \text{data}) = \frac{\mathbb{P}_D(\text{data})}{\max_D \mathbb{P}_D(\text{data})} \qquad (1.2)$$

A graph of $\mathscr{L}$ vs D provides a visual display of the relative merits of each value of D in explaining the observed data.

In addition we can find the values of D such that

$$\mathscr{L}(D; \text{data}) \geq \frac{1}{k}$$

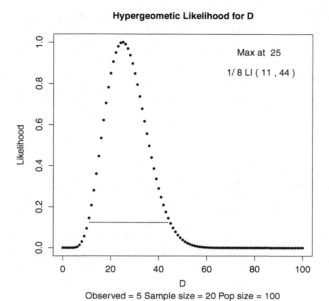

Fig. 1.1 1/8 likelihood interval for D

This interval is called a $\frac{1}{k}$ **likelihood interval**. Choice of the value of k will be explained later.

Here is the likelihood and the $\frac{1}{8}$ likelihood for this example (Fig. 1.1).

1.1.2 Bayesian Approach

Suppose now that I tell you that I selected D by drawing a number, at random between 0 and 100, i.e.,

$$\mathbb{P}(D = d) = \frac{1}{101} \text{ for } d = 0, 1, 2, \ldots, 100$$

This distribution is called a **prior** distribution for D.

By Bayes theorem we have

$$\mathbb{P}(D|X = 5) = \frac{\mathbb{P}(X = 5; D)\mathbb{P}(D)}{\sum_{d=0}^{100} \mathbb{P}X = 5; d)\mathbb{P}(d)} = \frac{\binom{D}{5}\binom{100-D}{20-5}}{\sum_{d=0}^{100} \binom{d}{x}\binom{100-d}{20-5}} \tag{1.3}$$

We can graph this density function which is called the **posterior distribution** of D.

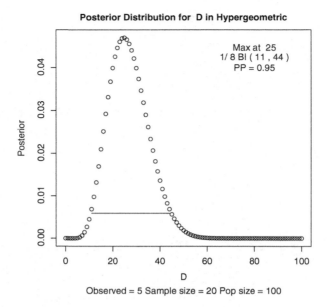

Posterior Distribution for D in Hypergeometric

Observed = 5 Sample size = 20 Pop size = 100

Fig. 1.2 Credible interval for D

We can also find an interval I such that the posterior probability that $D \in I$ is $100(1 - \alpha)\%$ and

$$\mathbb{P}(D_2|X = 5) \geq \mathbb{P}(D_1|X = 5) \ \ \text{if } D_2 \in I \text{ and } D_1 \notin I$$

This interval is called a **highest posterior density** (HPD) interval or posterior interval or Bayes or credible interval.

Here is the posterior distribution for this example and a 95 % posterior interval, called a 95 % **credible interval** (Fig. 1.2).

1.1.3 Frequentist Approach

Another approach to this problem is the frequentist confidence interval approach. The "logic" behind this approach is

(i) If D were large, observing 5 or less in the sample is unlikely. The upper confidence limit, $D_U(x)$, is the smallest D such that

$$\mathbb{P}_D(X \leq 5) \leq \frac{\alpha}{2}$$

Note that $\mathbb{P}(X \leq 5)$ decreases as D increases.

(ii) If D were small, observing 5 or more in the sample is unlikely. The lower confidence limit, $D_L(x)$, is the largest D such that

$$\mathbb{P}_D(X \geq 5) \leq \frac{\alpha}{2}$$

Note that $\mathbb{P}(X \geq 5)$ decreases as D decreases.

(iii) The interval $[D_L(x), D_U(x)]$ has the property that

$$\mathbb{P}_D \{[D_L(X), D_U(X)] \ni D\} \geq 1 - \alpha \ \text{ for any } D$$

(iv) The value of $\mathbb{P}_D \{[D_L(X), D_U(X)] \ni D\}$ is called the **coverage probability** of the interval which is called a **confidence interval**.

Choice of α will be discussed later.

Here is a graphical display of the confidence interval for this example (Fig. 1.3) .

1.1.4   Comments on the Example

The hypergeometric example shows the essence of the likelihood, Bayesian and frequentist approaches to statistical inference.

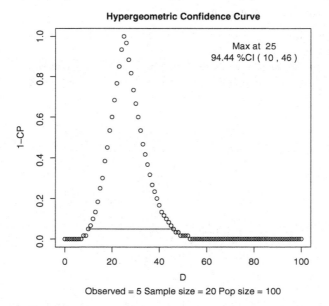

Fig. 1.3 Confidence interval for D

1. **Likelihood**

   (a) Easy to understand but doesn't suggest conclusions.
   (b) Turns out to be hard to use in complicated problems.
   (c) However, it does depend only on the data and the model.

2. **Bayesian**

   (a) Gives us what we want, probability statements about parameters.
   (b) However it requires prior probabilities which, for some, means it is not objective and thus not appropriate for science.
   (c) More later on "Objective Bayes" where priors are chosen so as to have minimal impact on the posterior.

3. **Frequentist**

   (a) Uses data not observed in the process of making inferences.
   (b) For decades it has been the approach of choice despite difficulty of interpretation.
   (c) Its use sometimes leads to "silly conclusions."

1.1.5   Choice of k and α

Choice of the values of k and α is somewhat arbitrary, but the following simple experiment provides some guidance:

1. I have two coins in my pocket: one is a normal quarter, and the other is a quarter with two heads.
2. I select a coin at random and toss it c times. Each toss is a head.
3. What is the probability that the quarter I am tossing is the two-headed one?

   By Bayes theorem

$$\mathbb{P}(\text{th}|c\text{ heads})$$

is given by

$$\frac{\mathbb{P}(c\text{ heads}|\text{th}\mathbb{P}(\text{th})}{\mathbb{P}(c\text{ heads}|\text{th})\mathbb{P}(\text{th}) + \mathbb{P}(c\text{ heads}|\text{n})\mathbb{P}(\text{n})}$$

which reduces to

$$\frac{\left(1 \times \frac{1}{2}\right)}{\left(1 \times \frac{1}{2}\right) + \left(\frac{1}{2^c} \times \frac{1}{2}\right)} = \frac{2^c}{2^c + 1}$$

1. If $c = 3$ this posterior probability is $8/9$ while the posterior probability that it was the normal quarter is $1/9$.
2. For $c = 4$ these probabilities are $16/17$ and $1/17$.

3. For $c = 5$ they are $32/33$ and $1/33$.
4. This suggests 8, 16, or 32 as values for k.

For the choice of α note that $c = 4$ gives a posterior probability of $1/17$ for the normal quarter which is a reasonable explanation of the reason α is often chosen to be 0.05, i.e., this value of α corresponds to being quite skeptical that the coin is really the normal coin.

1.2 What Is Statistics?

There are a variety of views of what constitutes statistical inference.

- "the purpose of inductive reasoning, based on empirical observations, is to improve our understanding of the systems from which these observations are drawn"
  Fisher [17]
- "A statistical inference will be defined for the purposes of the present paper to be a statement about statistical populations made from given observations with measured uncertainty."
  Cox [9]
- "statistics is concerned with decision making under uncertainty"
  Chernoff and Moses [7]
- "the problem of inference, or how degrees of belief are altered by data"
  Lindley [29]
- "By statistical inference I mean how we find things out—whether with a view to using the new knowledge as a basis for explicit action or not—and how it comes to pass that we often acquire practically identical opinions in the light of evidence"
  Savage [45]
- We aim, in fact, at methods of inference which should be equally convincing to all rational minds, irrespective of any intentions they may have in utilizing the knowledge inferred. We have the duty of formulating, of summarizing, and of communicating our conclusions, in intelligible form, in recognition of the right of other free minds to utilize them in making their own decisions.
  Fisher [16]

  - A statistical analysis of a data set, ..., is supposed to conclude what the data say and how far these conclusions can be trusted.
  - Statistics is the theory of accumulating information (evidence) especially information (evidence) that arrives a little bit at a time.
    Bradley Efron
  - Statistics is the study of algorithms for data analysis.
    Rudy Beran

- Its most important task is to provide objective quantitative alternatives to personal judgment for interpreting the evidence produced by experiments and observational studies.
  Royall [43]

With such a wide variety of different conceptions about what constitutes statistics it is not surprising that many have a distaste for the subject.

1.2.1 General Setup

The following pictures illustrate the statistical approach to scientific problems starting with the basic example.

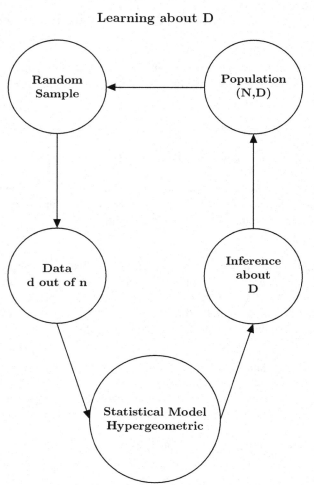

Learning about D

Scientific Learning

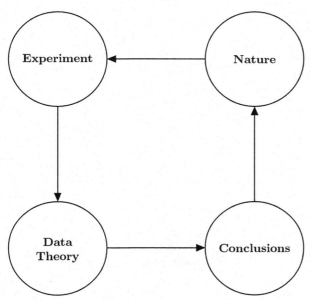

In this book we will concentrate on the inference part of the last diagram.

1.2.2   Scope of Statistical Inference

I will take the following as a working definition of statistical inference.

> Statistical inference is the process of learning about probability models using observed data.

To be more specific suppose we have observed data x assumed to be modeled by a probability density function f. The goal of statistical inference is then to learn about f.

Scientific Learning and Statistics

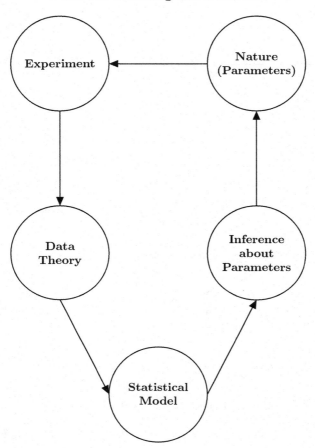

More precisely:

1. Given observed data what do we know about f?
2. How well do we know it?
3. How do we convey what we know?

or

1. Given observed data what evidence do we have about f?
2. How strong is the evidence?
3. How do we convey the evidence?

Chapter 2
The Statistical Approach

2.1 The Setup

Assume that we have observed data $D = x$ which was the result of a random experiment X (or can be approximated as such). The data are then modelled using

1. A sample space, $\mathcal{X}$ for the observed value of x
2. A probability density function for X at x, $f(x; \theta)$
3. A parameter space for θ, Θ

The **inference problem** is to use x to infer properties of θ.

2.2 Approaches to Statistical Inference

The major approaches to statistical inference are:

1. **Frequentist** or classical
2. **Bayesian**
3. **Likelihood**

2.3 Types of Statistical Inference

There are four major statistical inferences:

1. **Estimation:** Select one value of θ, the estimate, to be reported. Some measure of reliability is assumed to be reported as well.

© Springer International Publishing Switzerland 2014
C.A. Rohde, *Introductory Statistical Inference with the Likelihood Function*, DOI 10.1007/978-3-319-10461-4_2

2. **Testing:** Compare two values (or sets of values) of θ and choose one of them as better.
3. **Interval Estimation:** Select a region of θ values as being consistent, in some sense, with the observed data.
4. **Prediction:** Use the observed data to predict a new result of the experiment.

Note that the first three inferences can be defined as functions from the sample space to subsets of the parameter space. Thus estimation of θ is achieved by defining

$$\widehat{\theta} : \mathcal{X} \mapsto \Theta$$

Then the observation of x results in $\widehat{\theta}(x)$ as the estimated value of θ for the observed data. Similarly hypothesis testing maps $\mathcal{X}$ into $\{\Theta_0, \Theta_1\}$ and interval estimation maps $\mathcal{X}$ into subsets (intervals) of Θ.

2.4   Statistics and Combinants

2.4.1   Statistics and Sampling Distributions

Since inferences are defined by functions on the sample space it is convenient to have some nomenclature.

Definition 2.4.1. A **statistic** is a real or vector-valued function defined on the sample space of a statistical model.

The sample mean, sample variance, sample median, and sample correlation are all statistics.

Definition 2.4.2. The probability distribution of a statistic is called its **sampling distribution**.

A major problem in standard or frequentist statistical theory is the determination of sampling distributions:

1. Either exactly (using probability concepts)
2. Approximately (using large sample results)
3. By simulation (using R or similar statistical software)

2.4.2   Combinants

Definition 2.4.3. A **combinant** is a real or vector-valued function defined on the sample space and the parameter space such that for each fixed θ it is a statistic.

Thus a combinant is defined for pairs (x, θ) where x is in the sample space and θ is in the parameter space. For each θ it is required to be a statistic.

The density function $f(x; \theta)$ is a combinant, as are the likelihood and functions of the likelihood.

Definition 2.4.4. If $f(x; \theta)$ is the density of x the **score function** is the combinant defined by

$$s(\theta; x) = \frac{\partial f(x : \theta)}{\partial \theta}$$

(This assumes differentiation with respect to θ is defined.)

Definition 2.4.5. The **score equation** is the equation (in θ) defined by

$$s(\theta; x) = \frac{\partial f(x : \theta)}{\partial \theta} = 0$$

The solution to this equation gives the maximum likelihood estimate, MLE, of θ.

Combinants are used to determine estimates, interval estimates, and tests as well as to investigate the frequency properties of likelihood-based quantities.

2.4.3 Frequentist Inference

In the **frequentist paradigm** inference is the process of connecting the observed data and the inference (statements about the parameters) using the **sampling distribution** of a statistic. Note that the sampling distribution is determined by the density function $f(x; \theta)$.

2.4.4 Bayesian Inference

In the **Bayesian paradigm** inference is the process of connecting the observed data and the inference (statements about the parameters) using the **posterior distribution** of the parameter values. The **posterior distribution** is determined by the model density and the **prior distribution** of θ using Bayes theorem (this implicitly treats $f(x; \theta)$ as the conditional $f(x|\theta)$ of X given θ):

$$p(\theta|x) = \frac{f(x; \theta)\text{prior}(\theta)}{f(x)}$$

where $f(x)$ is the marginal distribution of X at x.

$$f(x) = \int_{\Theta} f(x;\theta)\mathrm{prior}(\theta)d\theta$$

2.4.5 Likelihood Inference

In the **likelihood paradigm** inference is the process of evaluating the statistical evidence for parameter values provided by the likelihood function.

The statistical evidence for θ_2 vis-a-vis θ_1 is defined by

$$\mathrm{Ev}(\theta_2 : \theta_1 ; x) = \frac{f(x;\theta_2)}{f(x;\theta_1)}$$

Values for this ratio of 8, 16, and 32 are taken as moderate, strong, and very strong evidence, respectively.

Note that if we define the **likelihood** of θ as

$$\mathscr{L}(\theta;x) = \frac{f(x;\theta)}{f(x;\widehat{\theta})}$$

where $\widehat{\theta}$ is the maximum likelihood estimate of θ, then the statistical evidence for θ_2 vs θ_1 can be expressed as

$$\mathrm{Ev}(\theta_2 : \theta_1 ; x) = \frac{\mathscr{L}(\theta_2;x)}{\mathscr{L}(\theta_1;x)}$$

and the posterior of θ can then be expressed as

$$p(\theta|x) = \frac{\mathscr{L}(\theta;x)\mathrm{prior}(\theta)}{f(x)}$$

i.e., the posterior is proportional to the product of the likelihood and the prior.

2.5 Exercises

As pointed out in the text if $f(\mathbf{x};\theta)$ is the density function of the observed data $(x_1, x_2, \ldots, x_n)$ and θ is the parameter, then

(a) The **likelihood**, $\mathscr{L}(\theta;\mathbf{x})$, is

$$\mathscr{L}(\theta) = \frac{f(\mathbf{x};\theta)}{f(\mathbf{x};\widehat{\theta})}$$

where $\widehat{\theta}$ maximizes $f(\mathbf{x};\theta)$ and is called the maximum likelihood estimate of θ.

(b) The **score function** is

$$\frac{\partial \ln[f(\mathbf{x}; \theta)]}{\partial \theta}$$

(c) The **observed Fisher information** is

$$J(\theta) = - \frac{\partial^2 \ln[f(\mathbf{x}; \theta)]}{\partial \theta^2}$$

evaluated at $\theta = \widehat{\theta}$.

(d) The **expected Fisher information**, $I(\theta)$, is the expected value of $J(\theta)$, i.e.,

$$I(\theta) = -\mathbb{E}\left\{ \frac{\partial^2 \ln[f(\mathbf{x}; \theta)]}{\partial \theta^2} \right\}$$

1. Find the likelihood, the maximum likelihood estimate, the score function, and the observed and expected Fisher information when $x_1, x_2, \ldots, x_n$ represent the results of a random sample from

    (i) A normal distribution with expected value θ and known variance σ^2
    (ii) A Poisson distribution with parameter θ
    (iii) A Gamma distribution with known parameter α and θ

2. For each of the problems in (1) generate a random sample of size 25, i.e.:

    (i) Take $\sigma^2 = 1$ and $\theta = 3$.
    (ii) Take $\theta = 5$.
    (iii) Take $\alpha = 3$ and $\theta = 2$.

    For (i)–(iii) plot the likelihood functions.

3. Suppose that Y_i for $i = 1, 2, \ldots, n$ are independent, each normal with expected value βx_i and variance σ^2 where σ^2 is known and the x_i are known constants.

    (i) Show that the joint density is

    $$f(\mathbf{y}; \beta) = (2\pi\sigma^2)^{-n/2} \exp\left\{ -\frac{1}{2\sigma^2} \sum_{i=1}^{n} (y_i - \beta\, x_i)^2 \right\}$$

    (ii) Find the score function.
    (iii) Show that the maximum likelihood estimate for β is

    $$\widehat{\beta} = \frac{\sum_{i=1}^{n} x_i y_i}{\sum_{i=1}^{n} x_i^2}$$

    (iv) Find the observed Fisher information.

(v)   Using (iii) find the likelihood for β.
(vi) Find the sampling distribution of $\widehat{\beta}$. Remember that the sum of independent normal random variables is also normal.
(vii) Show that the sampling distribution of $-2\ln[\mathcal{L}(\beta;\mathbf{y})]$ is chi-square with 1 degree of freedom.

Chapter 3
Estimation

3.1 Frequentist Concepts

As previously indicated the major problems of inference are estimation, testing, and interval estimation.

1. Of these estimation is the easiest to understand and in certain respects the most important.
2. Intuitively, a point estimate is simply a guess as to the value of a parameter of interest.
3. Along with this guess it is customary to provide some measure of reliability.

We assume a statistical model $(\mathcal{X}, f(x\,;\theta), \Theta)$ for X and an observed value x_{obs}. From the classical, frequentist, point of view an estimate is evaluated on the basis of its properties if used repeatedly, i.e., based on its sampling distribution.

To be precise in discussing estimation we often need to distinguish between:

1. The **true value** of the parameter being estimated, θ_0
2. The **estimator**, i.e., the rule by which we calculate the estimate
3. The **estimate**, i.e., the actual estimate determined by the estimator evaluated at a particular observed value of X, x_{obs}
4. Other values of the parameter, θ

Note that an **estimator** is a statistic, and its probability distribution is called its **sampling distribution**. We typically denote an estimator by $\widehat{\theta}_n$, neglecting the dependence on X but emphasizing the dependence on the sample size. Properties of the sampling distribution determine which of the several estimators is preferred in a given problem and whether an estimator is "good."

© Springer International Publishing Switzerland 2014
C.A. Rohde, *Introductory Statistical Inference with the Likelihood Function*, DOI 10.1007/978-3-319-10461-4_3

3.1.1   Bias, Unbiasedness, and Standard Errors

The most important properties of the sampling distribution of an estimator are

1. Its **location**, e.g., $E_{\theta_0}(\widehat{\theta}_n)$.
2. If $E_{\theta_0}(\widehat{\theta}_n) = \theta_0$. The estimator $\widehat{\theta}_n$ is said to be an **unbiased** estimator.
3. The **bias** of an estimator is

$$B_n(\theta_0) = E_{\theta_0}(\widehat{\theta}_n) - \theta_0$$

4. The **standard error** of an estimator is defined as

$$\text{s.e.}(\widehat{\theta}) = \sqrt{\text{var}(\widehat{\theta}_n)}$$

5. The standard error of an estimator is the natural measure of reliability for an estimator in frequentist statistics.
6. Note that the standard error of an estimator is the standard deviation of the sampling distribution of the estimator.

3.1.2   Consistency

Definition 3.1.1. If the true value of the parameter is θ_0 an estimator is **consistent** if

$$\widehat{\theta}_n \xrightarrow{p} \theta_0$$

Intuitively, an estimator is consistent if for large sample sizes the probability that the estimator is "close to" the true parameter value is near one. Recall that convergence in probability means that

$$\lim_{n \to \infty} \mathbb{P}(|\widehat{\theta}_n - \theta_0| < \epsilon) = 1$$

Most statisticians consider consistency a minimal requirement for an estimator. Unfortunately, consistency, as are most properties of sampling distributions, is of little help in evaluating a particular estimate. It is only a property which guarantees closeness with high probability but not for any particular sample.

Example. If $X_1, X_2, \ldots, X_n$ are independent and identically distributed with expected value θ and variance σ^2 then

$$\overline{X}_n \xrightarrow{p} \theta$$

by the weak law of large numbers so that $\overline{X}_n$ is a consistent estimator of θ.

If we define a new estimator, $\widetilde{\theta}_n$, as

$$\widetilde{\theta}_n = \begin{cases} -17 & n \leq n_1 \\ \overline{X}_n & n > n_1 \end{cases}$$

then $\widetilde{\theta}_n$ is also consistent. If, however, $n_1 = 10^{10^{10}}$ this estimator is of no practical use.

Use of consistency as a criterion should include some simulation to ensure at least some level of decent small-sample behavior. The same is true of other asymptotic properties.

Example. Consider the Bernoulli trial model, i.e., $X_1, X_2, \ldots, X_n$ are independent and

$$\mathbb{P}(X = x) = \begin{cases} p & \text{if } x = 1 \\ 1 - p & \text{if } x = 0 \end{cases}$$

This might represent the result of a sample of n individuals and recording their disease status, 1 being diseased, 0 disease free. The usual estimator is the observed frequency and is given by

$$\widehat{p}_n = \frac{X}{n}$$

where

$$X = X_1 + X_2 + \cdots + X_n$$

Note that

$$E_{p_0}(\widehat{p}_n) = p_0$$

so that $\widehat{p}_n$ is an **unbiased** estimator. Also note that

$$\text{var}(\widehat{p}_n) = \frac{p_0(1 - p_0)}{n}$$

and hence the standard error of $\widehat{p}_n$ is

$$\text{s.e.}(\widehat{p}_n) = \sqrt{\frac{p_0(1 - p_0)}{n}}$$

Recall that Markov's inequality states that if Y is a nonnegative random variable then for any $\delta > 0$

$$\mathbb{P}(Y \geq \delta) \leq \frac{\mathbb{E}(X)}{\delta}$$

By Markov's inequality we have that

$$\mathbb{P}_{p_0}(|\widehat{p}_n - p_0| < \epsilon) \geq 1 - \frac{p_0(1 - p_0)}{n\epsilon^2} \quad \rightarrow \quad 1 \ \text{ as } n \rightarrow \infty$$

so that $\widehat{p}_n$ is a consistent estimator.

3.1.3   Mean Square Error

Consistency is a large sample property. A criterion useful for small samples is mean square error.

Definition 3.1.2. The **mean square error** of an estimator is

$$\text{MSE} = \mathbb{E}_\theta(\widehat{\theta}_n - \theta)^2$$

It easy to show that

$$\text{MSE}(\widehat{\theta}_n) = \mathbb{V}_\theta(\widehat{\theta}_n) + [\text{Bias}(\widehat{\theta}_n)]^2$$

i.e., the mean square error equals the variance plus the bias squared.

Theorem 3.1.1. *If the mean square error of an estimator approaches 0 as $n \rightarrow \infty$, then it is consistent.*

Proof of this result simply uses Markov's inequality.

3.1.4   Asymptotic Distributions

Another useful property of estimators is their asymptotic distribution which can serve as a large sample approximation to their sampling distribution.

Definition 3.1.3. An estimator $\widehat{\theta}_n$ is **asymptotically normal** if

$$\frac{\widehat{\theta}_n - \theta_0}{v_n(\widehat{\theta}_n)} \xrightarrow{d} \text{N}(0, 1)$$

Note that the expected value of $\widehat{\theta}_n$ is not necessarily θ_0 and that $v_n(\widehat{\theta}_n)$ is not necessarily the standard error of $\widehat{\theta}_n$.

Example. For Bernoulli trials the central limit theorem implies that

$$\frac{\widehat{p}_n - p}{\sqrt{p(1-p)/n}} \xrightarrow{d} \text{N}(0,1)$$

We may replace p in the standard error by $\widehat{p}$ and still have asymptotic normality.

Example. Assume that we have a sample $\mathbf{x} = x_1, x_2, \ldots, x_n$ which is a realized value of $\mathbf{X} = (X_1, X_2, \ldots, X_n)$ where the X_i are iid N (μ, σ^2) and σ^2 is known. Of interest is inference on μ.

The joint density is given by

$$f(\mathbf{y}; \mu) = \prod_{i=1}^{n} (2\pi\sigma^2)^{-\frac{1}{2}} \exp\left\{ -\frac{(x_i - \mu)^2}{2\sigma^2} \right\}$$

A natural estimate of μ is $\overline{x}$ and this is also the maximum likelihood estimate. Since

$$\mathbb{E}_\mu(\overline{X}_n) = \mu$$

$\overline{X}_n$ is an unbiased estimator for μ. The variance of $\overline{X}_n$ is σ^2/n so that the mean square error is

$$\text{MSE}(\overline{X}_n) = \frac{\sigma^2}{n}$$

This tends to 0 as $n \to \infty$ so that $\overline{X}_n$ is a consistent estimator of μ.

We also know that the distribution of $\overline{X}_n$ is

$$\text{N}\left(\mu, \frac{\sigma^2}{n}\right)$$

It is trivially asymptotically normal since

$$\frac{\overline{X} - \mu}{\sigma/\sqrt{n}} \text{ is exactly normal } (0,1)$$

3.1.5 Efficiency

Comparison of estimators is achieved by considering the relative efficiency.

Definition 3.1.4. The **relative efficiency** of two estimators $\widehat{\theta}_n^{(1)}$ and $\widehat{\theta}_n^{(2)}$ of a parameter θ is

$$\frac{\mathrm{MSE}(\widehat{\theta}_n^{(2)})}{\mathrm{MSE}(\widehat{\theta}_n^{(1)})}$$

Generally speaking if the relative efficiency is less than one we prefer $\widehat{\theta}_n^{(2)}$ because it has smaller mean square error.

If the estimators are unbiased then the above criteria say to choose the estimator with the smallest variance.

Example (Dangers of Frequentist Statistics).. Suppose we observe X_1 and X_2 independent each with pdf given by

$$f(x;\theta) = \begin{cases} \frac{1}{2} \text{ if } x = \theta + 1 \\ \frac{1}{2} \text{ if } x = \theta - 1 \end{cases}$$

where θ is an integer.

Then the joint distribution of X_1 and X_2 is given by

$$\mathbb{P}_\theta(X_1 = \theta - 1, X_2 = \theta - 1) = 1/4$$
$$\mathbb{P}_\theta(X_1 = \theta - 1, X_2 = \theta + 1) = 1/4$$
$$\mathbb{P}_\theta(X_1 = \theta + 1, X_2 = \theta - 1) = 1/4$$
$$\mathbb{P}_\theta(X_1 = \theta + 1, X_2 = \theta + 1) = 1/4$$

Consider the estimator of θ defined by

$$\widehat{\theta} = \begin{cases} \frac{X_1 + X_2}{2} \ X_1 \neq X_2 \\ X_1 + 1 \ X_1 = X_2 \end{cases}$$

The sampling distribution of $\widehat{\theta}$ is given by

$$P_\theta(\widehat{\theta} = \theta) = \frac{3}{4} \ ; \ \mathbb{P}_\theta(\widehat{\theta} = \theta + 2) = \frac{1}{4}$$

It follows that

$$\mathbb{E}_\theta(\widehat{\theta}) = \theta + \frac{1}{2} \text{ and } \mathbb{E}_\theta(\widehat{\theta}^2) = \frac{3\theta^2}{4} + \frac{(\theta + 2)^2}{4} = \theta^2 + \theta + 1$$

and hence

$$\mathbb{V}_\theta(\widehat{\theta}) = \left\{\theta^2 + \theta + 1\right\} - \left\{\theta^2 + \theta + \frac{1}{4}\right\} = \frac{3}{4}$$

The mean square error of $\widehat{\theta}$ is

$$\mathbb{E}_\theta(\widehat{\theta} - \theta)^2 = \mathbb{V}_\theta(\widehat{\theta}) + \left(\text{Bias}(\widehat{\theta})\right)^2$$
$$= \frac{3}{4} + \frac{1}{4}$$
$$= 1$$

Consider the unbiased estimator $\widetilde{\theta} = \widehat{\theta} - 1/2$ which has mean square error

$$\mathbb{E}_\theta(\widetilde{\theta} - \theta)^2 = \mathbb{V}_\theta(\widehat{\theta} - 1/2) + [\text{Bias}(\widetilde{\theta})]^2 = \mathbb{V}_\theta(\widehat{\theta}) = \frac{3}{4}$$

Thus $\widetilde{\theta}$ has smaller mean square error than $\widehat{\theta}$ but is always wrong whereas $\widehat{\theta}$ is right 75 % of the time.

The moral is: blind adherence to frequentist criteria can lead to undesirable statements.

3.1.6 Equivariance

Definition 3.1.5. An estimating procedure or property is **equivariant** if the estimator of $g(\theta)$ is $g(\widehat{\theta}_n)$.

This is an appealing property but is not possessed by many popular estimators. We will prove in a later section that maximum likelihood estimators are equivariant.

We know that $\overline{X}_n$ is an unbiased estimator of μ. However $\overline{X}_n^2$ is not an unbiased estimator of μ^2 since

$$\mathbb{E}_\mu(\overline{X}_n^2) = [\mathbb{E}_\mu(\overline{X}_n)]^2 + \mathbb{V}_\mu(\overline{X}_n) = \mu^2 + \frac{\sigma^2}{n}$$

Thus unbiased estimators do not possess the equivariance property.

In the binomial we know that $\widehat{p} = X/n$ is unbiased. However, if we are interested in the odds, i.e., $\frac{p}{1-p}$, then the natural estimator $\frac{\widehat{p}}{1-\widehat{p}}$ does not even have an expected value since there is a positive probability that $\widehat{p} = 1$.

3.2 Bayesian and Likelihood Paradigms

We defer detailed discussion of the use of the Bayes and likelihood approaches to estimation in later chapters.

1. Essentially the Bayesian uses as an estimate a measure obtained from the posterior distribution of the parameter such as the posterior mean or median. Reliability is assessed by the posterior standard error of that estimate.
2. In the likelihood paradigm the focus is not directly on estimation. However, the maximum of the likelihood occurs at the parameter value which is most consistent with the observed data and is thus a natural estimate. The curvature of the likelihood function at the maximum can be used as a measure of reliability.

3.3   Exercises

1. Show that MSE $= \mathbb{V}(\widehat{\theta}) + [\mathbb{B}(\widehat{\theta})]^2$.
2. Suppose that $X_1, X_2, \ldots, X_n$ are independent each exponential, i.e., each X_i has pdf

$$f(x; \theta) = \frac{e^{-x/\theta}}{\theta} \quad x \geq 0$$

This pdf is often used to model response or survival times.

(a) Find the joint density of the X_i and hence find the score function.
(b) Using the score function show that the maximum likelihood estimator for θ is $\widehat{\theta} = \overline{X}$. Show that it is unbiased, consistent, and find its variance.
(c) Using the joint density you found in (a) and the maximum likelihood estimate you found in (b) show that the likelihood function for θ is

$$\mathscr{L}(\theta; \mathbf{x}) = \frac{f(\mathbf{x}; \theta)}{f(\mathbf{x}; \widehat{\theta})} = \left(\frac{\widehat{\theta}}{\theta}\right)^n \exp\left\{-n\left(\frac{\widehat{\theta}}{\theta} - 1\right)\right\}$$

(d) The exponential is a special case of the Gamma which has pdf

$$f(y; \theta) = \frac{y^{\alpha-1}e^{-y/\beta}}{\Gamma(\alpha)\beta^\alpha} \quad y \geq 0$$

(i.e., $\alpha = 1$ and $\beta = \theta$). It is known that if $X_1, X_2, \ldots, X_n$ are independent each gamma (α_i, β) then

$$S_n = X_1 + X_2 + \ldots + X_n$$

has a Gamma pdf with parameters

$$\alpha = \alpha_1 + \alpha_2 + \cdots + \alpha_n \quad \text{and} \quad \beta$$

Using this fact show that the pdf of $Y = n\widehat{\theta}$ is

$$f(y; \theta) = \frac{y^{n-1} \exp\left\{-\frac{y}{\theta}\right\}}{\Gamma(n)\theta^n}$$

3. A scientist needs to weigh three objects O_1, O_2, and O_3 each of which weighs between 0.5 and 1.0 g. Unfortunately she only has a scale which can weigh objects only if their weight exceeds 1 g.

    (a) Show that she can get a weight for each one by weighing them two at a time, i.e., she weighs O_1 and O_2 together and gets Y_1 and so on.
    (b) Find the variance of her estimated weights (assume weights are uncorrelated).

4. Suppose that $X_1, X_2, \ldots, X_n$ are independent with density function (continuous) f and distribution function F.

    (a) Find an expression for the density function of

$$Y_n = \max\{X_1, X_2, \ldots, X_n\}$$

    (b) Find an expression for the density function of

$$Y_1 = \min\{X_1, X_2, \ldots, X_n\}$$

5. Suppose that the density of X is

$$f(x) = \exp\left\{-(x - \theta)\right\} \quad \text{for } x \geq \theta$$

and that we have $X_1, X_2, \ldots, X_n$ independent each with density f.

    (a) Write down the joint density of $X_1, X_2, \ldots, X_n$.
    (b) Find the maximum likelihood estimator for θ. Note you cannot do this by differentiating (why?).

6. (Bonus Problem) Suppose that $X_1, X_2, \ldots, X_n$ are independent each uniform on the interval $[0, \theta]$ where $\theta > 0$.

    (a) Find the distribution of $Y_n = \max\{X_1, X_2, \ldots, X_n\}$.
    (b) Show that the limiting distribution of Z_n where

$$Z_n = n(\theta - Y_n)$$

is exponential θ, i.e.,

$$f(z; \theta) = \theta^{-1} e^{-z/\theta} \quad z \geq 0$$

Note that the limiting distribution is not normal.

(c) Generate 1,000 samples of size 50 from a uniform on $[0, 5]$ and plot the histogram of Z_{50}. Superimpose the plot of the limiting distribution.

(d) Show that the MLE of θ is Y_n.

(e) Discuss the asymptotic distribution of $2\overline{X}_n$ which is an unbiased estimator of θ.

(h) Compare the estimators in (d) and (e).

Chapter 4
Interval Estimation

4.1 The Problem

In this chapter we describe methods for finding interval or set estimators mainly illustrated using random samples from the normal distribution.

The importance of interval estimation is that it most clearly provides an answer to summarizing the information in the data about a parameter. Indeed, many professional journals now are suggesting that intervals be reported as opposed to the results of hypothesis tests.

4.2 Frequentist Approach

A general method of obtaining interval estimates for θ assumes that we have a statistic T_n such that

(i) small values of T_n are rare if θ is large
(ii) large values of T_n are rare if θ is small

where rare is defined by

$$P_\theta(T_n \leq t_{obs}) \leq \alpha/2 \ \text{ and } \ P_\theta(T_n \geq t_{obs}) \leq \alpha/2$$

and α is small (usually $\alpha = 0.05$).

Then a $100(1 - \alpha)\%$ confidence interval for θ has upper endpoint

$$\theta_U(t_{obs}) = \min_\theta \{\theta : \ P_\theta(T_n \leq t_{obs}) \leq \alpha/2\}$$

© Springer International Publishing Switzerland 2014
C.A. Rohde, *Introductory Statistical Inference with the Likelihood Function*, DOI 10.1007/978-3-319-10461-4__4

and lower endpoint

$$\theta_L(t_{obs}) = \max_{\theta}\{\theta : P_\theta(T_n \geq t_{obs}) \leq \alpha/2\}$$

1. The interval of θ values defined by

$$\theta_L(T_n) \leq \theta \leq \theta_U(T_n)$$

   is called a $100(1 - \alpha)\%$ **confidence interval** for θ.
2. $1 - \alpha$ is called the **coverage probability** of the interval.
3. A fundamental problem in using frequentist confidence intervals is the determination of coverage probabilities.
4. This can be done exactly using the distribution of T_n, asymptotically, approximately (using the bootstrap) or by simulation.

   The interval is a random interval. Once an observed value, t_{obs}, is substituted for T_n, the resulting interval, given by,

$$\theta_L(t_{obs}) \leq \theta \leq \theta_U(t_{obs})$$

either covers θ or it doesn't. We don't know which.

The fact that an interval estimate has little to do with a particular data set (the so-called single case) is well known but little appreciated. As Neyman himself put it:

"The available models are then used to deduce rules of behavior (or statistical decision functions) that, in a sense, minimize the frequency of wrong decisions. **It would be nice if something could be done to guard against errors in each particular case. However, as long as the postulate is maintained that the observations are subject to variation affected by chance (in the sense of the frequentist theory of probability), all that appears possible to do is to control the frequencies of errors in a sequence of situations $\{S_n\}$, whether similar, or all very different.**" Neyman [35]

4.2.1 Importance of the Long Run

As an example to illustrate the importance of the long-run concept suppose that we observe X_1 and X_2 independent each with pdf given by

$$f(x; \theta) = \begin{cases} \frac{1}{2} & \text{if } x = \theta + 1 \\ \frac{1}{2} & \text{if } x = \theta - 1 \end{cases}$$

where θ is an integer.

The "interval" defined by

$$\mathscr{I}(X_1, X_2) = \begin{cases} \frac{X_1 + X_2}{2} & X_1 \neq X_2 \\ X_1 + 1 & X_1 = X_2 \end{cases}$$

is a 75 % confidence "interval" for θ.

To see this note that

$$\mathbb{P}_\theta(\mathscr{I}(X_1, X_2) \supseteq \theta) =$$
$$= \mathbb{P}_\theta(\mathscr{I}(X_1, X_2) \supseteq \theta | X_1 \neq X_2)\mathbb{P}_\theta(X_1 \neq X_2)$$
$$+ \mathbb{P}_\theta(\mathscr{I}(X_1, X_2) \supseteq \theta | X_1 = X_2)\mathbb{P}_\theta(X_1 = X_2)$$
$$= (1) \times \left(\frac{1}{2}\right) + \left(\frac{1}{2}\right) \times \left(\frac{1}{2}\right)$$
$$= \frac{1}{2} + \frac{1}{4}$$
$$= 0.75$$

Suppose now that we observe

$$X_1 = 4 \text{ and } X_2 = 6$$

Then we know that

$$\theta - 1 = 4 \text{ and } \theta + 1 = 6$$

so that θ is exactly 5, i.e., there is no uncertainty left.

But a frequentist can only say that this is a 75 % confidence interval for θ i.e. beware the particular case as Neyman advised.

4.2.2 Application to the Normal Distribution

Given a random sample from a normal distribution with known variance σ^2 we let $T_n = \overline{X}_n$. Then

$$\mathbb{P}_\mu(\overline{X}_n \leq \overline{x}_{obs}) = \mathbb{P}\left(Z \leq \frac{\sqrt{n}(\overline{x}_{obs} - \mu)}{\sigma}\right)$$

where Z is a standard normal random variable.

It follows that for the upper endpoint we have

$$\frac{\sqrt{n}(\overline{x}_{obs} - \mu_U)}{\sigma} = -z_{1-\alpha/2}$$

or

$$\mu_U(x_{obs}) = \overline{x}_{obs} + z_{1-\alpha/2}\frac{\sigma}{\sqrt{n}}$$

Similarly the lower endpoint is given by

$$\mu_L(x_{obs}) = \overline{x}_{obs} - z_{1-\alpha/2}\frac{\sigma}{\sqrt{n}}$$

The interval

$$\overline{x}_{obs} \pm z_{1-\alpha/2}\frac{\sigma}{\sqrt{n}}$$

is called a $100(1 - \alpha)$ confidence interval for the parameter μ. Typically the value of α is taken to be 0.05 in which case $z_{1-\alpha/2} = 1.96$.

Since $\overline{X}$ is the natural estimator of μ which has variance σ^2/n the interval has the approximate form

$$\text{estimate} \pm 2 \text{ s.e.}$$

where s.e. is the standard error of the estimator (square root of the variance of the estimator).

The **random** interval defined by

$$[\mu_L(\overline{X}), \mu_U(\overline{X})]$$

has coverage probability $1 - \alpha$ since

$$\mathbb{P}_\mu\left\{\mu_L(\overline{X}) \leq \mu \leq \mu_U(\overline{X})\right\} = \mathbb{P}\left\{\overline{X} - z_{1-\alpha/2}\frac{\sigma}{\sqrt{n}} \leq \mu \leq \overline{X} + z_{1-\alpha/2}\frac{\sigma}{\sqrt{n}}\right\}$$

$$= \mathbb{P}_\mu\left\{-z_{1-\alpha/2} \leq \frac{\sqrt{n}(\mu - \overline{X})}{\sigma} \leq z_{1-\alpha/2}\right\}$$

$$= \mathbb{P}_\mu\left\{-z_{1-\alpha/2} \leq \frac{\sqrt{n}(\overline{X} - \mu)}{\sigma} \leq z_{1-\alpha/2}\right\}$$

$$= \mathbb{P}\left\{-z_{1-\alpha/2} \leq Z \leq z_{1-\alpha/2}\right\}$$

$$= 1 - \alpha$$

4.3 Pivots

Definition 4.3.1. A **pivot**, $t(X, \theta)$, is any combinant such that the distribution of $t(X, \theta)$ does not depend on θ.

Example. A simple, but important, example of a pivot is based on a random sample from the normal distribution with known variance σ^2. A pivot is

$$Z_n(\mu) = \frac{\sqrt{n}(\overline{X}_n - \mu)}{\sigma}$$

The distribution of $Z_n(\mu)$ is normal with mean 0 and variance 1 and does not depend on μ.

Example. Another pivot is

$$T_n(\mu) = \frac{\sqrt{n}(\overline{X}_n - \mu)}{s}$$

where the assumptions are the same as in the previous example, but now σ^2 is unknown. The distribution of $T_n(\mu)$ is known as Student's t distribution with $n - 1$ degrees of freedom. The quantity s is the square root of s^2 where

$$s^2 = \frac{1}{n-1} \sum_{i=1}^{n} (X_i - \overline{X}_n)^2$$

In both of the previous examples, we can find a confidence interval for μ by noting that

$$\mathbb{P}\left(-z_{1-\alpha/2} \leq \frac{\sqrt{n}(\overline{X}_n - \theta)}{\sigma} \leq z_{1-\alpha/2} \right) = 1 - \alpha$$

for the first example and

$$\mathbb{P}\left\{ -t_{1-\alpha/2}(n-1) \leq \frac{\sqrt{n}(\overline{X}_n - \theta)}{s} \leq t_{1-\alpha/2}(n-1) \right\} = 1 - \alpha$$

for the second example.

Thus the confidence intervals are

$$\overline{X}_n \pm z_{1-\alpha/2} \frac{\sigma}{\sqrt{n}} \quad \text{and} \quad \overline{X}_n \pm t_{1-\alpha/2}(n-1) \frac{s}{\sqrt{n}}$$

The process of converting the probability statement about the pivot to a statement about the parameter is called **inversion**. It is a very general method of obtaining confidence intervals when a pivot can be found. It is also the basis for the bootstrap to be discussed in a later chapter.

Example. Still another example of a pivot under the same setup with a normal distribution is

$$\frac{(n-1)s^2}{\sigma^2}$$

which has a chi-square distribution with $n-1$ degrees of freedom under the same assumptions as in the second example.

It follows that

$$\mathbb{P}\left(\chi^2_{\alpha/2}(n-1) \leq \frac{(n-1)s^2}{\sigma^2} \leq \chi^2_{1-\alpha/2}(n-1)\right) = 1-\alpha$$

so that a confidence interval for σ^2 is

$$\frac{(n-1)s^2}{\chi^2_{1-\alpha/2}(n-1)} \leq \sigma^2 \leq \frac{(n-1)s^2}{\chi^2_{\alpha/2}(n-1)}$$

4.4   Likelihood Intervals

Under the normal model, i.e., $X_1, X_2, \ldots, X_n$ independent, each with a $N(\mu, \sigma^2)$ distribution with σ^2 known, the maximum likelihood estimate for μ is $\overline{x}$ so that the likelihood is given by

$$\mathscr{L}(\mu; \mathbf{x}) = \frac{\exp\left\{-\sum_{i=1}^{n}(x_i - \mu)^2/2\sigma^2\right\}}{\exp\left\{-\sum_{i=1}^{n}(x_i - \overline{x})^2/2\sigma^2\right\}}$$

which reduces to

$$\mathscr{L}(\mu; \mathbf{x}) = \exp\left\{-\frac{n}{2\sigma^2}(\mu - \overline{x})^2\right\}$$

Note that $\mathscr{L}(\mu; \mathbf{x}) \geq 1/k$ if and only if

$$\mathscr{L}(\mu; \mathbf{x}) \geq \frac{1}{k}$$

or

$$\exp\left\{-\frac{n(\mu - \overline{x})^2}{2\sigma^2}\right\} \geq \frac{1}{k}$$

Taking logs yields

$$-\frac{n(\mu - \overline{x})^2}{2\sigma^2} \geq -\ln(k)$$

which is equivalent to

$$n(\mu - \overline{x})^2 \leq 2\ln(k)\sigma^2$$

and finally to

$$|\mu - \overline{x}| \leq \sqrt{\frac{2\ln(k)\sigma^2}{n}}$$

The interval

$$\left[\overline{x} - \sqrt{\frac{2\ln(k)\sigma^2}{n}} \;,\; \overline{x} + \sqrt{\frac{2\ln(k)\sigma^2}{n}}\right]$$

is called a $1/k$ **likelihood** or support interval for μ.

This interval represents

1. Those values of μ for which the likelihood, relative to the best supported value, is less than $1/k$.
2. Equivalently, values of μ outside of this interval have at least one value of μ, the MLE, which is k times better supported.

Likelihood intervals have not been widely used but the following indicates that maybe this is a mistake.

Fisher uses this normalized likelihood to evaluate the reasonableness of different values of the parameter and states (p. 76) that values for which the likelihood is less than 1/15 "are obviously open to grave suspicion." It is to be regretted that the use of this cutoff point of 1/15 has not become nearly as popular as Fisher's other famous proposal of using 0.05 as a cutoff point for the significance level of a test. Had this proposal become widely accepted, statistical practice would have been significantly changed for the better.

Bayarri et al. [2]

4.5 Bayesian Approach

The normal example can also be considered from a Bayesian perspective. Assume that prior knowledge about μ can be represented by a normal distribution centered at μ_p with variance σ_μ^2.

Then the posterior density of μ is the product of the density of $\mathbf{x}$ given μ

$$f(\mathbf{x}|\mu) = (2\pi\sigma^2)^{-n/2} \exp\left\{-\frac{1}{2\sigma^2}\sum_{i=1}^{n}(x_i - \overline{x})^2 + \frac{(n\overline{x} - \mu)^2}{2\sigma^2}\right\}$$

and the prior for μ

$$\pi(\mu) = (2\pi\sigma_\mu^2)^{-1/2} \exp\left\{-\frac{(\mu - \mu_0)^2}{2\sigma_\mu^2}\right\}$$

Thus the posterior density for μ is proportional to

$$\exp\left\{-\frac{1}{2}\left(\frac{n}{\sigma^2} + \frac{1}{\sigma_\mu^2}\right)\mu^2 + \left(\frac{n\overline{x}}{\sigma^2} + \frac{\mu_0}{\sigma_{mu}^2}\right)\mu\right\}$$

It follows that the posterior distribution for μ is normal with mean μ_* and variance σ_*^2 (see Chap. 21 for derivation)
    where

$$\mu_* = \left(\frac{n}{\sigma^2} + \frac{1}{\sigma_\mu^2}\right)^{-1}\left[\frac{n\overline{x}}{\sigma^2} + \frac{\mu_0}{\sigma_\mu^2}\right]$$

and

$$\sigma_*^2 = \left(\frac{n}{\sigma^2} + \frac{1}{\sigma_\mu^2}\right)^{-1}$$

The mean of the posterior can be written in a variety of ways. First note that it is a weighted average of the sample mean $\overline{x}$ and the prior mean μ_0

$$\mu_* = w\overline{x} + (1 - w)\mu_0$$

where

$$w = \frac{\frac{n}{\sigma^2}}{\frac{n}{\sigma^2} + \frac{1}{\sigma_\mu^2}}$$

i.e. weight the sample mean and the prior inversely proportional to their variances.
    It follows that the sample mean $\overline{x}$ "shrinks" toward the prior mean. This fact can be more precisely expressed by writing

$$\mu_* = \overline{x} + \frac{1}{\sigma_\mu^2}(\mu_0 - \overline{x})$$

1. If $\overline{x} > \mu_0$, then μ_* is less than $\overline{x}$.
2. If $\overline{x} < \mu_0$, then μ_* is greater than $\overline{x}$.

4.6 Objective Bayes

The "prior" distribution for μ which is uniform over the entire real line is an **improper prior** (does not have a finite integral) and corresponds to $\sigma_\mu^2 = \infty$. This "prior" is an example of a **reference prior**. Loosely speaking a reference prior allows the likelihood to dominate the prior in the calculation of the posterior.

For this prior the posterior mean and variance are $\overline{x}$ and σ^2/n.

The interval defined by

$$\mu_L(\overline{x}) = \overline{x} - z_{1-\alpha/2}\sigma/\sqrt{n} \ , \quad \mu_U(\overline{x}) = \overline{x} + z_{1-\alpha/2}\sigma/\sqrt{n}$$

is called a $100(1-\alpha)$ **Bayesian** or **credible** interval for μ. The credible interval satisfies

$$\mathbb{P}(\mu \geq \mu_U(\overline{x})) = \mathbb{P}\left(\frac{\sqrt{n}(\mu - \overline{x})}{\sigma} \geq \frac{\sqrt{n}(\mu_U(\overline{x}) - \overline{x})}{\sigma}\right) = \frac{\alpha}{2}$$

and

$$\mathbb{P}(\mu \leq \mu_L(\overline{x})) = \mathbb{P}\left(\frac{\sqrt{n}(\mu - \overline{x})}{\sigma} \leq \frac{\sqrt{n}(\mu_L(\overline{x}) - \overline{x})}{\sigma}\right) = \frac{\alpha}{2}$$

It follows that the credible interval satisfies

$$\mathbb{P}\left\{\overline{x} - z_{1-\alpha/2}\frac{\sigma}{\sqrt{n}} \leq \mu \leq \overline{x} + z_{1-\alpha/2}\frac{\sigma}{\sqrt{n}}\right\} = 1 - \alpha$$

Note that in the Bayesian formulation μ is **random** so that the above statement is a probability statement about μ for fixed **x**, i.e., the posterior probability that μ is in the credible interval is $1 - \alpha$.

Note, however, that this particular prior cannot represent prior belief because it is not a probability distribution.

4.7 Comparing the Intervals

The intervals for the normal distribution with known variance are

1. Frequentist: $\overline{x} \pm 1.96\sigma/\sqrt{n}$ ($\alpha = 0.05$)
2. Objective Bayes $\overline{x} \pm 1.96\sigma/\sqrt{n}$ ($\alpha = 0.05$)
3. Likelihood $\overline{x} \pm 2.04\sigma/\sqrt{n}$ ($k = 8$)

As Brad Efron said in a seminar at Johns Hopkins several years ago

estimate $\pm$ 2 standard error

has good credentials in any statistical theory.

4.8 Interval Estimation Example

In the case of a normal distribution the three approaches to interval estimation lead to virtually identical results with different interpretations so there appears to be no need to worry about the different interpretations from a practical perspective. As we will see good approximate confidence intervals are of this form for a wide variety of problems. However, only a small change to the experimental setup leads to considerable differences as the following example shows.

Example. This is a modified version of Cox's [9] example.

1. Two young investigators A and B are interested in the same problem.
2. A has sufficient funds to take 100 observations.
3. B thinks another approach might be better but doesn't have funds to investigate both. B decides to toss a coin, taking 4 observations if the coin falls heads and 100 observations if it falls tails. (If he takes 4 observations he would use the remaining funds to investigate something else.)

Techniques used by both investigators yield independent observations which are normal with mean μ and variance σ^2 where σ^2 is known. For investigator A the confidence interval is thus

$$\overline{x} \pm \frac{1.96\sigma}{10}$$

As luck would have it the coin toss by B resulted in a tail. After making 100 observations B observed the same sample mean as A. B thus reports the same interval as A

$$\overline{x} \pm \frac{1.96\sigma}{10}$$

To be certain about his methods B consults a statistician who, after hearing the experimental setup, tells him that his confidence interval should be

$$\overline{x} \pm \frac{2.58\sigma}{10}$$

because it is better, i.e., shorter on average.

The statistician reasoning is simple: we want a confidence interval for μ that has the right coverage probability (0.95) and is short.

Consider the following two confidence interval procedures:

(a) Always use $\overline{x} \pm 1.96\sigma/\sqrt{n}$ which implies that when $n = 4$ the interval is $\overline{x} \pm 1.96\sigma/2$ while if $n = 100$ the interval is $\overline{x} \pm 1.96\sigma/10$.
(b) If $n = 4$ use $\overline{x} \pm 1.68\sigma/2$ while if $n = 100$ use $\overline{x} \pm 2.58\sigma/100$.

Both of these intervals are "valid" 95 % confidence intervals in the sense that **before the experiment is performed** we can have 95 % confidence that the interval will contain μ:

1. For (a) the coverage probability is $\frac{1}{2}(0.95) + \frac{1}{2}(0.95) = 0.95$
2. For (b) the coverage probability is $\frac{1}{2}(0.91) + \frac{1}{2}(0.99) = 0.95$

Which of these two intervals is better? Consider the expected length.

1. For (a) the expected length is

$$\mathbb{E}(L) = \frac{1}{2}(2)(1.96)\sigma/2 + \frac{1}{2}(2)(1.96)\sigma/10 = 1.96\sigma\left(\frac{1}{2} + \frac{1}{10}\right) = 1.176\sigma$$

2. For (b) the expected length is

$$\mathbb{E}(L) = \frac{1}{2}(2)(1.68)\sigma/2 + \frac{1}{2}(2)(2.58/10)\sigma = \sigma\left(\frac{1.68}{2} + \frac{2.58}{10}\right) = 1.098\sigma$$

Thus (b) provides an interval with shorter expected length.

Although the statistician is right it is difficult to explain to investigator B why the evidence produced by his data set is not the same as that produced by A. After all, the same sample mean was observed with the same variance and the same number of observations. And yet the interval reported by B has length 0.516σ while that reported by A has length 0.392σ. Procedure (b) has a confidence coefficient of 0.95. It is probabilistically correct but does not seem logical.

1. In general frequentist procedures should take into account any and all aspects of the experimental setup even if it appears unrelated to the observed data. That is stopping rules, peeks at data before the experiment is finished, etc.
2. The fact is, most statisticians do not do this but still claim to be frequentists, i.e., they use the methods they want and interpret them how they want.

4.9 Exercises

1. Show that MSE $= \mathbb{V}(\widehat{\theta}) + [\mathbb{B}(\widehat{\theta})]^2$.
2. Suppose that $X_1, X_2, \ldots, X_n$ are independent each exponential, i.e., each X_i has pdf

$$f(x; \theta) = \frac{e^{-x/\theta}}{\theta} \quad x \geq 0$$

This pdf is often used to model response or survival times.

(a) Find the joint density of the X_i and hence find the score function.

(b) Using the score function show that the maximum likelihood estimator for θ is $\widehat{\theta} = \overline{X}$. Show that it is unbiased and consistent and finds its variance.

(c) Using the joint density you found in (a) and the maximum likelihood estimate you found in (b) show that the likelihood function for θ is

$$\mathcal{L}(\theta; \mathbf{x}) = \frac{f(\mathbf{x}; \theta)}{f(\mathbf{x}; \widehat{\theta})} = \left(\frac{\widehat{\theta}}{\theta}\right)^n \exp\left\{-n\left(\frac{\widehat{\theta}}{\theta} - 1\right)\right\}$$

(d) The exponential is a special case of the Gamma which has pdf

$$f(y; \theta) = \frac{y^{\alpha-1} e^{-y/\beta}}{\Gamma(\alpha)\beta^\alpha} \quad y \geq 0$$

(i.e., $\alpha = 1$ and $\beta = \theta$). It is known that if $X_1, X_2, \ldots, X_n$ are independent each gamma (α_i, β) then

$$S_n = X_1 + X_2 + \ldots + X_n$$

has a Gamma pdf with parameters

$$\alpha = \alpha_1 + \alpha_2 + \cdots + \alpha_n \text{ and } \beta$$

Using this fact show that the pdf of $Y = n\widehat{\theta}$ is

$$f(y; \theta) = \frac{y^{n-1} \exp\left\{-\frac{y}{\theta}\right\}}{\Gamma(n)\theta^n}$$

(e) Using the result of (d) show that $n\widehat{\theta}/\theta$ is a pivot and find the density of the pivot.

(f) Using the density of the pivot show how to find L and U such that

$$\mathbb{P}\left\{L \leq \frac{n\widehat{\theta}}{\theta} \leq U\right\} = 1 - \alpha$$

Note that R parametrizes the Gamma in terms of α and $1/\beta$.

(g) The following are the response times in milliseconds to a light stimulus for 10 animals.

$$\{70, 11, 66, 5, 20, 4, 35, 40, 29, 8\}$$

Using the result in (f) calculate the 95 % confidence interval for θ and interpret. Also calculate the $1/8$ likelihood interval for θ and interpret.

3. A scientist needs to weigh three objects O_1, O_2, and O_3 each of which weighs between 0.5 and 1.0 g. Unfortunately she only has a scale which can weigh objects only if their weight exceeds 1 g.

   (a) Show that she can get a weight for each one by weighing them two at a time, i.e., she weighs O_1 and O_2 together and gets Y_1 and so on.
   (b) Find the variance of her estimated weights (assume weights are uncorrelated).

4. Suppose that $X_1, X_2, \ldots, X_n$ are independent with density function (continuous) f and distribution function F.

   (a) Find an expression for the density function of

   $$Y_n = \max\{X_1, X_2, \ldots, X_n\}$$

   (b) Find an expression for the density function of

   $$Y_1 = \min\{X_1, X_2, \ldots, X_n\}$$

5. Suppose that the density of X is

   $$f(x) = \exp\left\{-(x - \theta)\right\} \quad \text{for } x \geq \theta$$

   and that we have $X_1, X_2, \ldots, X_n$ independent each with density f.

   (a) Write down the joint density of $X_1, X_2, \ldots, X_n$.
   (b) Find the maximum likelihood estimator for θ. Note you cannot do this by differentiating (why?).
   (c) Using the results of the previous problem or otherwise.

6. (Bonus Problem) Suppose that $X_1, X_2, \ldots, X_n$ are independent each uniform on the interval $[0, \theta]$ where $\theta > 0$.

   (a) Find the distribution of $Y_n = \max\{X_1, X_2, \ldots, X_n\}$.
   (b) Show that the limiting distribution of Z_n where

   $$Z_n = n(\theta - Y_n)$$

   is exponential θ, i.e.,

   $$f(z; \theta) = \theta^{-1} e^{-z/\theta} \quad z \geq 0$$

   Note that the limiting distribution is not normal.
   (c) Generate 1,000 samples of size 50 from a uniform on $[0, 5]$ and plot the histogram of Z_{50}. Superimpose the plot of the limiting distribution.
   (d) Show that the MLE of θ is Y_n.
   (e) Find a confidence interval for θ using the fact that Y_n/θ is a pivot.

(f) Compare to the exponential interval based on the large sample approximation you obtained in (b).
(g) Discuss the asymptotic distribution of $2\overline{X}_n$ which is an unbiased estimator of θ.
(h) Find a confidence interval for θ based on the results in (g) and compare to the interval in (e).

Chapter 5
Hypothesis Testing

5.1 Law of Likelihood

Suppose that hypothesis f specifies that the probability that the random variable X takes on the value x is $f(x)$ and hypothesis g specifies that the probability that the random variable X takes on the value x is $g(x)$.

Axiom 5.1.1. (Law of Likelihood). The observation x is statistical evidence supporting g over f if and only if

$$g(x) > f(x)$$

Moreover, the likelihood ratio

$$\mathscr{L}\mathscr{R} = \frac{g(x)}{f(x)}$$

measures the strength of the statistical evidence.

The Law of Likelihood provides a natural way of measuring evidence provided by data. It is almost a tautology and seems like a sensible way of defining support for one hypothesis vs another. It was not, however, formulated explicitly until the early 1960s. Rather less intuitive procedures were formulated and developed first.

Note that when we have a parametric statistical model $(\mathcal{X}, f(x;\theta), \Theta)$ the Law of Likelihood states that

$$\frac{\mathscr{L}(\theta_1; x)}{\mathscr{L}(\theta_0; \theta_0)}$$

measures the statistical evidence for θ_1 vs θ_0 provided by the data x.

© Springer International Publishing Switzerland 2014
C.A. Rohde, *Introductory Statistical Inference with the Likelihood Function*, DOI 10.1007/978-3-319-10461-4_5

5.2   Neyman-Pearson Theory

5.2.1   Introduction

Given the basic statistical model $(\mathcal{X}, f(x\,;\theta), \Theta)$ the inference called hypothesis testing is

"Based on data $X = x$ decide whether $\theta \in \Theta_0$ or whether $\theta \in \Theta_1$" where $\Theta = \Theta_0 \cup \Theta_1$ and $\Theta_0 \cap \Theta_1 = \emptyset$, i.e., the two hypotheses are incompatible:

1. The hypothesis $H_0 \,:\, \theta \in \Theta_0$ is called the **null hypothesis**.
2. The hypothesis $H_1 \,:\, \theta \in \Theta_1$ is called the **alternative hypothesis**.

The term null hypothesis arose because of the common experimental practice of investigating a control group and a treated group. If the treatment is ineffective then the difference between the treated group and the control group should be 0 or "null."

Since the null hypothesis is either true or not, and since we can either reject or retain the null hypothesis on the basis of the observed data, we see that we have the following possibilities:

	Action taken	
	Retain null	Reject null
H_0 true	✓	Type I error
H_1 true	Type II error	✓

where a ✓ indicates that a correct action has been taken.

The hypothesis testing problem is to use the data $X = x$ to determine which of the two actions to take. Typically this means that we select a region $\mathcal{C}$ such that if the observed data is in $\mathcal{C}$ we reject H_0 and otherwise we retain H_0 (do not reject H_0). The region $\mathcal{C}$ is called the **critical region** of the test.

A function φ such that

$$\varphi(x) = \begin{cases} 1 & x \in \mathcal{C} \\ 0 & \text{otherwise} \end{cases}$$

is called a **test function**.

We have a solution to the hypothesis testing problem if we can find $\mathcal{C}$ or equivalently the test function φ.

Neyman and Pearson focused on the probabilities of the two types of error. For a given critical region $\mathcal{C}$ we have

1. $\mathbb{P}(\text{Type I error}) = \mathbb{P}_{H_0}(X \in \mathcal{C}) = \mathbb{E}_{H_0}[\varphi(X)]$
2. $\mathbb{P}(\text{Type II error}) = 1 - \mathbb{P}_{H_1}(X \in \mathcal{C}) = 1 - \mathbb{E}_{H_1}[\varphi(X)]$

Note that using a "smaller" critical region $\mathcal{C}^* \subset \mathcal{C}$ decreases the probability of a Type I error but increases the probability of a Type II error since for $\mathcal{C}^* \subset \mathcal{C}$:

$$\mathbb{P}(\text{Type II error using } \mathcal{C}^*) = 1 - \mathbb{P}_{H_1}(X \in \mathcal{C}^*)$$
$$\geq 1 - \mathbb{P}_{H_1}(X \in \mathcal{C})$$
$$= \mathbb{P}(\text{Type II error using } \mathcal{C})$$

It follows that it is not possible to simultaneously reduce the probabilities of both types of errors. The Neyman–Pearson solution to this problem was to observe that one reasonable criterion is to

1. Fix the probability of a Type I error of the test so as not to exceed some value α, called the **significance level**. The maximum value of the Type I error probability when $\theta \in \Theta_0$ is called the **size** of the test.
2. Among all tests with size less than or equal to α choose the test that maximizes the **power**:

$$\text{power} = 1 - \mathbb{P}(\text{Type II error})$$

Equivalently choose that test which minimizes the probability of a Type II error subject to size less than or equal to α.

The hypothesis testing problem has thus been reduced to a formal maximization problem:
Choose $\mathcal{C}$ such that

$$\int_{\mathcal{C}} f(x; \theta)d\lambda(x) \text{ is maximized for } \theta \in \Theta_1$$

subject to

$$\int_{\mathcal{C}} f(x; \theta)d\lambda(x) \leq \alpha \text{ for } \theta \in \Theta_0$$

Note. I will write

$$\int g(x)d\lambda(x) = \begin{cases} \int g(x)dx & x \text{ continuous} \\ \sum g(x) & \text{discrete} \end{cases}$$

to avoid having to treat the continuous and discrete cases separately.

Definition 5.2.1. $\mathbb{P}_\theta(X \in \mathcal{C})$ is called the **power function** of the test based on $\mathcal{C}$.

As stated the problem cannot be solved for general Θ_0 and Θ_1.
There is a complete solution, however, when $\Theta_0 = \{\theta_0\}$ and $\Theta_1 = \{\theta_1\}$, i.e., when both the null and alternative hypotheses are **simple**, consisting of one point each.

5.2.2   Neyman-Pearson Lemma

Theorem 5.2.1 (Neyman–Pearson Lemma). *For testing the simple hypothesis* $H_0 : \theta = \theta_0$ *vs the simple alternative* $H_1 : \theta = \theta_1$ *the **likelihood ratio test**,* $\varphi(x)$*, defined by*

$$\varphi(x) = \begin{cases} 1 \ \text{if} \ \frac{f(x;\theta_1)}{f(x;\theta_0)} > c \\ 0 \ \text{otherwise} \end{cases}$$

where c is chosen so that

$$\mathbb{E}_{\theta_0}[\varphi(X)] = \alpha$$

is the most powerful test of size α*.*

Proof. A test of

$$H_0 : \theta = \theta_0 \quad \text{vs} \quad H_1 : \theta = \theta_1$$

is equivalent to using a test function $\varphi(x)$, where $\varphi(x) = 0$ if H_0 is not rejected and $\varphi(x) = 1$ if H_0 is rejected.   □

The size of the test can be written as

$$\alpha = \mathbb{P}_{\theta_0}[\varphi(X) = 1] = \mathbb{E}_{\theta_0}[\varphi(X)]$$

Similarly the power can be written as

$$\mathbb{P}_{\theta_1}[\varphi(X) = 1] = \mathbb{E}_{\theta_1}[\varphi(X)]$$

where $\mathbb{E}_\theta$ denotes expectation under the probability distribution specified by θ
   If $\varphi(x)$ corresponds to the likelihood ratio test then

$$\mathbb{E}_{\theta_0}[\varphi(X)] = \alpha$$

Let $\varphi^*(x)$ be another test satisfying

$$\mathbb{E}_{\theta_0}[\varphi^*(X)] = \mathbb{E}_{\theta_0}[\varphi(X)] = \alpha$$

We will show that

$$\text{Power of } \varphi^* = \mathbb{E}_{\theta_1}[\varphi^*(X)] \leq \mathbb{E}_{\theta_1}[\varphi(X)] = \text{Power of LR Test}$$

First note that

$$\varphi^*(x)[f(x; \theta_1) - cf(x; \theta_0)] \leq \varphi(x)[f(x; \theta_1) - cf(x; \theta_0)]$$

which holds since

1. If $\varphi(x) = 1$ then $f(x; \theta_1) - cf(x; \theta_0) > 0$
2. If $\varphi(x) = 0$ then $f_{\theta_1}(x) - cf_{\theta_0}(x) < 0$

Now integrating both sides of the above inequality with respect to x gives

$$\mathbb{E}_{\theta_1}[\varphi^*(X)] - c\mathbb{E}_{\theta_0}[\varphi^*(X)] \leq \mathbb{E}_{\theta_1}[\varphi(X)] - c\mathbb{E}_{\theta_0}[\varphi(X)]$$

and thus

$$c\{\mathbb{E}\theta_0[\varphi(X)] - \mathbb{E}_{\theta_0}[\varphi^*(X)]\} \leq \mathbb{E}_{\theta_1}[\varphi(X)] - \mathbb{E}_{\theta_1}[\varphi^*(X)]$$

The conclusion follows since the left-hand side of this inequality is 0 by assumption.

Example. In the vicinity of a nuclear reprocessing plant, four cases of childhood leukemia were observed over a certain period of time. From a national registry only 0.25 cases would have been expected. Of interest is whether the data are consistent with the national rates. This is a typical application of the Poisson distribution (rare independent events). The hypothesis testing approach is as follows.

Suppose that $X_1, X_2, \ldots, X_n$ are independent, each Poisson with parameter θ. We are interested in testing

$$H_0 : \theta = \theta_0 \quad vs \quad H_1 : \theta = \theta_1$$

where $\theta_1 > \theta_0$. The likelihood ratio is

$$\frac{\theta_1^{s_n} e^{-n\theta_1}}{\lambda_0^{s_n} e^{-n\theta_0}} = \left(\frac{\theta_1}{\theta_0}\right)^{s_n} e^{-n(\theta_1 - \theta_0)}$$

Rejecting when this ratio is "large" is equivalent to rejecting when s_n is "large" which is determined by requiring that c be such that

$$\mathbb{P}_{\theta_0}(S_n \geq c) \leq \alpha$$

Since S_n has a Poisson distribution with parameter $n\theta_0$ when H_0 is true this probability can be easily calculated. In our application $n = 1$ and $\theta_0 = 0.25$ and we find that $c = 1$. Thus we should reject $\theta_0 = 0.25$.

Here is the likelihood function for this example (Fig. 5.1):

Note that the ratio of the probability of observing four cases with $\theta = 0.76$ (the lower limit of the 1/32 likelihood interval) is given by R as

Poisson Likelihood 4 Observed Cases

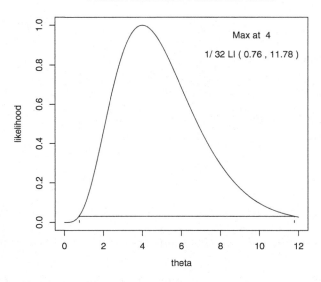

Fig. 5.1 Poisson likelihood

```
dpois(4,.76)/dpois(4,.25)
[1] 51.28663
```

which shows overwhelming evidence against $\theta = 0.25$ in favor of $\theta = 0.76$.

5.2.3   Using the Neyman-Pearson Lemma

The key idea is to find the critical region or test which satisfies two conditions:

1. The critical region consists of large values of the likelihood ratio, i.e.,

$$\mathcal{C} = \left\{ x \ : \ \frac{f(x; \theta_1)}{f(x; \theta_0)} \geq c \right\}$$

2. The critical value c is determined so that

$$\mathbb{P}_{\theta_0}(\mathcal{C}) \leq \alpha$$

If we can find a statistic t whose distribution is known when θ_0 is true and such that

$$\mathcal{C} = \{x \ : \ t(x) \in \mathcal{T}\}$$

where

$$\mathbb{P}_{\theta_0}(\mathcal{T}) \leq \alpha$$

then we can define the test in terms of t which is, in many cases, simpler.

Example. Suppose that $X_1, X_2, \ldots, X_n$ are independent each normal with mean μ and variance σ^2 where σ^2 is assumed known. We are interested in testing

$$H_0 : \mu = \mu_1 \;\; vs \;\; H_1 : \mu = \mu_2$$

where $\mu_2 > \mu_1$.

The likelihood ratio is

$$\frac{(2\pi\sigma^2)^{-n/2} \exp\left\{-\sum_{i=1}^{n}(x_i - \mu_2)^2/2\sigma^2\right\}}{(2\pi\sigma^2)^{-n/2} \exp\left\{-\sum_{i=1}^{n}(x_i - \mu_1)^2/2\sigma^2\right\}}$$

which reduces to

$$\exp\left\{\frac{n\bar{x}\mu_2}{\sigma^2} - \frac{n\bar{x}\mu_1}{\sigma^2} - \frac{n\mu_2^2}{2\sigma^2} + \frac{n\mu_1^2}{2\sigma^2}\right\}$$

where we have used the fact that for any μ

$$\sum_{i=1}^{n}(x_i - \mu)^2 = \sum_{i=1}^{n}x_i^2 - 2n\bar{x}\mu + n\mu^2$$

The likelihood ratio can be rewritten as

$$\exp\left\{\frac{n(\mu_2 - \mu_1)}{\sigma^2}\left[\bar{x} - \frac{\mu_1 + \mu_2}{2}\right]\right\}$$

Rejecting when the likelihood ratio is "large" is equivalent to rejecting when $\bar{x}$ is "large."

That is we choose d so that

$$\alpha = \mathbb{P}_{\mu_1}(\overline{X} \geq d)$$

$$= \mathbb{P}_{\mu_1}\left(\frac{\sqrt{n}(\overline{X} - \mu_1)}{\sigma} \geq \frac{\sqrt{n}(d - \mu_1)}{\sigma}\right)$$

$$= \mathbb{P}\left(Z \geq \frac{\sqrt{n}(d - \mu_1)}{\sigma}\right)$$

where Z has a (standard) normal distribution with mean 0 and variance 1.

Thus for any α we have

$$z_{1-\alpha} = \frac{(\sqrt{n}(d - \mu_1)}{\sigma} \quad \text{or} \quad d = \mu_1 + z_{1-\alpha}\frac{\sigma}{\sqrt{n}}$$

We thus reject H_0 in favor of H_1 whenever the observed value of $\overline{X}$, $\overline{x}_{obs}$ exceeds d.

5.2.4 Uniformly Most Powerful Tests

Sometimes the form of the test is the same for all values of the alternative parameter, e.g., for all values the parameter greater than θ_0. In such cases we call the test **uniformly most powerful**. Such tests arise mainly in one sided tests for the exponential family.

5.2.5 A Complication

In the previous example suppose that

$$\overline{x}_{obs} = \mu_1 + 2\frac{\sigma}{\sqrt{n}}$$

Then we would reject when $\alpha = 0.05$ since $z_{.95} = 1.645$.

Suppose now that $\mu_2 = \mu_1 + \sigma$. For these values of $\overline{x}_{obs}$ and μ_2 the likelihood ratio is given by

$$\exp\left\{ n\left(\frac{2}{\sqrt{n}} - \frac{1}{2} \right) \right\}$$

For $n = 16$ this ratio is exactly 1 and decreases rapidly as n increases (for $n = 30$ it is 0.02), indicating that even though H_0 is rejected in favor of H_1 the data are 50 times more likely under H_0 than under H_1.

That is, the use of the Neyman-Pearson Lemma is incompatible with the Law of Likelihood (Fig. 5.2).

5.2.6 Comments and Examples

The Neyman–Pearson Lemma is one of the great results in statistics and dominated statistics for most of the twentieth century. It paved the way for decision theory and other important advances in statistical theory. But is it all that useful or logical?

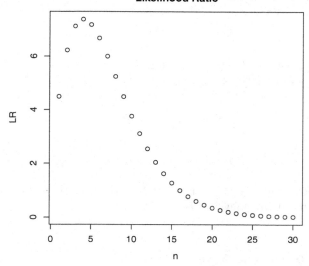

Fig. 5.2 Likelihood ratio

To be explicit consider the following situation:

$$n = 30 \quad \text{iid Bernoulli trials with parameter } \theta$$

and

$$H_0 : \ \theta = \frac{1}{4} \ , \quad H_1 : \ \theta = \frac{3}{4}$$

The most powerful test of size $\alpha = 0.05$ rejects H_0 in favor of H_1 if the observed x exceeds 12, i.e., the critical region is

$$\mathcal{C} = \{12, 13, 14, \ldots, 30\}$$

Note that, for a given x, the likelihood ratio for $\theta_1 = 3/4$ vs $\theta_0 = 1/4$ is given by

$$
\begin{aligned}
\mathscr{LR}(x) &= \frac{\mathscr{L}_1(x)}{\mathscr{L}_0(x)} \\[2mm]
&= \frac{\binom{30}{x} \left(\frac{3}{4}\right)^x \left(\frac{1}{4}\right)^{30-x}}{\binom{30}{x} \left(\frac{1}{4}\right)^x \left(\frac{3}{4}\right)^{30-x}} \\[2mm]
&= 3^x \left(\frac{1}{3}\right)^{30-x} \\[2mm]
&= 3^{2x-30}
\end{aligned}
$$

Thus if $x = 12$ the likelihood ratio is

$$\mathscr{LR} = 3^{2(12)-30} = 3^{-6} = \frac{1}{729}$$

Thus even though we reject $\theta = 1/4$ in favor of $\theta = 3/4$, $\theta = 1/4$ is 729 times more probable than $\theta = 3/4$ for the value $x = 12$.

Note also that we have the following:

$$\text{If } x = 13 \implies \mathscr{LR} = \tfrac{1}{81}$$
$$\text{If } x = 14 \implies \mathscr{LR} = \tfrac{1}{9}$$
$$\text{If } x = 15 \implies \mathscr{LR} = 1$$

Thus 15 leads to equal support for H_0 vis-a-vis H_1 even though Neyman-Pearson theory says to reject H_0 in favor of H_1.

5.2.7   A Different Criterion

Suppose, instead of minimizing the probability of a Type II error for fixed probability of a Type I error, we choose the test to minimize a linear combination of the two error probabilities. That is, we choose the critical region $\mathcal{C}$ so that

$$k \int_{\mathcal{C}} f(x; \theta_0) d\lambda(x) + \left[1 - \int_{\mathcal{C}} f(x; \theta_1) d\lambda(x) \right]$$

is minimized. Essentially this says that we view the Type I error probability as k times more important than the Type II error probability.

Note that the above expression can be written as

$$1 + \int_{\mathcal{C}} [k f(x; \theta_0) - f(x; \theta_1)] \, d\lambda(x)$$

This is clearly minimized whenever

$$[k f(x; \theta_0) - f(x; \theta_1)] \leq 0$$

i.e., $\mathcal{C}$ is given by

$$\mathcal{C} = \left\{ x \; : \; \frac{f(x; \theta_1)}{f(x; \theta_0)} \geq k \right\}$$

which is precisely the Law of Likelihood if $k > 1$.

In this formulation there is no need to fix the probability of a Type I error. The test depends only on the **value of the likelihood ratio at the observed value** x and not on unobserved values of x. Thus a simple change in the function to be minimized results in an entirely different methodology, one that does not depend on the unobserved values of x [8].

5.2.8   Inductive Behavior

Neyman and Pearson defended their solution to the hypothesis testing problem by means of the concept of **inductive behavior**.

> If a rule R unambiguously prescribes the selection of action for each possible outcome ..., then it is a rule of inductive behavior.

Neyman [34]

> (Mathematical) statistics is a branch of the theory of probability. It deals with problems relating to performance characteristics of rules of inductive behavior based on random experiments.

Neyman [34]

Performance characteristics relate to the properties of the sampling distribution of a statistic on which a test (or other inference) is based.

For testing problems the Neyman-Pearson theory assures us that if we use a test with significance level α, then, in repeated use, we will make a Type I error at most $100\alpha\%$ of the time.

5.2.9   Still Another Criterion

Suppose we have to make n tests of a simple H_0 vs a simple H_1 based on data $x_1, x_2, \ldots, x_n$ where the density under H_{i0} is f_{i0} and the density under H_{i1} is f_{i1} for $i = 1, 2, \ldots, n$.

Let the test function for the ith test be φ_i, i.e.,

$$\varphi_i(x_i) = \begin{cases} 1 \text{ Reject } H_{i0} \text{ when } x_i \text{ is observed} \\ 0 \text{ Retain } H_{i0} \text{ when } x \text{ is observed} \end{cases}$$

and let α_i denote the size of the ith test (probability of rejecting H_{i0} when H_{i0} is true) and let γ_i denote the power of the ith test (probability of rejecting H_{i0} when H_{i1} is true.

By the Neyman–Pearson Lemma we know that the best test function for the ith test is given by

$$\varphi(x_i) = \begin{cases} 1 & f_{i1}(x_i) \geq c_i f_{i0}(x_i) \\ 0 & f_{i1}(x_i) < c_i f_{i0}(x_i) \end{cases}$$

i.e., this choice of c_i maximizes the power for fixed size.

In the spirit of inductive behavior we could decide to choose a test which maximized the average power for a fixed average size. Pitman [37]

Theorem 5.2.2. *The test function which maximizes the average power of the n tests for fixed average size has $c = c_i$, i.e., the same value of c is used in all tests.*

As Pitman [37] says:

This result suggests that, to some extent, a particular numerical value of a likelihood ratio means the same thing, whatever the experiment. This is obvious when we have a priori probabilities for H_0 and H_1; for if the prior odds of H_1 vs H_0 are p_1/p_0, the posterior odds are $(p_1/p_0)(f_1/f_0)$, and all that comes from the experiment is the ratio f_1/f_0.

Pitman's result can be thought of as yet another justification of the Law of Likelihood.

5.3   p-Values

Scientifically, reporting that the hypothesis of a difference between a treatment and a control group is rejected, is not very interesting. Scientists demand a measure of the **strength of evidence** against a null hypothesis. The p-value of a test is supposed to fill this gap.

Definition 5.3.1. The p-value is the probability, under the null hypothesis, of a test statistic as or more extreme than actually observed.

We shall see that it **does not measure evidence** and in fact is a rather useless quantity.

Formally, if T is a test statistic for which large values lead to rejection of the hypothesis, the p-value is defined as

$$\text{p-value} = \mathbb{P}_0(T \geq t_{obs})$$

where t_{obs} is the observed value of the test statistic. Note that the p-value is computed under the null hypothesis. There is no explicit alternative (the alternative implicitly defines what values of the test statistic are extreme however).

The p-value can also be viewed as the smallest size at which we can reject the null hypothesis. The p-value originally arose as a result of a **test of significance** in which a null hypothesis is deemed unsupported by the data if the observed result or more extreme is unlikely (has low probability) under the null hypothesis.

In Fisher's words

> The force with which such a conclusion is supported is that of a simple disjunction: *Either* son theory developed test staurred, *or* the theory . . . is not true.

Fisher [17]

As the Neyman–Pearson theory developed test statistics it was natural that they were given a similar interpretation.

> In applications, there is usually available a nested family of rejection regions corresponding to different significance levels. It is then good practice to determine not only whether the hypothesis is accepted or rejected at the given significance level, but also determine the smallest significance level $\widehat{\alpha} = \widehat{\alpha}(x)$, the *critical level*, at which the hypothesis would be rejected for the given observation. This number gives an idea of how strongly the data contradict (or support) the hypothesis, and enables others to reach a verdict based on the significance level of their choice.

Lehmann [27]

But does the p-value provide a measure of how strongly the data contradict (or support) a hypothesis? Jeffreys wrote

> . . . a hypothesis which may be true may be rejected because it has not predicted observable results which have not occurred.

Jeffreys [24]

Example. The following example is taken from Royall [43]. Suppose we are interested in the null hypothesis that $\theta = 0.5$ in 20 Bernoulli trials and the implicit alternative is that $\theta < 0.5$. We use the test statistic x, the number of successes, and small values of x are extreme in the sense that they are not likely under the null hypothesis.

Suppose that the result is reported to you and I in a code. You have a code book and I do not. I only know the code for the number 6.

Suppose the result is reported as $x = 6$. Thus we both know that 6 successes occurred in 20 Bernoulli trials.

Your p-value is

$$\mathbb{P}(6 \text{ or less successes when } p = 0.5) = 0.06$$

Since I can observe only 6 or not 6, the observed value is the most extreme for me so that my p-value is

$$\mathbb{P}(6 \text{ successes when } p = 0.5) = 0.04$$

If it were true that the p-value measured evidence against the hypothesis that $p = 0.5$ then I have stronger evidence than you. Clearly this is illogical.

Example. This example comes from Good (1985). Consider the following "casino" game. There is an urn with 100 balls, W of which are white the remainder are black. Assume that $W > 0$ and that n balls are drawn at random with replacement. Of interest is the hypothesis that the proportion of white balls is $\frac{1}{2}$. For simplicity assume that n is a perfect square and is even. Note that the permissible parameter values are

$$\Theta = \{0.01, 0.02, \ldots, 0.99\}$$

Suppose that we observe

$$r_{obs} = \frac{n}{2} + \sqrt{n}$$

The P-value is then

$$P\text{-value(two-sided)} = 2\,\mathbb{P}_{\theta_0}\{R \geq r_{obs}\}$$

$$= 2\,\mathbb{P}_{\theta_0}\left\{R \geq \frac{n}{2} + \sqrt{n}\right\}$$

$$= 2\,\mathbb{P}_{\theta_0}\left\{\frac{R - \frac{n}{2}}{\sqrt{n/4}} \geq 2\right\}$$

$$\approx 2\,\mathbb{P}(Z \geq 2)$$

$$= 0.0455$$

According to traditional p-value concepts we have "evidence against the null that $\theta = 0.5$." But it is clear that the observed proportion is

$$\frac{r_{obs}}{n} = \frac{\frac{n}{2} + \sqrt{n}}{n} = \frac{1}{2} + \frac{1}{\sqrt{n}}$$

which for n large enough is arbitrarily close to $\frac{1}{2}$.

Thus we can be nearly certain that $\theta = 0.5$ (and in fact the observed proportion can be much closer to 0.5 than any other permissible value of the proportion) despite having evidence against it by P-value standards.

Thus the phrase "P-values provide evidence against the null" is nonsense. Note that the 0.05 cutoff is not the problem. Any other cutoff could be used with similar results (although larger sample sizes are needed). The following is a graph of the likelihood ratio at 0.51 to that of 0.50 plotted vs sample size (Fig. 5.3).

What we see from the graph is that the Law of Likelihood shows that the support for p=0.51 vs p=0.50 never reaches 8 (moderately strong evidence) and after a sample size of 40,000 shows that 0.50 is better supported than 0.51

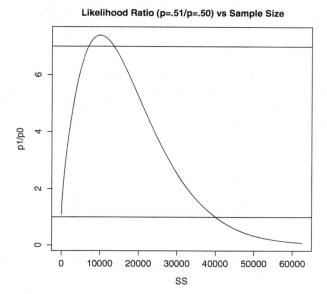

Fig. 5.3 Likelihood ratio for Good's example

5.4   Duality of Confidence Intervals and Tests

Consider a situation where we have data x consisting of an observed value of X which has a distribution depending on a parameter θ.

Assume that we have a test for θ with significance level α.

Define the **acceptance region** $\mathcal{A}(\theta_0)$ for this test as

$$\mathcal{A}(\theta_0) = \{x : \ H_0 : \theta_0 \ \text{is } \textbf{not} \text{ rejected}\}$$

i.e., $\mathcal{A}(\theta_0)$ is the collection of all values of x such that the hypothesis θ_0 is accepted.

By the definition of a test we have that

$$P_{\theta_0}[X \notin \mathcal{A}(\theta_0)] \leq \alpha$$

where α is the significance level of the test. Now define, for each x, the set $\mathcal{C}(\mathbf{x})$ by

$$\mathcal{C}(x) = \{\theta_0 : \ x \in \mathcal{A}(\theta_0)\}$$

Then we have that for all θ_0

$$P_{\theta_0}[\mathcal{C}(X)] \geq 1 - \alpha$$

i.e., $\mathcal{C}(X)$ is a $1 - \alpha$ confidence set for θ.

Conversely if we have a $1 - \alpha$ confidence set for θ and if we define

$$\mathcal{A}(\theta_0) = \{x : \theta_0 \in \mathcal{C}(x)\}$$

then $\mathcal{A}(\theta_0)$ is the acceptance region of an α level significance test for θ_0.

Loosely speaking, what we have is that to every test there is a corresponding confidence interval (all those parameter values not rejected by the test). Conversely to every confidence interval there is a test (values outside of the interval are rejected). Thus tests and confidence intervals are **dual**.

Example. Let $X_1, X_2, \ldots, X_n$ be IID each normal with mean μ and variance σ^2. The t-test for $\mu = \mu_0$ rejects μ_0 if

$$\left| \frac{\sqrt{n}(\overline{x} - \mu_0)}{s} \right| > t_{1-\alpha/2}(n-1)$$

where

$$s^2 = \frac{1}{n-1} \sum_{i=1}^{n} (x_i - \overline{x})^2$$

and $t_{1-\alpha/2}(n-1)$ is the $1 - \alpha/2$ percentile of the Student's t distribution with $n-1$ degrees of freedom.

It follows that

$$A(\mu_0) = \left\{ \mathbf{x} : \left| \frac{\sqrt{n}(\overline{x} - \mu_0)}{s} \right| \leq t_{1-\alpha/2}(n-1) \right\}$$

Hence the $1 - \alpha$ level confidence interval is given by

$$\overline{x} \pm t_{1-\alpha/2}(n-1) \frac{s}{\sqrt{n}}$$

5.5 Composite Hypotheses

In the case where the hypotheses are not simple many types of tests have been proposed. The most important of which is the likelihood ratio test.

Definition 5.5.1. The **likelihood ratio test** rejects for $x \in \mathcal{C}$ where

$$\mathcal{C} = \left\{ x : \mathscr{LR}(x) = \frac{\max_{\theta \in \Theta_0} f(x; \theta)}{\max_{\theta \in \Theta} f(x; \theta)} \leq c \right\}$$

and c is chosen so that

$$\mathbb{P}_\theta \left(X \in C \right) \leq \alpha \ \text{ for } \theta \in \Theta_0$$

Likelihood ratio tests are the natural generalization of the Neyman–Pearson Lemma to composite hypotheses. Most of the tests used in standard statistical packages such as analysis of variance tests, analysis of deviance tests, and chi-square tests are all likelihood ratio tests or are equivalent to likelihood ratio tests for large samples.

In typical applications the likelihood ratio is given by

$$\mathscr{LR}(x) = \frac{f(x; \widehat{\theta}_0)}{f(x; \widehat{\theta})}$$

where $\widehat{\theta}$ is the maximum likelihood estimate of θ in the (full) model and $\widehat{\theta}_0$ is the maximum likelihood estimate of θ when θ is constrained to lie in Θ_0.

The likelihood ratio test has the attractive property that under the null hypothesis and certain regularity conditions, the asymptotic distribution of

$$-2 \ln[\mathscr{LR}(X)] \ \text{ is chi-square}$$

with degrees of freedom equal to the number of parameters in the full model minus the number of parameters in the (reduced) constrained model.

5.5.1 One-Way Analysis of Variance

Consider a one-way analysis of variance problem. That is, we have p groups and r observations per group. We assume further that all observations are realized values of independent normal random variables with

$$\mathbb{E}(Y_{ij}) = \mu_i \ \text{ and } \ \mathbb{V}(Y_{ij}) = \sigma^2$$

To develop the likelihood ratio test we first find the maximum for the full model. The joint density is given by

$$\prod_{i=1}^{p} \prod_{j=1}^{r} (2\pi\sigma^2)^{-1/2} \exp\left\{ -\frac{(y_{ij} - \mu_i)^2}{2\sigma^2} \right\}$$

which has logarithm given by

$$-\frac{rp}{2} \ln(2\pi) - \frac{rp}{2} \ln(\sigma^2) - \frac{1}{2\sigma^2} \sum_{i=1}^{p} \sum_{j=1}^{r} (y_{ij} - \mu_i)^2$$

The partial derivative with respect to μ_i is thus

$$\frac{1}{2\sigma^2} \sum_{j=1}^{r} (y_{ij} - \mu_i)$$

and it follows that the maximum likelihood estimate of μ_i is

$$\widehat{\mu}_i = \overline{y}_{i+}$$

i.e., the mean of the ith group.

The partial derivative with respect to σ^2 is

$$-\frac{rp}{2\sigma^2} + \frac{1}{2\sigma^4} \sum_{i=1}^{p} \sum_{j=1}^{r} (y_{ij} - \mu_i)^2$$

and it follows that the maximum likelihood estimate of σ^2 is given by

$$\widehat{\sigma}^2 = \frac{1}{rp} \sum_{i=1}^{p} \sum_{j=1}^{r} (y_{ij} - \overline{y}_{i+})^2$$

For these values of μ_i and σ^2 the log of the joint density is given by

$$-\frac{rp}{2} \ln(2\pi) - \frac{rp}{2} \ln(\widehat{\sigma}^2) - \frac{n}{2}$$

and hence the denominator of the likelihood ratio test is given by

$$(2\pi)^{-rp/2} [\widehat{\sigma}^2]^{-rp/2} e^{-rp/2}$$

which is the maximum for the full model.

Now we obtain the maximum for the reduced model. If the composite hypothesis $H_0 : \mu_1 = \mu_2 = \cdots = \mu_p = \mu$ is true then the joint density, $f(\mathbf{y}, \mu, \sigma^2)$, is given by

$$\prod_{i=1}^{p} \prod_{j=1}^{r} (2\pi\sigma^2)^{-1/2} \exp\left\{ -\frac{(y_{ij} - \mu)^2}{2\sigma^2} \right\}$$

which has logarithm

$$-\frac{rp}{2} \ln(2\pi) - \frac{rp}{2} \ln(\sigma^2) - \frac{1}{2\sigma^2} \sum_{i=1}^{p} \sum_{j=1}^{r} (y_{ij} - \mu)^2$$

The partial derivatives with respect to μ and σ^2 are thus

$$\frac{1}{2\sigma^2} \sum_{i=1}^{p} \sum_{j=1}^{r} (y_{ij} - \mu)$$

and

$$-\frac{rp}{2\sigma^2} + \frac{1}{2\sigma^4} \sum_{i=1}^{p} \sum_{j=1}^{r} (y_{ij} - \mu)^2$$

It follows that

$$\tilde{\mu} = \overline{y}_{++} \quad \text{and} \quad \tilde{\sigma}^2 = \frac{1}{rp} \sum_{i=1}^{p} \sum_{j=1}^{r} (y_{ij} - \overline{y}_{++})^2$$

The maximized log of the joint density is thus

$$-\frac{rp}{2} \ln(2\pi) - \frac{rp}{2} \ln(\tilde{\sigma}^2) - \frac{rp}{2}$$

Hence the numerator of the likelihood ratio test is given by

$$(2\pi)^{-rp/2} [\tilde{\sigma}^2]^{-rp/2} e^{-rp/2}$$

which is the maximum over the reduced model.

Thus the likelihood ratio is

$$\mathscr{LR}(\mathbf{y}) = \left[\frac{\hat{\sigma}^2}{\tilde{\sigma}^2} \right]^{rp/2} = \left[\frac{\sum_{i=1}^{p} \sum_{j=1}^{r} (y_{ij} - \overline{y}_{i+})^2}{\sum_{i=1}^{p} \sum_{j=1}^{r} (y_{ij} - \overline{y}_{++})^2} \right]^{rp/2}$$

Since

$$\sum_{i=1}^{p} \sum_{j=1}^{r} (y_{ij} - \overline{y}_{++})^2$$

can be written as

$$\sum_{i=1}^{p} \sum_{j=1}^{r} (y_{ij} - \overline{y}_{i+})^2 + r \sum_{i=1}^{p} (y_{i+} - \overline{y}_{++})^2$$

the likelihood ratio is given by

$$\left\{ \frac{1}{1 + \frac{\text{SSB}}{\text{SSE}}} \right\}^{rp/2}$$

where

$$\text{SSB} = r \sum_{i=1}^{p} (\overline{y}_{i+} - \overline{y}_{++})^2 \text{ and } \text{SSE} = \sum_{i=1}^{p} \sum_{i=1}^{r} (y_{ij} - \overline{y}_{i+})^2$$

are the between-group sum of squares and the within-group sum of squares.

The hypothesis is rejected whenever

$$\frac{\text{SSB}}{\text{SSE}}$$

is too large, i.e., whenever the estimated variability between the sample means (SSB) is too large relative to the variability within the groups (SSE).

The test is formally based on rejecting whenever

$$F_{obs} = \frac{\text{SSB}/(p-1)}{\text{SSE}/p(r-1)} \geq F_{1-\alpha}(p-1, p(r-1))$$

because we know the distribution of F, under the null hypothesis, is F with $(p-1)$ and $p(r-1)$ degrees of freedom. This test is called the F-test, named after Fisher, although in this form it was first derived by Snedecor.

5.6   The Multiple Testing Problem

Consider a problem in which we have N hypotheses

$$H_{01}, H_{02}, \ldots, H_{0N}$$

where N may be large (as it is in microarray problems). We also have N corresponding alternative hypotheses

$$H_{A1}, H_{A2}, \ldots, H_{AN}$$

For each individual problem suppose that we have a "good" test procedure which has an appropriate α and good power against the alternative. Also assume that the tests are independent. It is tempting to use each test at level α and state a conclusion such as

$$x \text{ of the tests rejected } H_{0i}$$

and the significance level is α.

From a frequentist's point of view this is incorrect: the overall significance level is much larger than α. To see this note that

Overall $\alpha = \mathbb{P}(\text{Reject at least one of the } H_{0i} \text{ when all are true})$

$\qquad = 1 - \mathbb{P}(\text{Do not reject any of the } H_{0i} \text{ when all are true})$

$\qquad = 1 - (1 - \alpha)^N$

A small table indicates the problem:

N	$\alpha = 0.05$	$\alpha = 0.01$	$\alpha = 0.001$
1	0.050	0.010	0.001
2	0.098	0.020	0.002
5	0.226	0.049	0.005
10	0.401	0.096	0.010
25	0.723	0.222	0.025
50	0.923	0.395	0.049
100	0.994	0.634	0.095

Note that for the widely level of $\alpha = 0.05$, for ten tests, the actual level is 40 % as opposed to the nominal level of 5 %.

Many methods exist to "correct" this problem:

1. Bonferoni adjustment
2. False Discovery Rate
3. Dozens of others including Duncan's multiple range test, Fisher's LSD approach, Duncan's k ratio test, Tukey's HSD, etc.

The basic scientific logic does not seem right, however. Consider an investigator who carefully designs a study to see the impact of vitamin supplements on bone loss in the elderly. Several hundred people are monitored, some on the vitamin regimen, the others not. Each person's bone loss is measured along with lots of other covariates such as gender, socioeconomic status, ethnicity, diet histories, etc.

The analysis is carefully done, and as expected, vitamin supplementation is associated with a significant decrease ($p < 0.05$) in bone loss. The results are submitted to the New Science in Medicine Journal. A referee asks whether or not tests were done on the association of bone loss with the other covariates. The response from the investigator is "of course" why not take advantage of the information available from my well-done study?

The response from the referee, a traditional frequentist, is as expected: after you adjust for the multiple tests, your results are no longer significant and of no use to our audience. Thank you for your submission and better luck next time.

Scientifically it makes no sense not to look at other aspects of the study and this should have no impact on the strength of the conclusions for the primary variable of interest. The fact that traditional frequentist methods force this dependence seems illogical.

5.7   Exercises

1. Using the Neyman–Pearson Lemma develop a test for $\lambda = \lambda_0$ vs $\lambda = \lambda_1 > \lambda_0$ in the exponential distribution.

2. If $X_1, X_2, X_3, X_4, X_5 \overset{d}{\sim}$ Bernoulli$(5, \theta)$ to test $\theta = .$ vs $\theta > 0.5$ show that we have a $1/16$ level test if we reject if $\sum_{i=1}^{5} X_i = 5$ or if $X_1 = 0, X_2 = 1, X_3 = 1, X_4 = 1, X_5 = 1$. Comment on the reasonableness of this test.

Chapter 6
Standard Practice of Statistics

6.1 Introduction

Most commonly used statistical methods, interval estimation (confidence intervals), estimation, hypothesis tests, and significance tests have as justification their properties under repeated sampling. This is the frequency interpretation of statistical methods and is the basis for much (most) of the statistical methods commonly applied to data in research and practice. This chapter is based on Table 2.1 in Royall. What we have shown in Chaps. 3–5 is that many of the standard statistical results are misleading.

6.2 Frequentist Statistical Procedures

6.2.1 Estimation

- **Procedure**
  An estimator $t(X)$ depending on a random variable X
- **Property of Procedure**
  Determined by the distribution of X

The expected value of $t(X)$ is θ

The standard error of $t(X)$ is σ

$E[t(X)] = \theta \quad , \quad \text{var}\,[t(X)] = \sigma^2$

- **Observation** Realized value of a random variable X

$X = x$, assumed to be generated by f_θ

© Springer International Publishing Switzerland 2014
C.A. Rohde, *Introductory Statistical Inference with the Likelihood Function*, DOI 10.1007/978-3-319-10461-4_6

- **Result of Procedure:** Fixed by observing $X = x$

$$\text{An estimate, } t(x)$$
$$\text{an estimate of variability, } \sigma(x)$$

- **"Usual" Interpretation:** Property used to interpret results

1. The observation x provides evidence that θ is near $t(x)$.
2. The smaller $\sigma(x)$, the stronger the evidence.

6.2.2   Confidence Intervals

- **Procedure**
  An interval $[\ell(X) , \; u(X)]$ depending on a random variable X
- **Property of Procedure**
  Determined by the distribution of X

  1. We are 95 % confident that the random interval $[\ell(X), u(X)]$ will contain θ.
  2. The confidence coefficient is

$$P[\ell(X) \leq \theta \leq u(X)] = 0.95$$

- **Observation:** Realized value of a random variable X

$$X = x, \text{ assumed to be generated by } f_\theta$$

- **Result of Procedure:** Fixed by observing $X = x$

$$\text{An interval } [\ell(x), u(x)]$$

- **"Usual" Interpretation:** Property used to interpret results

  1. The observation x provides evidence that θ is in the interval $[\ell(x), u(x)]$.
  2. Large confidence coefficient means strong evidence.

6.2.3   Hypothesis Testing

- **Procedure**

$$\text{A test } \delta(X) \text{ depending on a random variable } X$$

- **Property of Procedure**
  Determined by the distribution of X

  1. The Type I error probability is α.
  2. The Type II error probability is β.

- **Observation:** Realized value of a random variable X

$$X = x, \text{ assumed to be generated by } f_\theta$$

- **Result of Procedure:** Fixed by observing $X = x$. A selected hypothesis:

$$H_1 \text{ if } \delta(x) = 1, H_0 \text{ if } \delta(x) = 0$$

- **"Usual" Interpretation:** Property used to interpret results

  1. The observation x provides evidence in favor of the selected hypothesis.
  2. Small α and β mean strong evidence.

6.2.4 Significance Tests

- **Procedure**
  A statistic $t(X)$ depending on a random variable X
- **Property of Procedure**
  Determined by the distribution of X
  The probability of extreme values of t
- **Observation:** Realized value of a random variable X

$$X = x, \text{ assumed to be generated by } f_\theta$$

- **Result of Procedure:** Fixed by observing $X = x$

  1. A P-value defined by $P[t(X) \geq t(x)]$.
  2. The P-value is calculated under the assumption that H_0 is true.

- **"Usual" Interpretation:** Property used to interpret results.

  1. The observation x provides evidence against the null hypothesis.
  2. The smaller the P-value the stronger the evidence.

Chapter 7
Maximum Likelihood: Basic Results

7.1 Basic Properties

As we have seen once we have an estimator and its sampling distribution we can easily obtain confidence intervals and tests regarding the parameter. We now develop the theory of estimation focusing on the method of maximum likelihood, which for parametric models is the most widely used method. This will also supply us with a collection of statistical methods for important problems.

For comparing two values of a parameter, θ_2 vs θ_2, a natural role is played by the likelihood ratio

$$\mathcal{LR}(\theta_2, \theta_1; x) = \frac{f(x; \theta_2)}{f(x; \theta_1)}$$

According to the Law of Likelihood the likelihood ratio represents the statistical evidence in the data for comparing θ_2 to θ_1.

The **score function** is defined by

$$s(\theta; x) = \frac{\partial \ln[f(x; \theta)]}{\partial \theta}$$

The score function plays a major role in the theory of maximum likelihood estimation.

Example. Consider n iid normal random variables with parameters θ, σ^2 where σ^2 is known. Then

$$f(x; \theta) = (2\pi\sigma^2)^{-n/2} \exp\left\{ -\frac{1}{2\sigma^2} \sum_{i=1}^{n}(x_i - \theta)^2 \right\}$$

© Springer International Publishing Switzerland 2014
C.A. Rohde, *Introductory Statistical Inference with the Likelihood Function*, DOI 10.1007/978-3-319-10461-4_7

and

$$f'(x;\theta) = f(x;\theta)\frac{1}{\sigma^2}\sum_{i=1}^{n}(x_i - \theta)$$

It follows that

$$\frac{f'(x;\theta)}{f(x;\theta)} = \frac{n(\overline{x} - \theta)}{\sigma^2}$$

As a random variable we have that the score function has expected value 0 and variance n/σ^2 when evaluated at the true θ.

Because of the Law of Likelihood a natural estimate of θ is that value of θ which maximizes the likelihood or the log of the likelihood.

Assuming that $\ln[f(x;\theta)]$ is differentiable with respect to θ the maximum likelihood estimate is then the solution to

$$\frac{\partial \ln[f(x;\theta)]}{\partial \theta} = 0$$

which is called the **likelihood** or **score** equation. If there are r parameters we differentiate with respect to each and equate to 0, obtaining r equations. Note that one needs to check the second derivative to ensure a maximum.

Example 1 (Binomial).. If X is binomial with parameter θ then

$$f(x;\theta) = \binom{n}{x}\theta^x(1 - \theta)^{n-x} \quad x = 0, 1, \ldots, n$$

First note that if $x = 0$ then $f(0;\theta) = (1 - \theta)^n$ and in this case $\widehat{\theta} = 0$. If $x = n$ then $f(n;\theta) = \theta^n$ and in this case $\widehat{\theta} = 1$.

For $x = 1, 2, \ldots, n - 1$ we have that

$$\ln[f(x;\theta)] = \ln[\binom{n}{x}] = x\ln(\theta) + (n - x)\ln(1 - \theta)$$

and

$$\frac{\partial \ln[f(x;\theta)]}{\partial \theta} = \frac{x}{\theta} - \frac{n - x}{1 - \theta} = \frac{x - n\theta}{\theta(1 - \theta)}$$

It follows that

$$\widehat{\theta} = \frac{x}{n} \quad \text{for } x = 0, 1, \ldots, n$$

Note that it is unbiased with variance $\theta(1 - \theta)/n$ so that it is also consistent.

Example 2.. Let $Y_1, Y_2, \ldots, Y_n$ be iid each normal with mean μ and variance σ^2. Then we have

$$f(y; \theta) = \prod_{i=1}^{n} (2\pi\sigma^2)^{-1/2} \exp\left\{ -\frac{(y_i - \mu_i)^2}{2\sigma^2} \right\}$$

$$= (2\pi\sigma^2)^{-n/2} \exp\left\{ -\frac{\sum_{i=1}^{n}(y_i - \mu)^2}{2\sigma^2} \right\}$$

It follows that the log likelihood is given by

$$\ln[f(y; \theta)] = -\frac{n}{2}\ln(2\pi) - \frac{n}{2}\ln(\sigma^2) - \frac{1}{2\sigma^2}\sum_{i=1}^{n}(y_i - \mu)^2$$

Thus we have that

$$\frac{\partial \ln[f(x; \theta)]}{\partial \mu} = \frac{1}{\sigma^2}n(\bar{y} - \mu)$$

and

$$\frac{\partial \ln[f(x; \theta)]}{\partial \sigma^2} = -\frac{n}{2\sigma^2} + \frac{\sum_{i=1}^{n}(y_i - \mu)^2}{2\sigma^4}$$

and it follows that

$$\hat{\mu} = \bar{y} \quad \text{and} \quad \hat{\sigma}^2 = \frac{1}{n}\sum_{i=1}^{n}(y_i - \bar{y})^2$$

7.2 Consistency of Maximum Likelihood

1. Consider the case where there are only two possible values of the parameter θ_2 and θ_1.
2. Also suppose that we have n observations which are realized values of independent and identically distributed random variables having density $f(x; \theta_2)$ or $f(x; \theta_1)$.

The maximum likelihood estimate is defined by

$$\hat{\theta} = \begin{cases} \theta_2 \text{ if } f(x_1, x_2, \ldots, x_n; \theta_2) \geq f(x_1, x_2, \ldots, x_n; \theta_1) \\ \theta_1 \text{ otherwise} \end{cases}$$

1. Assume with no loss of generality that θ_2 is the true value of the parameter.
2. The maximum likelihood estimator is consistent if

$$\mathbb{P}_{\theta_2}(\widehat{\theta} = \theta_2) \; \longrightarrow \; 1$$

We note that $\widehat{\theta} = \theta_2$ if and only if

$$\frac{f(x_1, x_2, \ldots, x_n; \theta_2)}{f(x_1, x_2, \ldots, x_n; \theta_1)} = \prod_{i=1}^{n} \frac{f(x_i; \theta_2)}{f(x_i; \theta_1)} > 1$$

Equivalently

$$\sum_{i=1}^{n} \ln \left[\frac{f(x_i; \theta_2)}{f(x_i; \theta_1)} \right] > 0$$

Now note that the random variables

$$Y_i = \ln \left[\frac{f(X_i; \theta_2)}{f(X_i; \theta_1)} \right] \quad i = 1, 2, \ldots, n$$

are independent and identically distributed.

Moreover

$$\mathbb{E}_{\theta_2}(Y_i) = \int \ln \left[\frac{f(x; \theta_2)}{f(x; \theta_1)} \right] f(x; \theta_2) \lambda(dx)$$

$$= - \int \ln \left[\frac{f(x; \theta_1)}{f(x; \theta_2)} \right] f(x; \theta_2) \lambda(dx)$$

$$> - \int \left[\frac{f(x; \theta_1)}{f(x; \theta_2)} - 1 \right] f(x; \theta_2) \lambda(dx)$$

$$= 0$$

By the law of large numbers we have that

$$\frac{1}{n} \sum_{i=1}^{n} Y_i \; \xrightarrow{p} \; \mathbb{E}_{\theta_2}(Y) > 0$$

and hence

$$\mathbb{P}_{\theta_2}(\widehat{\theta} = \theta_2) \; \longrightarrow \; 1$$

i.e., $\widehat{\theta}$ is consistent:

1. The same proof holds provided the parameter space Θ is finite.
2. The more general case where Θ is an interval requires more delicate arguments and is of technical, not statistical interest.

7.3   General Results on the Score Function

We know that

$$\int f(x;\theta)d\lambda(x) = 1$$

for any density function $f(x;\theta)$. Recall that for a function g we write

$$\int g(x;\theta)d\lambda(x) = \begin{cases} \int g(x;\theta)dx & g \text{ continuous} \\ \sum g(x;\theta) & g \text{ discrete} \end{cases}$$

Assuming that we can differentiate under the integral or summation sign, we have that

$$\int \frac{\partial f(x;\theta)}{\partial\theta}d\lambda(x) = 0$$

Now note that

$$\frac{\partial f(x;\theta)}{\partial\theta} = \frac{\partial \ln[f(x;\theta)]}{\partial\theta}f(x;\theta)$$

It follows that

$$\mathbb{E}_\theta\left\{\frac{\partial \ln[f(x;\theta)]}{\partial\theta}\right\} = 0$$

Thus the expected value of the score function is 0.

If we differentiate again we have that

$$\int \frac{\partial^2 f(x;\theta)}{\partial\theta^2}\lambda(x) = 0$$

Noting that

$$\frac{\partial^2 f(x;\theta)}{\partial\theta^2} = \frac{\partial}{\partial}\left[\frac{\partial f(x;\theta)}{\partial\theta}\right]$$

$$= \frac{\partial}{\partial}\left[\frac{\partial \ln[f(x;\theta)]}{\partial\theta}f(x;\theta)\right]$$

we see that

$$\frac{\partial^2 f(x;\theta)}{\partial\theta^2} = \left[\frac{\partial^2 \ln[f(x;\theta)]}{\partial\theta^2}\right]f(x;\theta)$$

$$+ \left[\frac{\partial \ln[f(x;\theta)]}{\partial \theta} \right] \frac{\partial f(x;\theta)}{\partial \theta}$$

The right-hand side may be written as

$$\left[\frac{\partial^2 \ln[f(x;\theta)]}{\partial \theta^2} \right] f(x;\theta) + \left[\frac{\partial \ln[f(x;\theta)]}{\partial \theta} \right]^2 f(x;\theta)$$

It follows that

$$\mathbb{E}_\theta \left\{ \left[\frac{\partial \ln[f(x;\theta)]}{\partial \theta} \right]^2 \right\} = -\mathbb{E}_\theta \left\{ \left[\frac{\partial^2 \ln[f(x;\theta)]}{\partial \theta^2} \right] \right\}$$

and hence

$$\mathbb{V}_\theta \left\{ \frac{\partial \ln[f(x;\theta)]}{\partial \theta} \right\} = -\mathbb{E}_\theta \left\{ \left[\frac{\partial^2 \ln[f(x;\theta)]}{\partial \theta^2} \right] \right\}$$

The quantity

$$-\mathbb{E}_\theta \left\{ \left[\frac{\partial^2 \ln[f(x;\theta)]}{\partial \theta^2} \right] \right\}$$

is called the (expected) **Fisher information** and

$$-\left[\frac{\partial^2 \ln[f(x;\theta)]}{\partial \theta^2} \right]$$

is called the (observed) **Fisher information**.

7.4   General Maximum Likelihood

1. Let X be a random variable with density $f(x;\theta)$.
2. Assume that the parameter space Θ is an interval and that $f(x;\theta)$ is sufficiently smooth so that derivatives with respect to θ are defined and that differentiation under a summation or integral is allowed.
3. Finally assume that the range of X does not depend on θ.

Under weak regularity conditions it follows from the previous section that

$$\mathbb{E}_\theta \left\{ \left[\frac{\partial \ln[f(X;\theta)]}{\partial \theta} \right] \right\} = 0$$

$$\mathbb{E}_\theta \left\{ \left[\frac{\partial \ln[f(X;\theta)]}{\partial \theta} \right]^2 \right\} = -\mathbb{E}_\theta \left\{ \left[\frac{\partial^2 \ln[f(X;\theta)]}{\partial \theta^2} \right] \right\}$$

Thus the random variable

$$U(\theta) = \left[\frac{\partial \ln[f(X;\theta)]}{\partial \theta}\right]$$

i.e., the **score function** has expected value and variance given by

$$\mathbb{E}_\theta[U(\theta)] = 0 \;\;, \mathbb{V}_\theta[U(\theta)] = i(\theta)$$

where

$$i(\theta) = -\mathbb{E}_\theta\left\{\left[\frac{\partial^2 \ln[f(X;\theta)]}{\partial \theta^2}\right]\right\}$$

is the expected Fisher information for a sample size of one.

Example. If X is normal with mean θ and variance σ^2 with σ^2 known then

$$\ln[f(x;\theta)] = -\frac{1}{2}\ln[2\pi\sigma^2] - \frac{1}{2\sigma^2}(x - \theta)^2$$

and hence

$$\frac{\partial \ln[f(x;\theta)]}{\partial \theta} = \frac{x - \theta}{\sigma^2}$$

and

$$\frac{\partial^2 \ln[f(x;\theta)]}{\partial \theta^2} = -\frac{1}{\sigma^2}$$

so Fisher's information is

$$i(\theta) = \frac{1}{\sigma^2}$$

Example. If X is Bernoulli θ then

$$f(x;\theta) = \theta^x(1 - \theta)^{1-x}$$

and hence

$$\ln[f(x;\theta)] = x\ln(\theta) + (1 - x)\ln(1 - \theta)$$

It follows that

$$\frac{\partial \ln[f(x;\theta)]}{\partial \theta} = \frac{x}{\theta} - \frac{1-x}{1-\theta}$$

and

$$\frac{\partial^2 \ln[f(x;\theta)]}{\partial \theta^2} = -\frac{x}{\theta^2} - \frac{1-x}{(1-\theta)^2}$$

so Fisher's information is

$$i(\theta) = \frac{1}{\theta} + \frac{1}{1-\theta} = \frac{1}{\theta(1-\theta)}$$

If we have a random sample $X_1, X_2, \ldots, X_n$ from $f(x;\theta)$ and if

$$u_i(\theta) = \frac{\partial \ln[f(x_i;\theta)]}{\partial \theta}$$

then

$$\overline{U}(\theta) = \frac{1}{n} \sum_{i=1}^{n} U_i(\theta)$$

is the sample mean of n iid random variables with expected value 0 and variance $i(\theta)$. It follows that

$$\sqrt{n}\,\overline{U} \xrightarrow{d} N[0, i(\theta)]$$

by the central limit theorem.

Define the maximum likelihood estimate of θ as that value of θ which maximizes $f(\mathbf{x};\theta)$ or equivalently $\ln[f(\mathbf{x};\theta)]$.

Thus we solve

$$\frac{\partial \ln[f(\mathbf{x};\theta)]}{\partial \theta} = 0$$

or when $f(\mathbf{x};\theta) = \prod_{i=1}^{n} f(x_i;\theta)$ we solve

$$u(\theta) = \sum_{i=1}^{n} u_i(\theta) = 0$$

Since we can write, using Taylor's theorem,

$$u(\widehat{\theta}) = u(\theta) + \frac{du(\theta)}{d\theta}(\widehat{\theta} - \theta) + v(\theta^*)\frac{(\widehat{\theta} - \theta)^2}{2}$$

where

$$v(\theta^*) = \frac{d^2 u(\theta)}{d\theta^2}\bigg|_{\theta=\theta^*}$$

and θ^* is between θ and $\widehat{\theta}$.

Since $u(\widehat{\theta}) = 0$ we have

$$(\widehat{\theta} - \theta)\left[\frac{du(\theta)}{d\theta} + v(\theta^*)\frac{(\widehat{\theta} - \theta)}{2}\right] = -u(\theta)$$

It follows that

$$\sqrt{n}(\widehat{\theta} - \theta) = \frac{\frac{1}{\sqrt{n}}u(\theta)}{\left[-\frac{1}{n}\frac{du(\theta)}{d\theta} - \frac{1}{n}v(\theta^*)\frac{(\widehat{\theta} - \theta)}{2}\right]}$$

Application of the results of the preceding section shows that

$$\sqrt{n}(\widehat{\theta} - \theta) \xrightarrow{d} N(0, [i(\theta)]^{-1})$$

where $i(\theta)$ is Fisher's information for a sample of size 1.

7.5 Cramer-Rao Inequality

If $t(x)$ is any unbiased estimator of θ i.e.

$$\mathbb{E}[t(X)] = \theta$$

then

$$\int t(x)f(x;\theta)d\lambda(x) = \theta$$

Assuming that we can differentiate under the integral or summation sign, we have that

$$\int t(x)\frac{\partial \ln[f(x;\theta)]}{\partial \theta}f(x;\theta)d\lambda(x) = 1$$

and hence

$$\mathbb{C}\left\{t(X), \left[\frac{\partial \ln[f(X;\theta)]}{\partial \theta}\right]\right\} = 1$$

It follows that

$$\mathbb{V}[t(X)]\mathbb{V}\left\{\frac{\partial \ln[f(X;\theta)]}{\partial \theta}\right\} \geq 1$$

or

$$\mathbb{V}[t(X)] \geq \frac{1}{I(\theta)}$$

where $I(\theta)$ is the expected Fisher information. Thus the smallest variance for an unbiased estimator is the inverse of Fisher's information. This result is called the Cramer–Rao inequality.

Since $1/I(\theta)$ is the large sample variance of the maximum likelihood estimator we have the result that the method of maximum likelihood produces estimators which are asymptotically efficient, i.e., have smallest variance.

7.6 Summary Properties of Maximum Likelihood

1. Maximum likelihood have the **equivariance** property: i.e., the maximum likelihood estimate of $g(\theta)$, $\widehat{g(\theta)}$, is $g(\widehat{\theta})$.
2. Under weak regularity conditions maximum likelihood estimators are **consistent**, i.e.,

$$\widehat{\theta} \xrightarrow{p} \theta$$

3. Maximum likelihood estimators are **asymptotically normal**:

$$\sqrt{n}(\widehat{\theta} - \theta_0) \xrightarrow{d} N(0, v(\theta_0))$$

where $v(\theta_0)$ is the inverse of **Fisher's information**.
4. Maximum likelihood estimators are **asymptotically efficient**, i.e., in large samples

$$\mathbb{V}(\widehat{\theta}) \leq \mathbb{V}(\widetilde{\theta})$$

where $\widetilde{\theta}$ is any other consistent estimator which is asymptotically normal.

The regularity conditions under which the results on maximum likelihood estimators are true consist of conditions of the form:

(i) The range of the distributions cannot depend on the parameter.
(ii) The first three derivatives of the log likelihood function with respect to θ exist are continuous and have finite expected values as functions of X.

7.7 Multiparameter Case

All of the results for maximum likelihood generalize to the case where there are p parameters $\theta_1, \theta_2, \ldots, \theta_p$. Let

$$\boldsymbol{\theta} = \begin{bmatrix} \theta_1 \\ \theta_2 \\ \vdots \\ \theta_p \end{bmatrix}$$

If the pdf is given by

$$f(\mathbf{x}; \boldsymbol{\theta})$$

the maximum likelihood or score equation is

$$\frac{\partial \ln[f(\mathbf{x}; \boldsymbol{\theta})]}{\partial \boldsymbol{\theta}} = \begin{bmatrix} \frac{\partial \ln[f(\mathbf{x};\boldsymbol{\theta})]}{\partial \theta_1} \\ \frac{\partial \ln[f(\mathbf{x};\boldsymbol{\theta})]}{\partial \theta_2} \\ \vdots \\ \frac{\partial \ln[f(\mathbf{x};\boldsymbol{\theta})]}{\partial \theta_p} \end{bmatrix} = \mathbf{0}$$

Fisher's information matrix

$$\mathcal{I}(\boldsymbol{\theta})$$

has $i - j$ element given by

$$-\frac{\partial^2 \ln[f(\mathbf{x}; \boldsymbol{\theta})]}{\partial \theta_i \partial \theta_j}$$

Note that it is a $p \times p$ matrix.

Under regularity conditions, similar to those for the single parameter case we have

1. The maximum likelihood estimate of $g(\boldsymbol{\theta})$, $\widehat{g(\boldsymbol{\theta})}$, is $g(\widehat{\boldsymbol{\theta}})$.
2. Maximum likelihood estimators are **consistent**, i.e.,

$$\widehat{\boldsymbol{\theta}} \xrightarrow{p} \boldsymbol{\theta}$$

3. Maximum likelihood estimators are **asymptotically normal**:

$$(\widehat{\boldsymbol{\theta}} - \boldsymbol{\theta}_0) \approx \mathrm{N}(0, \mathbf{V}_n(\boldsymbol{\theta}_0))$$

where $\mathbf{V}_n(\boldsymbol{\theta}_0)$ is the inverse of Fisher's information matrix. We can replace $\boldsymbol{\theta}_0$ by $\widehat{\boldsymbol{\theta}}$ to use this result to determine confidence intervals.

7.8   Maximum Likelihood in the Multivariate Normal

Let $\mathbf{y}_1, \mathbf{y}_2, \ldots, \mathbf{y}_n$ be independent each having a multivariate normal distribution with parameters $\boldsymbol{\mu}$ and $\boldsymbol{\Sigma}$, i.e.,

$$f_{\mathbf{Y}_i}(\mathbf{y}_i; \boldsymbol{\mu}, \boldsymbol{\Sigma}) = (2\pi)^{-\frac{p}{2}} [\det(\boldsymbol{\Sigma})]^{-\frac{1}{2}} \exp\left\{ -\frac{1}{2}(\mathbf{y}_i - \boldsymbol{\mu})^\top \boldsymbol{\Sigma}^{-1}(\mathbf{y}_i - \boldsymbol{\mu}) \right\}$$

The joint density is thus

$$f_{\mathbf{Y}}(\mathbf{y}; \boldsymbol{\mu}, \boldsymbol{\Sigma}) = (2\pi)^{-\frac{np}{2}} [\det(\boldsymbol{\Sigma})]^{-\frac{n}{2}} \exp\left\{ -\frac{1}{2}\sum_{i=1}^n (\mathbf{y}_i - \boldsymbol{\mu})^\top \boldsymbol{\Sigma}^{-1}(\mathbf{y}_i - \boldsymbol{\mu}) \right\}$$

We will show that the maximum likelihood estimates of $\boldsymbol{\mu}$ and $\boldsymbol{\Sigma}$ are

$$\widehat{\boldsymbol{\mu}} = \overline{\mathbf{y}} = \frac{1}{n}\sum_{i=1}^n \mathbf{y}_i$$

and

$$\boldsymbol{\Sigma} = \mathbf{S} = \frac{1}{n}\sum_{i=1}^n (\mathbf{y}_i - \overline{\mathbf{y}})(\mathbf{y}_i - \overline{\mathbf{y}})^\top$$

i.e., the $j - k$ element of $\mathbf{S}$ is

$$\frac{1}{n}\sum_{i=1}^n (y_{ij} - \overline{y}_j)(y_{ik} - \overline{y}_k)$$

essentially the sample covariance between the jth and kth variable.
  The first step is to note that

$$\sum_{i=1}^n (\mathbf{y}_i - \boldsymbol{\mu})^\top \boldsymbol{\Sigma}^{-1}(\mathbf{y}_i - \boldsymbol{\mu})$$

can be written as

$$\sum_{i=1}^n (\mathbf{y}_i - \overline{\mathbf{y}})^\top \boldsymbol{\Sigma}^{-1}(\mathbf{y}_i - \overline{\mathbf{y}}) + n(\overline{\mathbf{y}} - \boldsymbol{\mu})^\top \boldsymbol{\Sigma}^{-1}(\overline{\mathbf{y}} - \boldsymbol{\mu})$$

or

$$n\mathrm{tr}\left[\boldsymbol{\Sigma}^{-1}\mathbf{S}\right] + n(\overline{\mathbf{y}} - \boldsymbol{\mu})^\top \boldsymbol{\Sigma}^{-1}(\overline{\mathbf{y}} - \boldsymbol{\mu})$$

where the trace of a square matrix, $\text{tr}(A)$, is the sum of the diagonal elements, i.e.,

$$\text{tr}(A) = \sum_{i=1}^{p} a_{ii}$$

Thus the joint density $f_{\mathbf{Y}}(\mathbf{y}; \boldsymbol{\mu}, \boldsymbol{\Sigma}) =$ can be written as

$$(2\pi)^{-\frac{np}{2}} [\det(\boldsymbol{\Sigma})]^{-\frac{n}{2}} \exp\left\{-\frac{n}{2}\text{tr}\left[\boldsymbol{\Sigma}^{-1}\mathbf{S}\right] - \frac{n}{2}(\overline{\mathbf{y}} - \boldsymbol{\mu})^{\top}\boldsymbol{\Sigma}^{-1}(\overline{\mathbf{y}} - \boldsymbol{\mu})\right\}$$

It follows immediately that the maximum likelihood estimate of $\boldsymbol{\mu}$ is $\overline{\mathbf{y}}$ and the joint density at $\widehat{\boldsymbol{\mu}}$ and $\widehat{\boldsymbol{\Sigma}} = \mathbf{S}$ is thus

$$f_{\mathbf{Y}}(\mathbf{y}; \widehat{\boldsymbol{\mu}}, \widehat{\boldsymbol{\Sigma}}) = (2\pi)^{-\frac{np}{2}} [\det(\mathbf{S})]^{-\frac{n}{2}} \exp\left\{-\frac{np}{2}\right\}$$

The ratio

$$\frac{f_{\mathbf{Y}}(\mathbf{y}; \widehat{\boldsymbol{\mu}}, \widehat{\boldsymbol{\Sigma}})}{f_{\mathbf{Y}}(\mathbf{y}; \boldsymbol{\mu}, \boldsymbol{\Sigma})}$$

is thus equal to

$$\frac{[\det(\mathbf{S})]^{-\frac{n}{2}} \exp\left\{-\frac{np}{2}\right\}}{[\det(\boldsymbol{\Sigma})]^{-\frac{n}{2}} \exp\left\{-\frac{n}{2}\text{tr}\left[\boldsymbol{\Sigma}^{-1}\mathbf{S}\right] - \frac{n}{2}(\overline{\mathbf{y}} - \boldsymbol{\mu})^{\top}\boldsymbol{\Sigma}^{-1}(\overline{\mathbf{y}} - \boldsymbol{\mu})\right\}}$$

which is greater than or equal to

$$\det(\boldsymbol{\Sigma}^{-1}\mathbf{S})^{-\frac{n}{2}} \exp\left\{-\frac{np}{2} + \frac{n}{2}\text{tr}\left[\boldsymbol{\Sigma}^{-1}\mathbf{S}\right]\right\}$$

This ratio is greater than or equal to 1 if and only its logarithm is greater than or equal to 0. The logarithm is

$$\frac{n}{2}\left\{-\ln\left[\det(\boldsymbol{\Sigma}^{-1}\mathbf{S})\right] - p + \text{tr}\left[\boldsymbol{\Sigma}^{-1}\mathbf{S}\right]\right\}$$

If $\lambda_1, \lambda_2, \ldots, \lambda_p$ are the characteristic roots of $\boldsymbol{\Sigma}^{-1}\mathbf{S}$ then it can be shown that

1. $\lambda_i \geq 0$ for each i
2. $\det(\boldsymbol{\Sigma}^{-1}\mathbf{S}) = \prod_{i=1}^{p} \lambda_i$
3. $\text{tr}(\boldsymbol{\Sigma}^{-1}\mathbf{S}) = \sum_{i=1}^{p} \lambda_i$

It follows that the log of the ratio is greater than or equal to

$$\frac{n}{2}\left\{-\sum_{i=1}^{p} \ln(\lambda_i) - \frac{p}{2} + \sum_{i=1}^{p} \lambda_i\right\}$$

or

$$\frac{n}{2}\left\{\sum_{i=1}^{p}[\lambda_i - 1 - \ln(\lambda_i)]\right\}$$

which is greater than or equal to zero since

$$a - 1 - \ln(a) \geq 0 \text{ for any positive real number}$$

Thus the maximum likelihood estimators for the multivariate normal are

$$\widehat{\boldsymbol{\mu}} = \overline{\mathbf{y}} \text{ and } \widehat{\boldsymbol{\Sigma}} = \mathbf{S}$$

We usually use

$$\frac{n}{n-1}\mathbf{S}$$

as the estimator so that the estimated components of $\boldsymbol{\Sigma}$ are exactly the sample covariances and variances.

7.9   Multinomial

Suppose that $X_1, X_2, \ldots, X_k$ have a multinomial distribution, i.e.,

$$f(x_1, x_2, \ldots, x_k; \theta_1, \theta_2, \ldots, \theta_k) = n! \prod_{i=1}^{k} \frac{\theta_i^{x_i}}{x_i!}$$

where

$$0 \leq x_i \leq n \text{ each } i = 1, 2, \ldots, k \text{ and } \sum_{i=1}^{k} x_i = n$$

and

$$0 \leq \theta_i \leq 1 \text{ each } i = 1, 2, \ldots, k \text{ and } \sum_{i=1}^{k} \theta_i = 1$$

Note that

$$\theta_k = 1 - \sum_{i=1}^{k-1} \theta_i \text{ and } x_k = n - \sum_{i=1}^{k-1} x_i$$

The maximum likelihood estimates of the θ_i are found by taking the partial derivatives of the log likelihood with respect to θ_i for $i = 1, 2, \ldots, k - 1$ where the log likelihood is

$$\ln[f(\mathbf{x}, \boldsymbol{\theta}] = \ln(n!) - \sum_{i=1}^{k} \ln(x_i!) + \sum_{i=1}^{k} x_i \ln(\theta_i)$$

Since $\theta_k = 1 - \theta_1 - \theta_2 - \cdots - \theta_{k-1}$ we have

$$\frac{\partial \ln[f(\mathbf{x}, \boldsymbol{\theta})]}{\partial \theta_i} = \frac{x_i}{\theta_i} - \frac{x_k}{\theta_k}$$

for $i = 1, 2, \ldots, k - 1$. It follows that the maximum likelihood estimates satisfy

$$x_i \widehat{\theta}_k = \widehat{\theta}_i x_k \quad \text{for } i = 1, 2, \ldots, k - 1$$

Summing from $i = 1$ to $k - 1$ yields

$$(n - x_k)\widehat{\theta}_k = (1 - \widehat{\theta}_k)x_k$$

and hence

$$n\widehat{\theta}_k = x_k$$

so that

$$\frac{x_i x_k}{n} = \widehat{\theta}_i x_k \quad \text{or} \quad \widehat{\theta}_i = \frac{x_i}{n}$$

The second derivatives of the log likelihood are given by

$$\frac{\partial^2 \ln[f(\mathbf{x}, \boldsymbol{\theta})]}{\partial \theta_i^2} = -\frac{x_i}{\theta_i^2} - \frac{x_k}{\theta_k}$$

which has expected value

$$-\frac{n\theta_i}{\theta_i^2} - \frac{n\theta_k}{\theta_k^2} = -\frac{n}{\theta_i} - \frac{n}{\theta_k}$$

and

$$\frac{\partial^2 \ln[f(\mathbf{x}, \boldsymbol{\theta})]}{\partial \theta_i \partial \theta_j} = -\frac{x_k}{\theta_k^2}$$

which has expected value

$$-\frac{n\theta_k}{\theta_k^2} = -\frac{n}{\theta_k}$$

Thus Fisher's information matrix, $\mathcal{I}(\boldsymbol{\theta})$, is given by

$$\mathcal{I}(\boldsymbol{\theta}) = n \begin{bmatrix} \frac{1}{\theta_1} + \frac{1}{\theta_k} & \frac{1}{\theta_k} & \cdots & \frac{1}{\theta_k} \\ \frac{1}{\theta_k} & \frac{1}{\theta_2} + \frac{1}{\theta_k} & \cdots & \frac{1}{\theta_k} \\ \vdots & \vdots & \ddots & \vdots \\ \frac{1}{\theta_k} & \frac{1}{\theta_k} & \cdots & \frac{1}{\theta_{k-1}} + \frac{1}{\theta_k} \end{bmatrix}$$

Fisher's information can be written in matrix form as

$$n \left[\mathbf{D}(\boldsymbol{\theta})^{-1} + \frac{1}{\theta_k} \mathbf{1}\mathbf{1}^\top \right]$$

where $\mathbf{D}(\boldsymbol{\theta})$ is a $k - 1 \times k - 1$ matrix with diagonal elements $\theta_1, \theta_2, \ldots, \theta_{k-1}$ and $\mathbf{1}$ is a $k - 1$ column vector with each element equal to 1.

The general theory of maximum likelihood then implies that

$$\sqrt{n}(\widehat{\boldsymbol{\theta}} - \boldsymbol{\theta}) \xrightarrow{d} \mathrm{N}\left(\mathbf{0}, [i(\boldsymbol{\theta})]^{-1}\right)$$

where $i(\boldsymbol{\theta})$ is Fisher's information matrix with $n = 1$.

It is easy to check that

$$[i(\boldsymbol{\theta})]^{-1} = \mathbf{D}(\boldsymbol{\theta}) - \boldsymbol{\theta}\boldsymbol{\theta}^\top$$

or

$$[i(\boldsymbol{\theta})]^{-1} = \begin{bmatrix} \theta_1(1-\theta_1) & -\theta_1\theta_2 & \cdots & -\theta_1\theta_{k-1} \\ -\theta_2\theta_1 & \theta_2(1-\theta_2) & \cdots & -\theta_2\theta_{k-1} \\ \vdots & \vdots & \ddots & \vdots \\ \theta_{k-1}\theta_1 & -\theta_{k-1}\theta_2 & \cdots & \theta_{k-1}(1-\theta_{k-1}) \end{bmatrix}$$

which we recognize as the variance covariance matrix of $X_1, X_2, \ldots, X_{k-1}$

Standard maximum likelihood theory implies that

$$n(\widehat{\boldsymbol{\theta}} - \boldsymbol{\theta})^\top [i(\boldsymbol{\theta}] (\widehat{\boldsymbol{\theta}} - \boldsymbol{\theta}) \xrightarrow{d} \chi^2(k-1)$$

Now note that

$$n(\widehat{\boldsymbol{\theta}} - \boldsymbol{\theta})^\top [i(\boldsymbol{\theta}](\widehat{\boldsymbol{\theta}} - \boldsymbol{\theta})$$

is equal to

$$n(\widehat{\boldsymbol{\theta}} - \boldsymbol{\theta})^{\top} \left[\mathbf{D}(\boldsymbol{\theta})^{-1} + \frac{1}{p_k} \mathbf{1}\mathbf{1}^{\top} \right] (\widehat{\boldsymbol{\theta}} - \boldsymbol{\theta})$$

and hence to

$$n(\widehat{\boldsymbol{\theta}} - \boldsymbol{\theta})^{\top} \mathbf{D}(\boldsymbol{\theta})^{-1} (\widehat{\boldsymbol{\theta}} - \boldsymbol{\theta}) + \frac{n}{\theta_k} (\widehat{\boldsymbol{\theta}} - \boldsymbol{\theta})^{\top} \mathbf{1}\mathbf{1}^{\top} (\widehat{\boldsymbol{\theta}} - \boldsymbol{\theta})$$

This last expression simplifies to

$$n \sum_{i=1}^{k-1} \frac{(\widehat{\theta}_i - \theta_i)^2}{\theta_i} + \frac{n}{\theta_k} \left[\sum_{i=1}^{k-1} (\widehat{\theta}_i - \theta_i) \right]^2$$

which in turn simplifies to

$$\sum_{i=1}^{k-1} \frac{(x_i - n\theta_i)^2}{n\theta_i} + \frac{n}{\theta_k} (\theta_k - \widehat{\theta}_k)^2$$

and to

$$\sum_{i=1}^{k-1} \frac{(x_i - n\theta_i)^2}{n\theta_i} + \frac{(x_k - n\theta_k)^2}{n\theta_k}$$

This finally reduces to

$$\sum_{i=1}^{k} \frac{(x_i - n\theta_i)^2}{n\theta_i}$$

Noting that $\mathbb{E}(X_i) = n\theta_i = E_i$ this last formula may be written as

$$\sum_{i=1}^{k} \frac{(X_i - E_i)^2}{E_i}$$

which is called Pearson's chi-square statistic. For large n, it has a chi-square distribution with $k - 1$ degrees of freedom.

Chapter 8
Linear Models

8.1 Introduction

There is no doubt that the linear model is one of the most important and useful models in statistics. In this chapter we discuss the estimation problem in linear models and discuss interpretations of standard results.

While some of the detailed formulas appear complex they are based on two simple ideas:

1. The Pythagorean theorem
2. Solving two or three linear equations

8.2 Basic Results

Suppose we have a response $\mathbf{y}$, an $n \times 1$ vector, and a set of covariates

$$\mathbf{1}, \mathbf{x}_1, \ldots, \mathbf{x}_p$$

which we collect in an $n \times (p+1)$ matrix $\mathbf{Z}$.

If we represent y_i as a linear combination of the covariates we have

$$y_i = \sum_{j=0} z_{ij}\alpha_j \ \text{ or } \ \mathbf{y} = \mathbf{Z}\boldsymbol{\alpha}$$

where $z_{i0} \equiv 1$ for all i.

Assumption 1. $\mathbf{y}$ is a realized value of a random vector $\mathbf{Y}$ where

$$\mathbb{E}(\mathbf{Y}) = \mathbf{Z}\boldsymbol{\alpha} \ \text{ and } \ \text{Var}(\mathbf{Y}) = \mathbf{I}\sigma^2$$

© Springer International Publishing Switzerland 2014
C.A. Rohde, *Introductory Statistical Inference with the Likelihood Function*, DOI 10.1007/978-3-319-10461-4_8

Assumption 2. $\mathbf{y}$ is a realized value of a random vector $\mathbf{Y}$ where

$$\mathbf{Y} \stackrel{d}{\sim} \mathrm{MVN}(\mathbf{Z}\boldsymbol{\alpha}, \mathbf{I}\sigma^2)$$

Definition 8.2.1. The **least squares** estimate of $\boldsymbol{\alpha}$ is the minimizer over $\boldsymbol{\alpha}$ of

$$\mathrm{SSE}(\boldsymbol{\alpha}; \mathbf{y}) = \sum_{i=1}^{n} \left(y_i - \sum_{j=0}^{p} z_{ij}\alpha_j \right)^2 = (\mathbf{y} - \mathbf{Z}\boldsymbol{\alpha})^\top (\mathbf{y} - \mathbf{Z}\boldsymbol{\alpha})$$

Theorem 8.2.1. *The least squares estimate of $\boldsymbol{\alpha}$ is given by*

$$\widehat{\boldsymbol{\alpha}} = (\mathbf{Z}^\top \mathbf{Z})^{-1}\mathbf{Z}^\top \mathbf{y}$$

Moreover the minimum value can be expressed as

$$(\mathbf{y} - \mathbf{Z}\widehat{\boldsymbol{\alpha}})^\top (\mathbf{y} - \mathbf{Z}\widehat{\boldsymbol{\alpha}}) = \mathbf{y}^\top \mathbf{y} - \widehat{\boldsymbol{\alpha}}^\top \mathbf{Z}^\top \mathbf{Z}\widehat{\boldsymbol{\alpha}} = \mathbf{y}^\top \mathbf{y} - \mathbf{y}^\top \mathbf{Z}(\mathbf{Z}^\top \mathbf{Z})^{-1}\mathbf{Z}^\top \mathbf{y} = \mathbf{y}^\top \mathbf{D}_Z \mathbf{y}$$

where

$$\mathbf{D}_Z =: \mathbf{I} - \mathbf{Z}(\mathbf{Z}^\top \mathbf{Z})^{-1}\mathbf{Z}^\top$$

Proof.

$$\begin{aligned}
\mathrm{SSE}(\boldsymbol{\alpha}; \mathbf{y}) &= (\mathbf{y} - \mathbf{Z}\boldsymbol{\alpha})^\top (\mathbf{y} - \mathbf{Z}\boldsymbol{\alpha}) \\
&= [(\mathbf{y} - \mathbf{Z}\widehat{\boldsymbol{\alpha}}) + (\mathbf{Z}\widehat{\boldsymbol{\alpha}} - \mathbf{Z}\boldsymbol{\alpha})]^\top [(\mathbf{y} - \mathbf{Z}\widehat{\boldsymbol{\alpha}}) + (\mathbf{Z}\widehat{\boldsymbol{\alpha}} - \mathbf{Z}\boldsymbol{\alpha})] \\
&= (\mathbf{y} - \mathbf{Z}\widehat{\boldsymbol{\alpha}})^\top (\mathbf{y} - \mathbf{Z}\widehat{\boldsymbol{\alpha}}) + (\mathbf{Z}\widehat{\boldsymbol{\alpha}} - \mathbf{Z}\boldsymbol{\alpha})^\top (\mathbf{Z}\widehat{\boldsymbol{\alpha}} - \mathbf{Z}\boldsymbol{\alpha}) \\
&\quad + 2(\mathbf{Z}\widehat{\boldsymbol{\alpha}} - \mathbf{Z}\boldsymbol{\alpha})^\top (\mathbf{y} - \mathbf{Z}\widehat{\boldsymbol{\alpha}}) \\
&= (\mathbf{y} - \mathbf{Z}\widehat{\boldsymbol{\alpha}})^\top (\mathbf{y} - \mathbf{Z}\widehat{\boldsymbol{\alpha}}) + (\widehat{\boldsymbol{\alpha}} - \boldsymbol{\alpha})^\top \mathbf{Z}^\top \mathbf{Z}(\widehat{\boldsymbol{\alpha}} - \boldsymbol{\alpha})
\end{aligned}$$

The conclusion follows if the "cross-product" term vanishes.

To show that the "cross-product" term vanishes we note that

$$2(\mathbf{Z}\widehat{\boldsymbol{\alpha}} - \mathbf{Z}\boldsymbol{\alpha})^\top (\mathbf{y} - \mathbf{Z}\widehat{\boldsymbol{\alpha}}) = 2(\widehat{\boldsymbol{\alpha}} - \boldsymbol{\alpha})^\top \mathbf{Z}^\top (\mathbf{y} - \mathbf{Z}(\mathbf{Z}^\top \mathbf{Z})^{-1}\mathbf{Z}^\top \mathbf{y}) = 0$$

For the minimum value note that

$$\begin{aligned}
(\mathbf{y} - \mathbf{Z}\widehat{\boldsymbol{\alpha}})^\top (\mathbf{y} - \mathbf{Z}\widehat{\boldsymbol{\alpha}}) &= \mathbf{y}^\top \mathbf{y} - 2\mathbf{y}^\top \mathbf{Z}\widehat{\boldsymbol{\alpha}} + \widehat{\boldsymbol{\alpha}}^\top \mathbf{Z}^\top \mathbf{Z}\widehat{\boldsymbol{\alpha}} \\
&= \mathbf{y}^\top \mathbf{y} - \widehat{\boldsymbol{\alpha}}^\top \mathbf{Z}^\top \mathbf{Z}\widehat{\boldsymbol{\alpha}} \\
&= \mathbf{y}^\top \mathbf{y} - \mathbf{y}^\top \mathbf{Z}(\mathbf{Z}^\top \mathbf{Z})^{-1}\mathbf{Z}^\top \mathbf{y} \\
&= \mathbf{y}^\top [\mathbf{I} - \mathbf{Z}(\mathbf{Z}^\top \mathbf{Z})^{-1}\mathbf{Z}^\top]\mathbf{y} \\
&= \mathbf{y}^\top \mathbf{D}_Z \mathbf{y}
\end{aligned}$$

Under Assumption 2 the density of $\mathbf{y}$ is given by

$$f(\mathbf{y}; \boldsymbol{\alpha}, \sigma^2) = (2\pi\sigma^2)^{-n/2} \exp\left\{ -\frac{1}{2\sigma^2}(\mathbf{y} - \mathbf{Z}\boldsymbol{\alpha})^\top (\mathbf{y} - \mathbf{Z}\boldsymbol{\alpha}) \right\}$$

$$= (2\pi\sigma^2)^{-n/2} \exp\left\{ -\frac{1}{2\sigma^2} \sum_{i=1}^{n} \left(y_i - \sum_{j=0}^{p} z_{ij}\alpha_j \right)^2 \right\}$$

It is obvious that the least squares and maximum likelihood estimates are equal:

1. $\widehat{\boldsymbol{\alpha}}$ is unbiased since

$$\mathbb{E}(\widehat{\boldsymbol{\alpha}}) = \mathbb{E}[(\mathbf{Z}^\top \mathbf{Z})^{-1} \mathbf{Z}^\top \mathbf{Y}$$
$$= (\mathbf{Z}^\top \mathbf{Z})^{-1} \mathbf{Z}^\top \mathbb{E}[\mathbf{Y}]$$
$$= (\mathbf{Z}^\top \mathbf{Z})^{-1} \mathbf{Z}^\top \mathbf{Z}\boldsymbol{\alpha}$$
$$= \boldsymbol{\alpha}$$

2. The variance of $\widehat{\boldsymbol{\alpha}}$ is $(\mathbf{Z}^\top \mathbf{Z})^{-1}\sigma^2$ since

$$\mathrm{Var}(\widehat{\boldsymbol{\alpha}}) = \mathrm{Var}[(\mathbf{Z}^\top \mathbf{Z})^{-1} \mathbf{Z}^\top \mathbf{Y}]$$
$$= (\mathbf{Z}^\top \mathbf{Z})^{-1} \mathbf{Z}^\top \mathrm{Var}(\mathbf{Y})\mathbf{Z}(\mathbf{Z}^\top \mathbf{Z})^{-1}$$
$$= (\mathbf{Z}^\top \mathbf{Z})^{-1}\sigma^2$$

3. If Assumption 2 is satisfied then since $\widehat{\boldsymbol{\alpha}}$ is a linear combination of normally distributed random variables it follows that

$$\widehat{\boldsymbol{\alpha}} \stackrel{d}{\sim} \mathrm{MVN}[\boldsymbol{\alpha}, (\mathbf{Z}^\top \mathbf{Z})^{-1}\sigma^2]$$

8.2.1   The Fitted Values and the Residuals

The fitted values are defined as

$$\widehat{\mathbf{y}} = \mathbf{Z}\widehat{\boldsymbol{\alpha}} = \mathbf{Z}(\mathbf{Z}^\top \mathbf{Z})^{-1}\mathbf{Z}^\top \mathbf{y} = \mathbf{H}_Z \mathbf{y}$$

where

$$\mathbf{H}_Z =: \mathbf{Z}(\mathbf{Z}^\top \mathbf{Z})^{-1}\mathbf{Z}^\top \quad \text{is called the hat matrix}$$

and the residuals are defined as

$$\mathbf{e} = \mathbf{y} - \widehat{\mathbf{y}} = [\mathbf{I} - \mathbf{H}_Z]\mathbf{y} = \mathbf{D}_Z\mathbf{y}$$

where

$$\mathbf{D}_Z =: \ \mathbf{I} - \mathbf{Z}(\mathbf{Z}^\top\mathbf{Z})^{-1}\mathbf{Z}^\top$$

Note that $\mathbf{H}_Z$ and $\mathbf{D}_Z$ are symmetric and idempotent and that

$$\mathbf{H}_Z\mathbf{D}_Z = \mathbf{O}$$

Note that

$$\mathbf{y} = \mathbf{e} + \widehat{\mathbf{y}} \ \text{ and } \ \mathbf{e}^\top\widehat{\mathbf{y}} = 0$$

so that

$$\mathbf{y}^\top\mathbf{y} = \widehat{\mathbf{y}}^\top\widehat{\mathbf{y}} + \mathbf{e}^\top\mathbf{e}$$

which is just the Pythagorean theorem.
    Note that

$$\text{SSE} = \mathbf{Y}^\top\mathbf{D}_Z\mathbf{y}$$

so that the residual or error sum of squares is a quadratic form.
If $\mathbf{Y}^\top\mathbf{Q}\mathbf{Y}$ is a quadratic form then it is known that

$$\mathbb{E}(\mathbf{Y}^\top\mathbf{Q}\mathbf{Y}) = \text{tr}[Q\text{Var}(\mathbf{Y})] + \mathbb{E}(\mathbf{Y})^\top\mathbf{Q}\mathbb{E}(\mathbf{Y})$$

where $\text{tr}(\mathbf{A})$ is the trace of $\mathbf{A}$, i.e., $\sum_{i=1}^{n} a_{ii}$.
    Since the error sum of squares is a quadratic form we have that

$$\mathbb{E}[\text{SSE}] = \text{tr}[\mathbf{D}_Z\mathbf{I}\sigma^2] + (\mathbf{Z}\boldsymbol{\alpha})^\top\mathbf{D}_Z\mathbf{Z}\boldsymbol{\alpha}$$

Clearly

$$\text{tr}[\mathbf{D}_Z\mathbf{I}\sigma^2] = \sigma^2\text{tr}[\mathbf{I} - \mathbf{Z}(\mathbf{Z}^\top\mathbf{Z})^{-1}\mathbf{Z}^\top] = \sigma^2[\text{tr}(\mathbf{I}) - \text{tr}\{\mathbf{Z}(\mathbf{Z}^\top\mathbf{Z})^{-1}\mathbf{Z}^\top\}]$$
$$= (n - p - 1)\sigma^2$$

and since

$$\mathbf{D}_Z\mathbf{Z} = \mathbf{O}$$

we have that

$$\frac{\text{SSE}}{n - p - 1}$$

is an unbiased estimator of σ^2

8.3 The Basic "Regression" Model

If we write $\mathbf{Z} = [\mathbf{1}, \mathbf{X}]$, $\alpha_0 = \beta_0$, and $\alpha_j = \beta_j$ then the equations $\mathbf{Z}^\top \mathbf{Z} \widehat{\alpha} = \mathbf{Z}^\top \mathbf{y}$ become

$$\begin{bmatrix} n & \mathbf{1}^\top \mathbf{X} \\ \mathbf{X}^\top \mathbf{1} & \mathbf{X}^\top \mathbf{X} \end{bmatrix} \begin{bmatrix} \widehat{\beta}_0 \\ \widehat{\beta} \end{bmatrix} = \begin{bmatrix} \mathbf{1}^\top \mathbf{y} \\ \mathbf{X}^\top \mathbf{y} \end{bmatrix}$$

It follows that

$$\widehat{\beta}_0 = \frac{1}{n} \mathbf{1}^\top (\mathbf{y} - \mathbf{X}\widehat{\beta})$$

Substituting into the second equation we get

$$\mathbf{X}^\top \mathbf{1} \left\{ \frac{1}{n} \mathbf{1}^\top (\mathbf{y} - \mathbf{X}\widehat{\beta}) \right\} + \mathbf{X}^\top \mathbf{X} \widehat{\beta} = \mathbf{X}^\top \mathbf{y}$$

or

$$\mathbf{X}^\top \mathbf{D}_1 \mathbf{X} \widehat{\beta} = \mathbf{X}^\top \mathbf{D}_1 \mathbf{y}$$

where $D_1 = \mathbf{I} - \frac{1}{n} \mathbf{1} \mathbf{1}^\top$

Thus

$$\widehat{\beta} = (\mathbf{X}^\top \mathbf{D}_1 \mathbf{X})^{-1} \mathbf{X}^\top \mathbf{D}_1 \mathbf{y}$$

Note that for any vectors $\mathbf{z}$ and $\mathbf{w}$ we have

$$\mathbf{z}^\top \mathbf{D}_1 \mathbf{w} = \mathbf{z}^\top \left[\mathbf{I} - \frac{1}{n} \mathbf{1} \mathbf{1}^\top \right] \mathbf{w}$$

$$= \mathbf{z}^\top \mathbf{w} - \frac{1}{n} \mathbf{z}^\top \mathbf{1} \mathbf{w}^\top \mathbf{1}$$

$$= \sum_{i=1}^{n} z_i w_i - n \overline{z} \overline{w}$$

$$= \sum_{i=1}^{n} (z_i - \overline{z})(w_i - \overline{w})$$

i.e., $\mathbf{z}^\top \mathbf{D}_1 \mathbf{w}$ is $n - 1$ times the sample covariance of $\mathbf{z}$ and $\mathbf{w}$. It follows that the estimates of the regression coefficients are determined by the sample covariances (correlations) of the covariates and the sample covariances (correlations) of the covariates with the response.

If $\mathbf{X} = \mathbf{x}$, i.e., $p = 1$, we have a simple linear regression model and

$$\widehat{\beta} = \frac{\mathbf{x}^\top \mathbf{D}_1 \mathbf{y}}{\mathbf{x}^\top \mathbf{x}} = \frac{\sum_{i=1}^{n}(x_i - \overline{x})(y_i - \overline{y})}{\sum_{i=1}^{n}(x_i - \overline{x})^2}$$

Note that

$$\mathbf{y} - \mathbf{1}\widehat{\beta}_0 - \mathbf{X}\widehat{\beta} = \mathbf{y} - \mathbf{1}\overline{y} - \mathbf{D}_1 \mathbf{X}\widehat{\beta} = \mathbf{D}_1 \mathbf{y} - \mathbf{D}_1 \mathbf{X}\widehat{\beta}$$

so that

$$(\mathbf{y} - \mathbf{1}\widehat{\beta}_0 - \mathbf{X}\widehat{\beta})^\top (\mathbf{y} - \mathbf{1}\widehat{\beta}_0 - \mathbf{X}\widehat{\beta}) = \mathbf{y}^\top \mathbf{D}_1 \mathbf{y} - \widehat{\beta}^\top \mathbf{X}^\top \mathbf{D}_1 \mathbf{X}\widehat{\beta} = \mathbf{y}^\top \mathbf{D}_{1X} \mathbf{y}$$

where

$$\mathbf{D}_{1X} = \mathbf{D}_1 - \mathbf{D}_1 \mathbf{X}(\mathbf{X}^\top \mathbf{D}_1 \mathbf{X})^{-1}\mathbf{X}^\top \mathbf{D}_1$$

The previous equation may be written as

$$\mathrm{SSE} = \mathbf{y}^\top \mathbf{D}_1 \mathbf{y} - \widehat{\beta}^\top \mathbf{X}^\top \mathbf{D}_1 \mathbf{X}\widehat{\beta}$$

so that

$$\sum_{i=1}^{n}(y_i - \overline{y})^2 = \mathrm{SSE} + \widehat{\beta}^\top \mathbf{X}^\top \mathbf{D}_1 \mathbf{X}\widehat{\beta}$$

It follows that

$$R^2 =: \frac{\widehat{\beta}^\top \mathbf{X}^\top \mathbf{D}_1 \mathbf{X}\widehat{\beta}}{\sum_{i=1}^{n}(y_i - \overline{y})^2}$$

is the proportion of variability in $\mathbf{y}$ "explained by" regression on $\mathbf{X}$. It is called R^2. Recall that $\mathbf{y}$ has mean $\overline{y}$ and that $\widehat{\mathbf{y}}$ has mean $\overline{\mathbf{y}}$ since

$$\widehat{\mathbf{y}} = \mathbf{1}\widehat{\beta}_0 + \mathbf{X}\widehat{\beta} = \mathbf{1}\overline{y} + \mathbf{D}_1 \mathbf{X}\widehat{\beta}$$

It follows that

$$\mathbf{y}^\top \mathbf{D}_1 \mathbf{y} = \sum_{i=1}^n (y_i - \overline{y})^2$$

$$\mathbf{y}^\top \mathbf{D}_1 \widehat{\mathbf{y}} = \widehat{\boldsymbol{\beta}}^\top \mathbf{X}^\top \mathbf{D}_1 \mathbf{X} \widehat{\boldsymbol{\beta}}$$

$$\widehat{\mathbf{y}}^\top \mathbf{D}_1 \widehat{\mathbf{y}} = \widehat{\boldsymbol{\beta}}^\top \mathbf{X}^\top \mathbf{D}_1 \mathbf{X} \widehat{\boldsymbol{\beta}}$$

Thus the square of the sample correlation between $\mathbf{y}$ and $\widehat{\mathbf{y}}$ is

$$\frac{[\mathbf{y}^\top \mathbf{D}_1 \widehat{\mathbf{y}}]^2}{\mathbf{y}^\top \mathbf{D}_1 \mathbf{y} \widehat{\mathbf{y}}^\top \mathbf{D}_1 \widehat{\mathbf{y}}} = \frac{[\widehat{\boldsymbol{\beta}}^\top \mathbf{X}^\top \mathbf{D}_1 \mathbf{X} \widehat{\boldsymbol{\beta}}]^2}{[\widehat{\boldsymbol{\beta}}^\top \mathbf{X}^\top \mathbf{D}_1 \mathbf{X} \widehat{\boldsymbol{\beta}}] \sum_{i=1}^n (y_i - \overline{y})^2} = R^2$$

which is the reason for the expression R^2.

8.3.1   Adding Covariates

Suppose now that we add some covariates $\mathbf{c}_1, \mathbf{c}_2, \ldots, \mathbf{c}_q$ to the model. Then we have

$$\mathbf{Z} = [\mathbf{1}, \mathbf{c}_1, \mathbf{c}_2, \ldots, \mathbf{c}_q, \mathbf{x}_1, \mathbf{x}_2, \ldots, \mathbf{x}_p] = [\mathbf{1}, \mathbf{C}, \mathbf{X}]$$

and

$$\boldsymbol{\alpha}^\top = [\beta_0, \boldsymbol{\gamma}, \boldsymbol{\beta}]$$

The equations $\mathbf{Z}^\top \mathbf{Z} \widehat{\boldsymbol{\alpha}} = \mathbf{Z}^\top \mathbf{y}$ become

$$\begin{bmatrix} \mathbf{1}^\top \mathbf{1} & \mathbf{1}^\top \mathbf{C} & \mathbf{1}^\top \mathbf{X} \\ \mathbf{C}^\top \mathbf{1} & \mathbf{C}^\top \mathbf{C} & \mathbf{C}^\top \mathbf{X} \\ \mathbf{X}^\top \mathbf{1} & \mathbf{X}^\top \mathbf{C} & \mathbf{X}^\top \mathbf{X} \end{bmatrix} \begin{bmatrix} \widehat{\beta}_0 \\ \widehat{\boldsymbol{\gamma}} \\ \widehat{\boldsymbol{\beta}} \end{bmatrix} = \begin{bmatrix} \mathbf{1}^\top \mathbf{y} \\ \mathbf{C}^\top \mathbf{y} \\ \mathbf{X}^\top \mathbf{y} \end{bmatrix}$$

Solving for $\widehat{\beta}_0$ gives

$$\widehat{\beta}_0 = \frac{1}{n} \mathbf{1}^\top [\mathbf{y} - \mathbf{C}\widehat{\boldsymbol{\gamma}} - \mathbf{X}\widehat{\boldsymbol{\beta}}]$$

Substituting into the second equation gives

$$\mathbf{C}^\top \mathbf{1} \left\{ \frac{1}{n} \mathbf{1}^\top [\mathbf{y} - \mathbf{C}\widehat{\boldsymbol{\gamma}} - \mathbf{X}\widehat{\boldsymbol{\beta}}] \right\} + \mathbf{C}^\top \mathbf{C}\widehat{\boldsymbol{\gamma}} + \mathbf{C}^\top \mathbf{X}\widehat{\boldsymbol{\beta}} = \mathbf{C}^\top \mathbf{y}$$

or

$$\mathbf{C}^\top \mathbf{D}_1 \mathbf{C}\widehat{\gamma} + \mathbf{C}^\top \mathbf{D}_1 \mathbf{X}\widehat{\beta} = \mathbf{C}^\top \mathbf{D}_1 \mathbf{y}$$

Substituting into the third equation gives

$$\mathbf{X}^\top \mathbf{1} \left\{ \frac{1}{n} \mathbf{1}^\top [\mathbf{y} - \mathbf{C}\widehat{\gamma} - \mathbf{X}\widehat{\beta}] \right\} + \mathbf{X}^\top \mathbf{C}\widehat{\gamma} + \mathbf{X}^\top \mathbf{X}\widehat{\beta} = \mathbf{X}^\top \mathbf{y}$$

or

$$\mathbf{X}^\top \mathbf{D}_1 \mathbf{C}\widehat{\gamma} + \mathbf{X}^\top \mathbf{D}_1 \mathbf{X}\widehat{\beta} = \mathbf{X}^\top \mathbf{D}_1 \mathbf{y}$$

Thus the equations to be solved for $\widehat{\gamma}$ and $\widehat{\beta}$ are

$$\mathbf{C}^\top \mathbf{D}_1 \mathbf{C}\widehat{\gamma} + \mathbf{C}^\top \mathbf{D}_1 \mathbf{X}\widehat{\beta} = \mathbf{C}^\top \mathbf{D}_1 \mathbf{y}$$
$$\mathbf{X}^\top \mathbf{D}_1 \mathbf{C}\widehat{\gamma} + \mathbf{X}^\top \mathbf{D}_1 \mathbf{X}\widehat{\beta} = \mathbf{X}^\top \mathbf{D}_1 \mathbf{y}$$

Solving for $\widehat{\gamma}$ yields

$$\widehat{\gamma} = (\mathbf{C}^\top \mathbf{D}_1 \mathbf{C})^{-1} \mathbf{C}^\top \mathbf{D}_1 [\mathbf{y} - \mathbf{X}\widehat{\beta}]$$

Substituting into the second equation yields

$$\mathbf{X}^\top \mathbf{D}_1 \mathbf{C} \left\{ (\mathbf{C}^\top \mathbf{D}_1 \mathbf{C})^{-1} \mathbf{C}^\top \mathbf{D}_1 [\mathbf{y} - \mathbf{X}\widehat{\beta}] \right\} + \mathbf{X}^\top \mathbf{D}_1 \mathbf{X}\widehat{\beta} = \mathbf{X}^\top \mathbf{D}_1 \mathbf{y}$$

or

$$\mathbf{X}^\top \mathbf{D}_{1C} \mathbf{X}\widehat{\beta} = \mathbf{X}^\top \mathbf{D}_{1C} \mathbf{y}$$

where

$$\mathbf{D}_{1C} = \mathbf{D}_1 - \mathbf{D}_1 \mathbf{C}(\mathbf{C}^\top \mathbf{D}_1 \mathbf{C})^{-1} \mathbf{C} \mathbf{D}_1$$

It follows that

$$\widehat{\beta} = (\mathbf{X}^\top \mathbf{D}_{1C} \mathbf{X})^{-1} \mathbf{X}^\top \mathbf{D}_{1C} \mathbf{y}$$

8.3.2   *Interpretation of Regression Coefficients*

Suppose now that $\mathbf{X} = \mathbf{x}$, i.e., we are interested in one covariate in the presence of some other covariates $\mathbf{C}$. The estimate is given above and is

$$\widehat{\beta} = (\mathbf{x}^\top \mathbf{D}_{1C} \mathbf{x})^{-1} \mathbf{x}^\top \mathbf{D}_{1C} \mathbf{y} = \frac{\mathbf{x}^\top \mathbf{D}_{1C} \mathbf{y}}{\mathbf{x}^\top \mathbf{D}_{1C} \mathbf{x}}$$

The residuals for the model which has just $\mathbf{C}$ are given by $\mathbf{e}_C = \mathbf{D}_{1C}\mathbf{y}$ and if we fit $\mathbf{x}$ onto $[\mathbf{1}, \mathbf{C}]$ the residuals are $\mathbf{x}_C = \mathbf{D}_{1C}\mathbf{x}$.

The simple linear regression coefficient of a regression of $\mathbf{e}_C$ onto $\mathbf{X}_C$ is then

$$\frac{\mathbf{e}_C^\top \mathbf{x}_C}{\mathbf{x}_C^\top \mathbf{x}_C} = \frac{\mathbf{y}^\top \mathbf{D}_{1C}\mathbf{D}_{1C}\mathbf{x}}{\mathbf{x}^\top \mathbf{D}_{1C}\mathbf{D}_{1C}\mathbf{x}} = \frac{\mathbf{y}^\top \mathbf{D}_{1C}\mathbf{x}}{\mathbf{x}^\top \mathbf{D}_{1C}\mathbf{x}} = \widehat{\beta}$$

Thus the regression coefficient in a model can be interpreted as follows:

1. Fit (regress) the response $\mathbf{y}$ onto $[\mathbf{1}, \mathbf{C}]$ and obtain the residuals $\mathbf{e}_C$.
2. Fit (regress) the covariate $\mathbf{x}$ onto $[\mathbf{1}, \mathbf{C}]$ and obtain the residuals $\mathbf{x}_C$.
3. The regression coefficient of $\mathbf{X}$ in the full model based on $[\mathbf{1}, \mathbf{C}, \mathbf{x}]$ is the simple linear regression coefficient in a model which fits $\mathbf{e}_C$ onto $\mathbf{x}_C$.

Thus we "adjust", remove the effect of $\mathbf{C}$ on both $\mathbf{y}$ and $\mathbf{x}$. The association which remains is what is measured by the regression coefficient of $\mathbf{x}$ in the full model.

8.3.3 Added Sum of Squares

Now note that

$$\begin{aligned}
\mathbf{y} - \mathbf{1}\widehat{\beta}_0 - \mathbf{C}\widehat{\gamma} - \mathbf{X}\widehat{\beta} &= \mathbf{y} - \mathbf{1}\left\{\frac{1}{n}\mathbf{1}^\top[\mathbf{y} - \mathbf{C}\widehat{\gamma} - \mathbf{X}\widehat{\beta}]\right\} - \mathbf{C}\widehat{\gamma} - \mathbf{X}\widehat{\beta} \\
&= \mathbf{D}_1\mathbf{y} - \mathbf{D}_1\mathbf{C}\widehat{\gamma} - \mathbf{D}_1\mathbf{X}\widehat{\beta} \\
&= \mathbf{D}_1\mathbf{y} - \mathbf{D}_1\mathbf{C}\left\{(\mathbf{C}^\top\mathbf{D}_1\mathbf{C})^{-1}\mathbf{C}^\top\mathbf{D}_1[\mathbf{y} - \mathbf{X}\widehat{\beta}]\right\} - \mathbf{D}_1\mathbf{X}\widehat{\beta} \\
&= \mathbf{D}_1\mathbf{y} - \mathbf{D}_1\mathbf{C}(\mathbf{C}^\top\mathbf{D}_1\mathbf{C})^{-1}\mathbf{C}\mathbf{D}_1\mathbf{y} - \mathbf{D}_{1C}\mathbf{X}\widehat{\beta} \\
&= [\mathbf{D}_{1C} - \mathbf{D}_{1C}\mathbf{X}(\mathbf{X}^\top\mathbf{D}_{1C}\mathbf{X})^{-1}\mathbf{X}^\top\mathbf{D}_{1C}]\mathbf{y}
\end{aligned}$$

It follows that

$$(\mathbf{y} - \mathbf{1}\widehat{\beta}_0 - \mathbf{C}\widehat{\gamma} - \mathbf{X}\widehat{\beta})^\top(\mathbf{y} - \mathbf{1}\widehat{\beta}_0 - \mathbf{C}\widehat{\gamma} - \mathbf{X}\widehat{\beta}) = \mathbf{y}^\top\mathbf{D}_{1C}\mathbf{y} - \widehat{\beta}^\top\mathbf{X}^\top\mathbf{D}_{1C}\mathbf{X}\widehat{\beta}$$

Note that $\mathbf{y}^\top\mathbf{D}_{1C}\mathbf{y}$ is the error sum of squares for the model which has only the covariates $\mathbf{C}$. Thus

$$\widehat{\beta}^\top\mathbf{X}^\top\mathbf{D}_{1C}\mathbf{X}\widehat{\beta}$$

is the additional sum of squares explained by the covariates $\mathbf{X}$ in the presence of $\mathbf{C}$.

8.3.4 Identity of Regression Coefficients

Also note that the estimates of β are the same without $\mathbf{C}$ in the model if and only if $\mathbf{C}^\top \mathbf{D}_1 \mathbf{X} = \mathbf{O}$, i.e., the covariates in $\mathbf{C}$ are uncorrelated with the covariates in $\mathbf{X}$.

8.3.5 Likelihood and Bayesian Results

The likelihood for α is given by

$$
\mathscr{L}(\alpha; \mathbf{y}) = \frac{f(\mathbf{y}; \alpha, \sigma^2)}{f(\mathbf{y}; \widehat{\alpha}, \sigma^2)} = \frac{(2\pi\sigma^2)^{-n/2} \exp\left\{-\frac{1}{2\sigma^2}(\mathbf{y} - \mathbf{Z}\alpha)^\top(\mathbf{y} - \mathbf{Z}\alpha)\right\}}{(2\pi\sigma^2)^{-n/2} \exp\left\{-\frac{1}{2\sigma^2}(\mathbf{y} - \mathbf{Z}\widehat{\alpha})^\top(\mathbf{y} - \mathbf{Z}\widehat{\alpha})\right\}}
$$

This reduces to

$$
\mathscr{L}(\alpha; \mathbf{y}) = \exp\left\{-\frac{1}{2\sigma^2}(\alpha - \widehat{\alpha})^\top \mathbf{Z}^\top \mathbf{Z}(\alpha - \widehat{\alpha})\right\}
$$

It can be shown that the likelihood for, say, α_q is

$$
\exp\left\{-\frac{(\alpha_q - \widehat{\alpha}_q)^2 \mathbf{z}_q^\top \mathbf{D}_{Z_1} \mathbf{z}_q}{2\sigma^2}\right\}
$$

It follows that the likelihood function for any regression coefficient is of the form

$$
\exp\left\{-\frac{(\beta - \widehat{\beta})^2}{2\mathrm{var}(\widehat{\beta})}\right\}
$$

which is simply based on the sampling distribution of $\widehat{\beta}$.

This result holds exactly for the linear regression model but only approximately for other generalized linear models.

For Bayesian inference on regression parameters the likelihood result just obtained along with the assumption that the priors are relatively flat yields the result that the posterior distribution of β is normal with center at $\widehat{\beta}$ and variance equal to the sampling variance of $\widehat{\beta}$.

The last two results explain why there is little numerical difference in the results obtained for frequentist, likelihood, and Bayesian approaches to linear models despite the enormous conceptual and interpretation differences.

8.4 Interpretation of the Coefficients

Consider a regression model with just two covariates, x_1 and x_2, and an intercept, i.e.,

$$\mathbb{E}(Y) = \beta_0 + \beta_1 x_1 + \beta_2 x_2$$

If x_2 is increased by 1 unit the expected response is

$$\mathbb{E}(Y) = \beta_0 + \beta_1 x_1 + \beta_2 (x_2 + 1)$$

and hence the difference between the expected responses is β_2. A similar result holds for β_1.

Thus the interpretation of the coefficient of covariate x in a regression model is that it represents the change in the expected response if that covariate is increased by one unit and **all other covariates are unchanged**.

8.5 Factors as Covariates

A special role in regression models is played by covariates which define a categorization of the response variable, i.e., gender, ethnicity, income level, disease status, exposure status, etc.

In such cases it makes no sense to fit the covariate as is. Instead we assume that the covariate has been coded so that its values are $1, 2, \ldots, q$.

The covariate in this case is called a **factor** and the values $1, 2, \ldots, q$ are called its **levels**. q new covariates $f_{1x}, f_{2x}, \ldots, f_{qx}$ are now constructed of the form

$$\mathbf{f}_{1x} = \begin{cases} 1 & x_i = 1 \\ 0 & \text{otherwise} \end{cases}, \quad \mathbf{f}_{2x} = \begin{cases} 1 & x_i = 2 \\ 0 & \text{otherwise} \end{cases}, \quad \cdots \quad \mathbf{f}_{qx} = \begin{cases} 1 & x_i = q \\ 0 & \text{otherwise} \end{cases}$$

Obviously if an intercept is included in the model we need only include $q - 1$ of these covariates. It is customary and useful in subsequent interpretations to let level 1 of the factor be the control against which all other levels will be compared. Under the model with x coded as a factor the expected response for observations at level 1 of the factor is

$$\mathbb{E}(Y) = \beta_0$$

and the expected response for observations at level j of the factor is

$$\mathbb{E}(Y) = \beta_0 + \gamma_j$$

Hence the coefficient of a covariate corresponding to a level of a factor represents the difference between the expected response at level j and the expected response at level 1; all other covariates held constant.

If we have two covariates x_1 and x_2, both of which are factors with q_1 levels for x_1 and q_2 levels for x_2, the situation is slightly more complicated. We first set up q_1 new covariates for x_1 and q_2 covariates for x_2. We use in the model only $q_1 - 1$ of the covariates for x_1 and $q_2 - 1$ covariates for x_2.

In addition we recognize that the difference between the expected response for the jth level of factor x_1 and the first level of factor x_1 may depend on the level of x_2. For example, the effect of a hormone supplement (high or low) may differ between males and females. This is called **interaction** and is captured in the model by defining $(q_1 - 1)(q_2 - 1)$ new covariates as the product of the covariates for each factor. The regression coefficients of these covariates are called **interaction coefficients**.

The resulting model can be summarized in the following table of expected responses.(In the table α's indicate factor x_1, the γ's indicate factor x_2, and the $\alpha\gamma$'s indicate the interaction coefficients.)

Level of	Level of factor x_2			
factor x_1	1	2	$\cdots$	q_2
1	β_0	$\beta_0 + \gamma_2$	$\cdots$	$\beta_0 + \gamma_{q_2}$
2	$\beta_0 + \alpha_2$	$\beta_0 + \alpha_2 + \gamma_2 + (\alpha\gamma)_{22}$	$\cdots$	$\beta_0 + \alpha_2 + \gamma_{q_2} + (\alpha\gamma)_{2q_2}$
$\vdots$	$\vdots$	$\vdots$	$\ddots$	$\vdots$
q_1	$\beta_0 + \alpha_{q_1}$	$\beta_0 + \alpha_{q_1} + \gamma_2 + (\alpha\gamma)_{22}$	$\cdots$	$\beta_0 + \alpha_{q_1} + \gamma_{q_2} + (\alpha\gamma)_{q_1 q_2}$

It is obvious that the interaction coefficients are the difference between two differences, i.e.,

$$(\alpha\gamma)_{jk} = [\mathbb{E}(Y)_{jk} - \mathbb{E}(Y_{1k})] - [\mathbb{E}(Y_{j1}) - \mathbb{E}(Y_{11})]$$

and measures the extent to which the effect of x_1 differs between level k of factor x_2 and level 1 of factor x_2.

Example. For two factors x_1 and x_2, each at two levels with x_1 representing disease status and x_2 representing exposure status, we the table of expected responses is

Disease	Exposure status	
status	Not exposed	Exposed
No disease	β_0	$\beta_0 + \gamma_2$
Disease	$\beta_0 + \alpha_2$	$\beta_0 + \alpha_2 + \gamma_2 + (\alpha\gamma)_{22}$

In this table the effect of exposure in the no disease group is

$$\mathbb{E}(Y|E, ND) - \mathbb{E}(Y|NE, ND) = [\beta_0 + \gamma_2] - [\beta_0] = \gamma_2$$

The effect of exposure in the diseased group is

$$\mathbb{E}(Y|E, D) - \mathbb{E}(Y|NE, D) = [\beta_0 + \alpha_2 + \gamma_2 + (\alpha\gamma)_{22}] - [\beta_0 + \alpha_2] = \gamma_2 + (\alpha\gamma)_{22}$$

It follows that the difference is

$$\text{exposure effect in } D - \text{exposure effect in } ND = (\alpha\gamma)_{22}$$

The interaction coefficient $(\alpha\gamma)_{22}$ thus measures whether exposure has the same effect in the diseased group as it does in the not diseased group.

8.6 Exercises

1. Let $Y_1, Y_2, \ldots, Y_n$ be normal with

$$\mathbb{E}(Y_i) = \mu \; ; \quad i = 1, 2, \ldots, n$$

and

$$\mathbb{C}(Y_i, Y_j) = \begin{cases} \sigma^2 & j = i \\ \rho\sigma^2 & j \neq i \end{cases}$$

where $\rho > -1/(n-1)$.

   (a) Find the expected value and variance of $\overline{Y}$.
   (b) What implications does this have for confidence intervals, on μ, etc.?
   (c) Why does ρ, the correlation between Y_i and Y_j, have to be larger than $-1/(n-1)$?

2. In a regression model it is commonly said that the interpretation of β_2 is the change in the expected response if the covariate x_2 changes by 1 unit with all other covariates held fixed.

   (a) Suppose that the regression model is

$$\mathbb{E}(Y_i) = \beta_0 + \beta_1 x_i + \beta_2 x_i^2$$

   i.e., $x_1 = x$ and $x_2 = x^2$. Obviously we can't hold x fixed and change x^2 by 1 unit. How do we interpret β_2 in this case?
   (b) Suppose the regression model is

$$\mathbb{E}(Y_i) = \beta_0 + \beta_1 x_{1i} + \beta_2 x_{2i} + \beta_3 x_{1i} x_{2i}$$

   Obviously we can't hold x_1 and x_2 fixed and change $x_1 x_2$ by 1 unit. How do we interpret β_3 in this case?

3. Let $Y_1, Y_2, \ldots, Y_n$ be independent and normally distributed with

$$\mathbb{E}(Y_i) = \mu_i \ \text{ and } \ \mathbb{V}(Y_i) = \sigma^2$$

Let $x_{11}, x_{22}, \ldots, x_{n1}$ and $x_{12}, x_{22}, \ldots, x_{n2}$ be the values of two covariates x_1 and x_2.

(a) Let the **large model** be defined by

$$\mu_i = \beta_0 + \beta_1 x_{i1} + \beta_2 x_{i2}$$

Show that the maximum likelihood estimates of $\beta_0, \beta_1, \beta_2$ and σ^2 in the large model are given by

$$\widehat{\beta}_0^{lm} = \overline{y} - \widehat{\beta}_1^{lm} \, \overline{x}_1 - \widehat{\beta}_2^{lm} \, \overline{x}_2$$

$$\widehat{\sigma}_{lm}^2 = \sum_{i=1}^{n} (y_i - \widehat{\beta}_0^{lm} - \widehat{\beta}_1^{lm} \, x_{i1} - \widehat{\beta}_2^{lm} \, x_{i2})^2 / n$$

where $\widehat{\beta}_1^{lm}$ and $\widehat{\beta}_2^{lm}$ satisfy

$$c_{11}\widehat{\beta}_1^{lm} + c_{12}\widehat{\beta}_2^{lm} = c_{1y}$$
$$c_{12}\widehat{\beta}_1^{lm} + c_{22}\widehat{\beta}_2^{lm} = c_{2y}$$

and

$$c_{11} = \sum_{i=1}^{n} (x_{i1} - \overline{x}_1)^2$$
$$c_{22} = \sum_{i=1}^{n} (x_{i2} - \overline{x}_2)^2$$
$$c_{12} = \sum_{i=1}^{n} (x_{i1} - \overline{x}_1)(x_{i2} - \overline{x}_2)$$
$$c_{1y} = \sum_{i=1}^{n} (x_{i1} - \overline{x}_1)(y_i - \overline{y})$$
$$c_{2y} = \sum_{i=1}^{n} (x_{i2} - \overline{x}_1)(y_i - \overline{y})$$

Hence show that the maximized likelihood for the large model is given by

$$(2\pi\widehat{\sigma}_{lm}^2)^{-n/2} \exp\left\{ -\frac{n}{2} \right\}$$

(b) Now consider the **small model** defined by

$$\mu_i = \beta_0 + \beta_1 x_{i1}$$

Show that the maximum likelihood estimates of $\beta_0, \beta_1,$ and σ^2 under the small model are given by

$$\widehat{\beta}_0^{sm} = \overline{y} - \widehat{\beta}_1^{sm} \, \overline{x}_1$$

$$\widehat{\sigma}_{sm}^2 = \sum_{i=1}^{n} (y_i - \widehat{\beta}_0^{sm} - \widehat{\beta}_1^{sm} \, x_{i1})^2 / n$$

where $\widehat{\beta}_1^{sm}$ satisfies

$$c_{11}\widehat{\beta}_1^{sm} = c_{1y}$$

Hence show that the maximized likelihood for the small model is given by

$$(2\pi\widehat{\sigma}_{sm}^2)^{-n/2} \exp\left\{-\frac{n}{2}\right\}$$

(c) From parts (a) and (b) show that the likelihood ratio for the small model vs the large model is given by

$$\left(\frac{\widehat{\sigma}_{lm}^2}{\widehat{\sigma}_{sm}^2}\right)^{n/2}$$

(d) From (a) show that

$$\widehat{\beta}_1^{lm} = \widehat{\beta}_1^{sm} - \frac{c_{12}}{c_{11}}\,\widehat{\beta}_2^{lm}$$

(e) Also from (a) show that

$$\widehat{\beta}_2^{lm} = \frac{c_{2y} - \frac{c_{12}}{c_{11}}c_{1y}}{c_{22} - \frac{c_{12}^2}{c_{11}}}$$

(f) Using (d) and (e) show that

$$r_i^{lm} =: y_i - \widehat{\beta}_0^{lm} - \widehat{\beta}_1^{lm}x_{i1} - \widehat{\beta}_2^{lm}x_{i2}$$

reduce to

$$r_i^{lm} = y_i - \bar{y} - \widehat{\beta}_1^{lm}(x_{i1} - \bar{x}_1) - \widehat{\beta}_2^{lm}(x_{i2} - \bar{x}_2)$$

$$= y_i - \bar{y} - \widehat{\beta}_1^{sm}(x_{i1} - \bar{x}_1) + \widehat{\beta}_2^{lm}\left[x_{i2} - \bar{x}_2 - \frac{c_{12}}{c_{11}}(x_{i1} - \bar{x}_1)\right]$$

Thus show that

$$\text{SSE}_{lm} =: \sum_{i=1}^{n}[r_i^{lm}]^2 = \sum_{i=1}^{n}(y_i - \bar{y})^2 - [\widehat{\beta}_1^{sm}]^2 c_{11} - [\widehat{\beta}_2^{lm}]^2\left[c_{22} - \frac{c_{12}^2}{c_{11}}\right]$$

(g) Show that

$$y_i - \widehat{\beta}_0^{sm} - \widehat{\beta}_1^{sm}x_{i1} = y_i - \bar{y} - \widehat{\beta}_1^{sm}(x_{i1} - \bar{x}_1)$$

and hence that

$$\mathrm{SSE}_{sm} =: \sum_{i=1}^{n} (y_i - \widehat{\beta}_0^{sm} - \widehat{\beta}_1^{sm} x_{i1})^2 = \sum_{i=1}^{n} (y_i - \overline{y})^2 - [\widehat{\beta}_1^{sm}]^2 c_{11}$$

(h) From (f) and (g) it follows that

$$\frac{\widehat{\sigma}_{lm}^2}{\widehat{\sigma}_{sm}^2} = \frac{\mathrm{SSE}_{lm}}{\mathrm{SSE}_{sm}} = \frac{\mathrm{SSE}_{lm}}{\mathrm{SSE}_{lm} + [\widehat{\beta}_2^{lm}]^2 \left[c_{22} - \frac{c_{12}^2}{c_{11}} \right]}$$

Explain why rejecting when the likelihood ratio is small is equivalent to rejecting when $\widehat{\beta}_2^{lm}$ is large relative to $\widehat{\sigma}_{lm}^2$.

(i) Find the expected value, variance, and distribution of $\widehat{\beta}_2^{lm}$

(j) It can be shown that

$$\frac{\mathrm{SSE}_{lm}}{(n-3)\sigma^2} \overset{d}{\sim} \chi^2(n-3)$$

and is independent of $\widehat{\beta}_{lm}$. Explain why the likelihood ratio test of $\beta_2 = 0$ is equivalent to rejecting using a Student's t statistic with $n - 3$ degrees of freedom.

Chapter 9
Other Estimation Methods

9.1 Estimation Using Empirical Distributions

9.1.1 Empirical Distribution Functions

Suppose that we have sample data $x_1, x_2, \ldots, x_n$ assumed to be observed values of independent random variables each having the same distribution function F where

$$F(x) = \mathbb{P}(X \leq x)$$

Define new random variables Z_i as the indicator functions of the interval $(-\infty, x]$, i.e.,

$$Z_i(x) = \begin{cases} 1 & X_i \leq x \\ 0 & \text{otherwise} \end{cases}$$

Note that the $Z_i(x)$ are independent and are Bernoulli random variables with parameter $F(x)$, i.e.,

$$\mathbb{P}(Z_i(x) = 1) = \mathbb{P}(X_i \leq x) = F(x)$$

It follows that, for any fixed x, we have that

$$S_n(x) = \sum_{i=1}^{n} Z_i(x)$$

has a binomial distribution with parameters $F(x)$ and n.

© Springer International Publishing Switzerland 2014
C.A. Rohde, *Introductory Statistical Inference with the Likelihood Function*, DOI 10.1007/978-3-319-10461-4_9

Definition 9.1.1. The **empirical distribution function**, $\widehat{F}_n(x)$ is defined as

$$\widehat{F}_n(x) = \frac{S_n(x)}{n}$$

The empirical distribution function is the natural estimator of F, the population distribution function, for the following reasons:

1. $\widehat{F}_n(x)$ is **unbiased**, i.e.,

$$\mathbb{E}[\widehat{F}_n(x)] = F(x) \text{ for any } x$$

2. The variance of $\widehat{F}_n(x)$ is given by

$$\mathbb{V}\left[\widehat{F}_n(x)\right] = \frac{F(x)[1 - F(x)]}{n}$$

3. $\widehat{F}_n(x)$ is **consistent**, i.e.,

$$\widehat{F}_n(x) \xrightarrow{p} F(x) \text{ for any } x$$

The above results follow from the fact that $n\widehat{F}_n(x) = S_n$ is binomial with parameters n and $F(x)$.

There are two important additional properties of $\widehat{F}_n(x)$:

1. **Glivenko–Cantelli Theorem**
   Under the assumption of iid X_i's we have

   $$\sup_x \left|\widehat{F}_n(x) - F(x)\right| \xrightarrow{p} 0$$

   i.e., the maximum difference between $\widehat{F}_n(x)$ and $F(x)$ is small for large n.

2. **Dvoretzky–Kiefer–Wolfowitz (DKW) Inequality**
   Under the assumption that the X_i's are iid

   $$\mathbb{P}\left(\sup_x |\widehat{F}_n(x) - F(x)| > \epsilon\right) \leq 2e^{-2n\epsilon^2} \text{ for any } \epsilon > 0$$

The implication of the last result is that if we define

$$L(x) = \max\{\widehat{F}_n(x) - \epsilon_n, \, 0\} \text{ and } U(x) = \min\{\widehat{F}_n(x) + \epsilon_n, \, 1\}$$

where

$$\epsilon_n = \sqrt{\frac{\ln(2/\alpha)}{2n}}$$

then we have that

$$\mathbb{P}\left\{L(x) \leq F(x) \leq U(x) \ \text{ for all } x\right\} \geq 1 - \alpha$$

i.e., we have a $100(1 - \alpha)\%$ confidence interval for $F(x)$.

1. The previous two results, particularly the first, have been called the fundamental theorems of mathematical statistics because they show that we can, with high probability, learn about F using a random sample from a population assumed to have distribution F.
2. In most statistical applications we can do better (use smaller n) since we assume that F is specified by a small number of parameters.
3. In fact, in many cases, we are not interested in F itself but some other function such as the mean or variance of the population.

9.1.2   Statistical Functionals

In mathematics a **functional** is a function whose domain is a set of functions.

Definition 9.1.2. A **statistical functional**, $\theta = T(F)$, is any function of the distribution function F.

Almost any parameter of interest is a statistical functional, e.g., the mean, median, and quantiles. Since the sample distribution function is the natural estimate of the distribution function the following gives the natural estimates of statistical functionals.

Definition 9.1.3. The **plug-in estimator** of the statistical functional $\theta = T(F)$ is

$$\widehat{\theta}_n = T(\widehat{F}_n)$$

i.e., to estimate $T(F)$ plug in (substitute) $\widehat{F}_n$ for F.

9.1.3   Linear Statistical Functionals

One important class of statistical functionals are the linear statistical functionals.

Definition 9.1.4. A **linear statistical functional** is a statistical functional of the form

$$T(F) = \int r(x)dF(x) \ \text{ for some function } r$$

where by $\int r(x)dF(x)$ we mean

$$\sum_{x \in \mathcal{X}} r(x)f(x) \quad \text{or} \quad \int_{x \in \mathcal{X}} r(x)f(x)dx$$

depending on whether F is discrete or continuous.

For linear functionals we have the following two important results:

(i) The plug-in estimator for a linear functional is

$$T(\widehat{F}_n) = \frac{1}{n} \sum_{i=1}^{n} r(X_i)$$

(ii) Assuming that we can find an estimate, $\widehat{s.e.}$, of the standard error of $T(\widehat{F}_n)$, an approximate $100(1 - \alpha)$ confidence interval for $T(F)$ is given by

$$T(\widehat{F}_n) \pm z_{1-\alpha/2}\widehat{s.e.}$$

The reason for the second statement is that it is often true that

$$\frac{T(\widehat{F}_n - T(F))}{\widehat{se}} \xrightarrow{d} N(0, 1)$$

We then use the standard pivotal argument for the normal distribution to obtain the approximate confidence interval for $T(F)$.

9.1.4 Quantiles

One other class of statistical functionals is of major importance, the quantiles of a distribution.

Definition 9.1.5. If F has a density function f then the pth **quantile** of F is defined by

$$T(F) = F^{-1}(p)$$

The plug-in estimate of the p quantile is

$$T(\widehat{F}_n) = \inf_x \{x : \widehat{F}_n(x) \geq p\}$$

and is called the pth **sample quantile**.

The following are important quantiles:

p	Name	Estimate
$\frac{1}{10} - \frac{9}{10}$	Deciles	Sample deciles
$\frac{1}{4}, \frac{3}{4}$	Quartiles	Sample quartiles
$\frac{1}{2}$	Median	Sample median

9.1.5 Confidence Intervals for Quantiles

Let $X_1, X_2, \ldots, X_n$ be independent with distribution function F. Suppose that we want a confidence interval for η_p, the pth quantile of F, i.e.,

$$p = F(\eta_p) = \mathbb{P}(X_i \le \eta_p)$$

Define $Z_1, Z_2, \ldots, Z_n$ by

$$Z_i = \begin{cases} 1 \text{ if } X_i < \eta_p \\ 0 \text{ otherwise} \end{cases}$$

The Z_i are independent Bernoulli with

$$\mathrm{P}(Z_i = 1) = \mathbb{P}(X_i < \eta_p) = p$$

It follows that

$$S_n = \sum_{i=1}^{n} Z_i \text{ is binomial } (n, p)$$

Now define the **order statistics**, $X_{n1}, X_{n2}, \ldots, X_{nn}$, as the ordered values of $X_1, X_2, \ldots, X_n$ from smallest to largest.

Note that

$$S_n \ge j \iff X_{nj} < \eta_p$$

and

$$S_n \le k - 1 \iff X_{nk} \ge \eta_p$$

These last two facts allow us to determine confidence limits for η_p since

$$\mathbb{P}(X_{nj} < \eta_p \le X_{nk}) = \mathbb{P}(j \le S_n \le k - 1)$$

The last probability can be obtained from the binomial distribution with parameter p, i.e.,

$$\mathbb{P}(j \leq S_n \leq k - 1) = \mathbb{P}(S_n \leq k - 1) - \mathbb{P}(S_n \leq j - 1)$$

Thus all we need to do is find j and k such that

$$\mathbb{P}(S_n \leq k - 1) - \mathbb{P}(S_n \leq j - 1) \geq 1 - \alpha$$

and we will have a $100(1 - \alpha)\%$ confidence interval for η_p.

This interval is **nonparametric** since we do not need to assume the specific form of F. In cases where we are willing to assume a specific form for F we can do better, i.e., have a shorter confidence interval.

Where to start for j and k? Note that

$$\frac{S_n - np}{\sqrt{np(1 - p)}} \approx \text{N}(0, 1)$$

so that

$$\mathbb{P}(S_n \leq k - 1) \approx \mathbb{P}\left(Z \leq \frac{k - 1 - np}{\sqrt{np(1 - p)}}\right)$$

i.e.,

$$k - 1 \approx np + z_{1-\alpha/2}\sqrt{np(1 - p)}$$

Similarly

$$j - 1 \approx np - z_{1-\alpha/2}\sqrt{np(1 - p)}$$

Start with this j and k and iterate.

9.2   Method of Moments

The **method of moments** is related to the plug-in method. If

$$\alpha_j = \mathbb{E}(X^j)$$

the plug-in method of estimation equates α_j to the sample moment

$$\widehat{\alpha}_j = \frac{1}{n}\sum_{i=1}^{n} x_i^j$$

where x_i denotes the ith observation from a random sample. This defines the estimate of α_j

The method of moments uses the fact that the population moments are functions of the parameters θ and solves the equations

$$\alpha_j(\theta) = \widehat{\alpha}_j \quad \text{for } j = 1, 2, \ldots, k$$

assuming that there are k parameters

$$\theta_1, \theta_2, \ldots, \theta_k$$

The method of moments enjoys some reasonable properties in the frequentist paradigm:

1. Consistency, i.e., $\widehat{\theta}_n \xrightarrow{p} \theta$
2. Asymptotic normality, i.e.,

$$\sqrt{n}(\widehat{\theta}_n - \theta) \xrightarrow{d} N(0, \Sigma)$$

where Σ is determined by the solution to the equations defining the estimates.

9.2.1   Technical Details of the Method of Moments

Consider n iid random variables $X_1, X_2, \ldots, X_n$ and define the sample moments by

$$\overline{X}^1 = \frac{1}{n}\sum_{i=1}^{n} X_i, \quad \overline{X}^2 = \frac{1}{n}\sum_{i=1}^{n} X_i^2, \quad \ldots, \quad \overline{X}^k = \frac{1}{n}\sum_{i=1}^{n} X_i^k$$

and let

$$\alpha_r = E(X^r) \quad \text{and} \quad \mu_r = E(X - \mu)^r \quad \text{where } \mu = E(X)$$

be the corresponding population moments (moments of the distribution of X).
    Provided that the expected value of X^{2k} exists the central limit theorem guarantees that

$$\mathbf{Y} = (\overline{X}^1, \overline{X}^2, \ldots, \overline{X}^k)$$

are jointly asymptotically normal. More precisely,

$$\sqrt{n}[\mathbf{Y} - \mathbb{E}(\mathbf{Y})] \xrightarrow{d} N(\mathbf{0}, \Sigma)$$

where

$$\mathbb{E}(\mathbf{Y}) = \begin{bmatrix} E(X) \\ E(X^2) \\ \vdots \\ E(X^k) \end{bmatrix}$$

and Σ is given by

$$\begin{bmatrix} \mathrm{var}(X) & \mathrm{cov}(X, X^2) & \cdots & \mathrm{cov}(X, X^k) \\ \mathrm{cov}(X^2, X) & \mathrm{var}(X^2) & \cdots & \mathrm{cov}(X^2, X^k) \\ \vdots & \vdots & \ddots & \vdots \\ \mathrm{cov}(X^k, X) & \mathrm{cov}(X^k, X^2) & \cdots & \mathrm{var}(X^k) \end{bmatrix}$$

To obtain approximations to the sampling distributions of method of moment estimators we use the Delta method. Let g be a continuous and differentiable function and define

$$\nabla_g(\boldsymbol{\alpha}) = \begin{bmatrix} \frac{\partial g(y_1, y_2, \ldots, y_k)}{\partial y_1} \\ \frac{\partial g(y_1, y_2, \ldots, y_k)}{\partial y_2} \\ \vdots \\ \frac{\partial g(y_1, y_2, \ldots, y_k)}{\partial y_k} \end{bmatrix}_{y_1 = \alpha_1, y_2 = \alpha_2, \ldots, y_k = \alpha_k}$$

then the Delta method applies and we have that

$$\sqrt{n}[g(\overline{X}^1, \overline{X}^2, \ldots, \overline{X}^k) - g(\alpha_1, \alpha_2, \ldots, \alpha_k)]$$

converges in distribution to a

$$\mathrm{N}\left(0, \theta^2\right)$$

distribution where

$$\theta^2 = \nabla_g^\top(\boldsymbol{\alpha}) \Sigma \nabla_g(\boldsymbol{\alpha})$$

More generally if $g_1, g_2, \ldots, g_r$ are continuous and differentiable functions let $\mathbf{g} = (g_1, g_2, \ldots, g_r)$ and let

$$\nabla_g(\mathbf{y}) = \frac{\partial \mathbf{g}(\mathbf{y})}{\partial \mathbf{y}} = \begin{bmatrix} \frac{\partial g_1(\mathbf{y})}{\partial y_1} & \frac{\partial g_2(\mathbf{y})}{\partial y_1} & \cdots & \frac{\partial g_r(\mathbf{y})}{\partial y_1} \\ \frac{\partial g_1(\mathbf{y})}{\partial y_2} & \frac{\partial g_2(\mathbf{y})}{\partial y_2} & \cdots & \frac{\partial g_r(\mathbf{y})}{\partial y_2} \\ \vdots & \vdots & \ddots & \vdots \\ \frac{\partial g_1(\mathbf{y})}{\partial y_k} & \frac{\partial g_2(\mathbf{y})}{\partial y_k} & \cdots & \frac{\partial g_r(\mathbf{y})}{\partial y_k} \end{bmatrix}$$

be evaluated at

$$y_1 = \alpha_1, y_2 = \alpha_2, \ldots, y_k = \alpha_k$$

to obtain $\nabla_g(\boldsymbol{\alpha})$, then

$$\sqrt{n} \begin{bmatrix} g_1(\overline{X}_n^1, \overline{X}_n^2, \ldots, \overline{X}_n^k) - g_1(\alpha_1, \alpha_2, \ldots, \alpha_k) \\ g_2(\overline{X}_n^1, \overline{X}_n^2, \ldots, \overline{X}_n^k) - g_2(\alpha_1, \alpha_2, \ldots, \alpha_k) \\ \vdots \\ g_r(\overline{X}_n^1, \overline{X}_n^2, \ldots, \overline{X}_n^k) - g_r(\alpha_1, \alpha_2, \ldots, \alpha_k) \end{bmatrix}$$

converges in distribution to a

$$\mathrm{N}\,(\mathbf{0}, \mathbf{V})$$

distribution where

$$\mathbf{V} = \nabla_g^\top(\boldsymbol{\alpha}) \boldsymbol{\Sigma} \nabla_g(\boldsymbol{\alpha})$$

9.2.2 Application to the Normal Distribution

The following are some general relationships between the central moments (the μ's) and the moments (the α's) which are valid for any distribution.

$$\mu_1 = 0$$
$$\alpha_1 = \mu$$
$$\mu_2 = \alpha_2 - \mu^2$$
$$\alpha_2 = \mu_2 + \mu^2$$
$$\mu_3 = \alpha_3 - 3\alpha_2 + \mu^3$$
$$\alpha_3 = \mu_3 + 3\alpha^2\mu - \mu^3$$
$$\mu_4 = \alpha_4 - 4\alpha_3\mu + 6\alpha_2\mu^2 - 3\mu^4$$
$$\alpha_4 = \mu_4 + 4\alpha_3\mu - 6\alpha_2\mu^2 + 3\mu^4$$

Suppose now that X is normal with mean μ and variance σ^2. Then we have

$$\mu_1 = 0$$
$$\mu_2 = \sigma^2$$
$$\mu_3 = 0$$
$$\mu_4 = 3\sigma^4$$

and hence for the normal distribution

$$\begin{aligned}
\alpha_1 &= \mu \\
\alpha_2 &= \sigma^2 + \mu^2 \\
\alpha_3 &= 3\sigma^2\mu + \mu^3 \\
\alpha_4 &= \mu^4 + 6\mu^2\sigma^2 + 3\sigma^4
\end{aligned}$$

It follows that

$$\begin{aligned}
\mathrm{var}(X) &= \sigma^2 \\
\mathrm{cov}(X, X^2) &= E(X^3) - E(X^2)E(X) \\
&= 3\sigma^2\mu + \mu^3 - (\sigma^2 + \mu^2)\mu \\
&= 2\mu\sigma^2 \\
\mathrm{var}(X^2) &= E(X^4) - [E(X^2)]^2 \\
&= \mu^4 + 6\mu^2\sigma^2 + 3\sigma^4 - (\sigma^2 + \mu^2)^2 \\
&= 2\sigma^4 + 4\mu^2\sigma^2
\end{aligned}$$

Thus

$$\sqrt{n} \begin{bmatrix} \overline{X}^1 - E(X) \\ \overline{X}^2 - E(X^2) \end{bmatrix}$$

converges in distribution to

$$\mathrm{N}\left(\begin{bmatrix} 0 \\ 0 \end{bmatrix}, \begin{bmatrix} \sigma^2 & 2\mu\sigma^2 \\ 2\mu\sigma^2 & 2\sigma^4 + 4\mu^2\sigma^2 \end{bmatrix} \right)$$

Example 1. Asymptotic distribution of s^2. If we let

$$g(\overline{x}^1, \overline{x}^2) = \overline{x}^2 - [\overline{x}^1]^2$$

Then

$$g(\overline{x}^1, \overline{x}^2) = \frac{1}{n} \sum_{i=1}^n x_i^2 - (\overline{x})^2 = \frac{1}{n} \sum_{i=1}^n (x_i - \overline{x})^2$$

and hence

$$\frac{\partial g(\overline{x}^1, \overline{x}^2)}{\partial \overline{x}^1} = -2\overline{x}^1$$

$$\frac{\partial g(\overline{x}^1, \overline{x}^2)}{\partial \overline{x}^2} = 1$$

Evaluating at $\overline{x}^1 = \mu$ and $\overline{x}^2 = \sigma^2 + \mu^2$ yields

$$\frac{\partial g(\mu, \sigma^2)}{\partial \mu} = -2\mu$$

and

$$\frac{\partial g(\mu, \sigma^2)}{\partial \sigma^2} = 1$$

It follows that the asymptotic distribution of S^2 satisfies

$$\sqrt{n}(S^2 - \sigma^2) \xrightarrow{d} \mathrm{N}(0, v^2)$$

where

$$v^2 = [-2\mu, 1] \begin{bmatrix} \sigma^2 & 2\mu\sigma^2 \\ 2\mu\sigma^2 & 2\sigma^4 + 4\mu^2\sigma^2 \end{bmatrix} \begin{bmatrix} -2\mu \\ 1 \end{bmatrix}$$

$$= [0, 2\sigma^4] \begin{bmatrix} -2\mu \\ 1 \end{bmatrix}$$

$$= 2\sigma^4$$

Since $\overline{X}^1 = \overline{X}$ and S^2 are independent it follows that their joint distribution satisfies

$$\sqrt{n} \begin{bmatrix} \overline{X} - \mu \\ S^2 - \sigma^2 \end{bmatrix} \xrightarrow{d} \mathrm{N} \left(\begin{bmatrix} 0 \\ 0 \end{bmatrix}, \begin{bmatrix} \sigma^2 & 0 \\ 0 & 2\sigma^4 \end{bmatrix} \right)$$

Example 2 (Effect size). The **effect size** is defined as

$$\frac{\mu}{\sigma}$$

It is a widely used measure of the importance of a variable. If we let

$$g(\overline{x}, s^2) = \overline{x}_1(s^2)^{-1/2}$$

then we have a natural estimate of the effect size based on the method of moments.
   Note that

$$\frac{\partial g(\overline{x}, s^2)}{\partial \overline{x}} = (s^2)^{-1/2}$$

$$\frac{\partial g(\overline{x}, s^2)}{\partial s^2} = -\overline{x}(s^2)^{-3/2}/2$$

Evaluating these at $\overline{x} = \mu$ and $s^2 = \sigma^2$ we have

$$\frac{\partial g(\mu, \sigma^2)}{\partial \mu} = \frac{1}{\sigma}$$

and

$$\frac{\partial g(\mu, \sigma^2)}{\partial \sigma^2} = -\frac{\mu}{2\sigma^3}$$

It follows that

$$\sqrt{n} \left(\frac{\overline{x}}{s} - \frac{\mu}{\sigma} \right) \xrightarrow{d} N(0, v^2)$$

where

$$v^2 = \begin{bmatrix} \frac{1}{\sigma} & -\frac{\mu}{2\sigma^3} \end{bmatrix} \begin{bmatrix} \sigma^2 & 0 \\ 0 & 2\sigma^4 \end{bmatrix} \begin{bmatrix} \frac{1}{\sigma} \\ -\frac{\mu}{2\sigma^3} \end{bmatrix}$$

which reduces to

$$v^2 = 1 + \frac{\mu^2}{2\sigma^2}$$

Example 3 (Coefficient of variation). The **coefficient of variation** is defined as

$$\frac{\sigma}{\mu}$$

and is a widely used measure of variability.

If we let $cv = \frac{1}{\overline{x}/s}$ then we have a natural estimate of the coefficient of variation. It follows that

$$\sqrt{n} \left(\frac{s}{\overline{x}} - \frac{\sigma}{\mu} \right) \xrightarrow{d} N(0, v_1^2)$$

where

$$v_1^2 = \left(-\frac{\sigma^2}{\mu^2} \right) \left(1 + \frac{\mu^2}{2\sigma^2} \right) \left(-\frac{\sigma^2}{\mu^2} \right)$$

which reduces to

$$v_1^2 = \frac{\sigma^2}{\mu^2} \left(\frac{1}{2} + \frac{\sigma^2}{\mu^2} \right)$$

9.3 Estimating Functions

The method of moments and maximum likelihood are examples of obtaining estimates using estimating functions.

Definition 9.3.1. A function g such that the equation

$$\mathbf{g}(\mathbf{y}; \widehat{\boldsymbol{\theta}}) = \mathbf{0}$$

defines $\widehat{\boldsymbol{\theta}}$ as an estimate of $\boldsymbol{\theta}$ is called an **estimating function**. The equation itself is called an **estimating equation**.

Definition 9.3.2. The estimating function g is an unbiased estimating function if

$$E[\mathbf{g}(\mathbf{Y}; \boldsymbol{\theta})] = \mathbf{0} \quad \text{for all } \boldsymbol{\theta}$$

9.3.1 General Linear Model

Example 1. In a general linear model, i.e.,

$$E(\mathbf{Y}) = \mathbf{X}\boldsymbol{\beta} \;\; ; \;\; \text{var}\,(\mathbf{Y}) = \sigma^2 \mathbf{I}$$

where $\mathbf{Y}$ is $n \times 1$, $\mathbf{X}$ is $n \times (p+1)$, the estimating function

$$\mathbf{g}(\mathbf{y}; \boldsymbol{\beta}) = \mathbf{X}^\top (\mathbf{y} - \mathbf{X}\boldsymbol{\beta})$$

defines the **least squares estimate** of $\boldsymbol{\beta}$.

9.3.2 Maximum Likelihood

Example 2. If $\mathbf{Y}$ has density $f(\mathbf{y}\,;\,\boldsymbol{\theta})$ the estimating function

$$\mathbf{g}(\mathbf{y}\,;\,\boldsymbol{\theta}) = \frac{\partial \ln[f(\mathbf{y}\,;\,\boldsymbol{\theta})]}{\partial \boldsymbol{\theta}}$$

defines the **maximum likelihood estimate** of $\boldsymbol{\theta}$.

9.3.3   Method of Moments

Example 3. Let $Y_1, Y_2, \ldots, Y_n$ be iid $f(y \; ; \; \boldsymbol{\theta})$ and define

$$\bar{y}^r = \frac{\sum_{i=1}^n y_i}{n} \; ; \; \mu_r(\boldsymbol{\theta}) = E_{\boldsymbol{\theta}}(Y^r)$$

Then the estimating function $\mathbf{g}(\mathbf{y}; \boldsymbol{\theta})$ with rth component equal to

$$\bar{y}^r - \mu_r(\boldsymbol{\theta})$$

defines the **moment estimator** of θ.

9.3.4   Generalized Linear Models

Example 4. Let $Y_1, Y_2, \ldots, Y_n$ be independent where f_i is of the exponential type, i.e.,

$$f_i(y_i \; ; \; \boldsymbol{\theta}) = \exp\left\{\left[\frac{y_i\theta_i - b(\theta_i)}{a_i(\phi)}\right] + c_i(y_i \; ; \; \phi)\right\}$$

Then it is easy to show that

$$\mu_i = \mathbb{E}(Y_i) = b^{(1)}(\theta_i)$$

A function h such that

$$h(\mu_i) = h[b^{(1)}(\theta_i)] = \mathbf{x}_i^\top \boldsymbol{\beta}$$

is called a **link function** and $\eta_i = h(\mu_i)$ is called a **linear predictor**.
The link is called canonical if

$$\eta_i = \mathbf{x}_i^T \boldsymbol{\beta} = \theta_i$$

and in this case

$$\mu_i(\boldsymbol{\beta}) = b^{(1)}(\theta_i)$$

For canonical links the maximum likelihood estimating equations are given by

$$\sum_{i=1}^n \left[\frac{y_i - \mu_i(\boldsymbol{\beta})}{a_i(\phi)}\right] \frac{\partial \theta_i}{\partial \beta_j} = 0$$

for $j = 1, 2, \ldots, p$

Note that

$$\frac{\partial \mu_i(\boldsymbol{\beta})}{\partial \beta_j} = b^{(2)}(\theta_i)\frac{\partial \theta_i}{\partial \beta_j}$$

so that

$$\frac{\partial \theta_i}{\partial \beta_j} = \frac{\frac{\partial \mu_i(\boldsymbol{\beta})}{\partial \beta_j}}{b^{(2)}(\theta_i)}$$

Thus the maximum likelihood equations are

$$\sum_{i=1}^{n}\left[\frac{y_i - \mu_i(\boldsymbol{\beta})}{v_i}\right]\frac{\partial \mu_i(\boldsymbol{\beta})}{\partial \beta_j} \quad \text{for } j = 1, 2, \ldots, p$$

where v_i is the variance of Y_i. In matrix form the maximum likelihood equations are

$$\sum_{i=1}^{n}\left[\frac{\partial \mu_i(\boldsymbol{\beta})}{\partial \boldsymbol{\beta}}\right]^{\top}\left[\frac{y_i - \mu_i(\boldsymbol{\beta})}{v_i}\right] = \boldsymbol{0}$$

These equations specialize to the general linear model, the logistic regression model, the log linear model, and many other commonly used models.

Each of the above examples yields an unbiased estimating function. In R we have the packages LM and GLM.

9.3.5 Quasi-Likelihood

Example 5. The estimating function

$$\sum_{i=1}^{n}\left[\frac{\partial \mu_i(\boldsymbol{\beta})}{\partial \boldsymbol{\beta}}\right]^{\top} v_i^{-1}(y_i - \mu_i(\boldsymbol{\beta}))$$

where v_i is the variance of Y_i defines the **quasi-likelihood estimator** and it can be used regardless of whether the family is of the exponential type since it depends only on the mean and variance of Y_i.

9.3.6 Generalized Estimating Equations

Example 6. Consider clustered data (either defined as repeated measures over time on the same individual or as clusters defined by family or environmental facts). Specifically let the observations (responses) from the ith cluster be

$$(y_{i1}, y_{i2}, \ldots, y_{in_i}) \text{ for } i = 1, 2, \ldots, m$$

Let

$$\mathbb{E}(Y_{ij}) = \mu_{ij} \text{ where } h(\mu_{ij}) = \mathbf{x}_{ij}^\top \theta$$

where h is a link function and let

$$\mu_i(\theta)^\top = (\mu_{i1}(\theta), \mu_{i2}(\theta), \ldots, \mu_{in_i}(\theta))$$

for $i = 1, 2, \ldots, m$.

The **GEE** estimating equations are defined by

$$\sum_{i=1}^m \left[\frac{\partial \mu_i(\theta)}{\partial \theta}\right]^\top [\mathbb{V}(\mathbf{Y}_i)]^{-1} [\mathbf{y}_i - \mu_i(\theta)] = \mathbf{0}$$

In R there is a package GEEpack (and others). These methods were introduced by Liang and Zeger. See Diggle et al. [11] for details.

9.4   Generalized Method of Moments

Suppose there exists a function $g \, \mathcal{X} \times \Theta \mapsto \mathbb{R}^p$ such that

$$\mu_g(\theta_0) = \mathbb{E}\{g(\mathbf{X}, \theta_0)\} = \mathbf{0}$$

where $\mu_g(\theta_0) \neq \mathbf{0}$ for $\theta \neq \theta_0$.

The **generalized method of moments** replaces $\mathbb{E}$ by $\widehat{E}$, the sample average, to obtain

$$\widehat{\mu}_g(\theta) = \frac{1}{n} \sum_{i=1}^n g(X_i, \theta)$$

Then $\widehat{\theta}$ is chosen to minimize

$$\widehat{\mu}_g(\theta)^\top \mathbf{W} \widehat{\mu}_g(\theta)$$

where W is a weighting matrix (assumed positive definite). The optimum choice of $\mathbf{W}$ is Σ where

$$\Sigma = \text{Var}_{\theta_0}\left\{\frac{\partial g(Y, \theta)}{\partial \theta}\right\}$$

Under weak conditions, such a $\widehat{\theta}$ satisfies:

- Consistency
- Asymptotic normality, i.e.,

$$\sqrt{n}(\widehat{\theta} - \theta_0) \overset{d}{\longrightarrow} \text{MVN}(\mathbf{0}, \mathbf{G}^\top \mathbf{\Sigma} \mathbf{G})$$

where

$$\mathbf{G} = \frac{\partial g(Y, \theta)}{\partial \theta}$$

All of these facts arise from routine Taylor's expansions. In R there is a package GMM.

9.5 The Bootstrap

Most estimation methods have the property that they produce estimators which have the property that

$$\frac{\widehat{\theta}_n - \theta}{\text{s.e.}(\widehat{\theta}_n)} \overset{d}{\to} \text{N}(0, 1)$$

so that

$$\widehat{\theta}_n \pm z_{1-\alpha/2}\text{s.e.}(\widehat{\theta}_n)$$

is an approximate $100(1 - \alpha)\%$ confidence interval for θ.

9.5.1 Basic Ideas

The bootstrap, developed by Bradley Efron, is a method which can be used, with few assumptions, to estimate the standard error of a statistic and to calculate approximate confidence intervals for the parameter the statistic estimates.

Assume that T_n is a statistic, that is, T_n is some function of the observed data which is a random sample from F. The variance of T_n and distribution of T_n is of interest.

We write

$$\mathbb{V}_F(T_n)$$

to denote this variance and note that it depends on the unknown F.

The Bootstrap

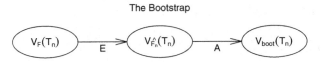

Fig. 9.1 The bootstrap

The following two steps constitute the basis of the bootstrap (Fig. 9.1):

1. **Estimate** $\mathbb{V}_F(T_n)$ by $\mathbb{V}_{\widehat{F}_n}(T_n)$
2. **Approximate** $\mathbb{V}_{\widehat{F}_n}(T_n)$ by **simulation**

1. The approximation error of F by the sample distribution function is the most likely of the approximations to be large since it requires that the sample distribution function be close, in some sense, to the true distribution function.
2. Thus it will work well if the sample is "representative" and if n is not too small.
3. The approximation error of the sampling distribution of T_n, assuming that $\widehat{F}_n$ is the true distribution function, by simulation is expected to be small.

9.5.2   Simulation Background

1. If $Y_1, Y_2, \ldots, Y_B$ is a random sample from a population with distribution G then the law of large numbers implies that

$$\frac{1}{B} \sum_{i=1}^{B} Y_j \xrightarrow{p} \mathbb{E}(Y)$$

i.e., if we draw a (large) sample from population G we can approximate $\mathbb{E}(Y)$ by the sample mean.

2. This result is easily generalizable to any function of Y, say $h(Y)$, which has finite mean, i.e.,

$$\frac{1}{B} \sum_{i=1}^{B} h(Y_i) \xrightarrow{p} \mathbb{E}[h(Y)]$$

3. Assuming that variances exist it follows that

$$\frac{1}{B} \sum_{i=1}^{B} (Y_i - \overline{Y}_B)^2 = \frac{1}{B} \sum_{i=1}^{B} Y_i^2 - (\overline{Y}_B)^2$$

converges in probability to $\mathbb{E}(Y^2) - [\mathbb{E}(Y)]^2$, i.e., to $\mathbb{V}(Y)$.

4. Thus the sample variance of the Y_i's can be used to approximate the variance of G. It follows that if we can simulate random samples from a population with distribution G, then we can get a good approximation to the expected value and variance of G.

R and other computer packages provide functions which allow selection of random samples from a variety of distributions, e.g., rnorm, rgamma, rbinom, etc. For other distributions and to understand how random samples are generated recall the following basic result from probability theory.

If X is a random variable with a continuous distribution function F then the random variable $U = F(X)$ has a uniform distribution on the interval $[0, 1]$.

Proof.

$$
\begin{aligned}
F_U(u) &= \mathbb{P}(U \le u) \\
&= \mathbb{P}(\{x \ : \ F(x) \le u\}) \\
&= \mathbb{P}(\{x \ : \ x \le F^{-1}(u)\}) \\
&= F[F^{-1}(u)] \\
&= u
\end{aligned}
$$

This result is called the **probability integral transformation** and provides, among other things, a method of obtaining a random observation from any continuous distribution. Simply generate a random uniform, then, $F^{-1}(U)$ has distribution F. More generally, generate $u_1, u_2, \ldots, u_n$, independent with each observation on a uniform on $[0, 1]$. Then

$$
x_1 = F^{-1}(u_1), x_2 = F^{-1}(u_2), \ldots, x_n = F^{-1}(u_n)
$$

is a random sample from F.

Computer scientists have discovered much more efficient ways to generate such samples, but the above result is important because it shows that we can always simulate from any distribution function.

9.5.3 Variance Estimation Using the Bootstrap

It is clear from the previous section that we can use simulation to approximate $\mathbb{V}_{\widehat{F}_n}(T_n)$. This requires the simulation of the distribution of T_n when the data are assumed to have population distribution $\widehat{F}_n$.

Note that $\widehat{F}_n$ puts probability mass $1/n$ on each sample point. Thus, drawing an observation from $\widehat{F}_n$ is equivalent to drawing one point at random from the original data set, i.e., to simulate

$$X_1^*, X_2^*, \ldots, X_n^*$$

from $\widehat{F}_n$ it is sufficient to draw n observations from the original data set $x_1, x_2, \ldots, x_n$ **with replacement**.

Assuming that $\widehat{F}_n$ adequately estimates F we thus have one sample from the original distribution function. Hence we can, by simulation, approximate the sampling variance of the statistic T_n.

Here is the bootstrap method for variance estimation.

1. Draw n observations $x_1^*, x_2^*, \ldots, x_n^*$ at random, with replacement from the original data set.
2. Compute the statistic $T_n^* = g(x_1^*, x_2^*, \ldots, x_n^*)$.
3. Repeat steps 1 and 2 a large number, B, of times to obtain

$$T_{n1}^*, T_{n2}^*, \ldots, T_{nB}^*$$

called the **bootstrap replicates** and their sample mean.

$$\overline{T}_n^* = \frac{1}{B} \sum_{i=1}^n T_{ni}^*$$

4. The bootstrap estimate of the variance of T_n is then given by

$$\mathrm{var}_{bs} = \frac{1}{B} \sum_{i=1}^B (T_{ni}^* - \overline{T}_n^*)^2$$

Note that $T_{n1}^*, T_{n2}^*, \ldots, T_{nB}^*$ can be used to estimate the distribution function of T_n (Fig. 9.2).

9.6   Confidence Intervals Using the Bootstrap

9.6.1   Normal Interval

There are many ways to find confidence intervals using the bootstrap.

If the distribution of $T_n = \widehat{\theta}_n$ is approximately normal, then use

$$\widehat{\theta}_n \pm z_{1-\alpha/2} \widehat{s.e.}_{bs}$$

In the R function **boot.ci** this method is called "norm."

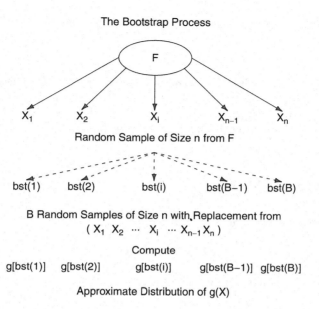

Fig. 9.2 The bootstrap process

9.6.2 Pivotal Interval

Recall that a **pivot**, $p(Y, \theta)$, is any function of a random variable Y and a parameter θ such that the distribution of $p(Y, \theta)$ does not depend on θ.

Example. The best known example of a pivot is

$$Z_n = \frac{\sqrt{n}(\overline{Y}_n - \theta)}{\sigma}$$

where

$$\overline{Y}_n = \frac{1}{n} \sum_{i=1}^{n} Y_i$$

and the Y_i's are iid each normal with mean μ and known variance σ^2. The distribution of Z_n is normal with mean 0 and variance 1 and does not depend on μ.

The standard inversion shows that

$$\overline{y}_n \pm z_{1-\alpha/2}\mathrm{se}$$

is a $100(1 - \alpha)\%$ confidence interval for μ.

The pivotal method for the bootstrap defines

$$R_n(\widehat{\theta}, \theta) = \widehat{\theta}_n - \theta$$

and assumes that it is a pivot with distribution function H. If H is known, standard inversion gives the confidence interval. Since H is unknown, it is estimated from the quantiles of the bootstrap.

In the R function **boot.ci**, this interval is called "basic."

9.6.3   Percentile Interval

Given the bootstrap replicates

$$\widehat{\theta}^*_{n1}, \widehat{\theta}^*_{n2}, \ldots, \widehat{\theta}^*_{nB}$$

The percentile interval is simply defined as

$$\left[\theta^*_{\alpha/2}, \theta^*_{1-\alpha/2}\right]$$

where $\theta^*_{\alpha/2}$ is the $\alpha/2$ quantile of the set of bootstrap replicates and $\theta^*_{1-\alpha/2}$ is the $1 - \alpha/2$ quantile of the set of bootstrap replicates.

In the R function **boot.ci** this interval is called "perc."

The R library **boot** has a wide variety of bootstrap functions.

9.6.4   Parametric Version

There is also a parametric version of the bootstrap in which we

1. Assume the model density is known.
2. Estimate parameters by maximum likelihood or some other methods.
3. Use the estimates to draw random bootstrap samples from the known distribution, substituting the estimated parameter values for the parameters.
4. Use the resulting bootstrap distribution to assess standard errors, confidence limits, etc.
5. This version is particularly useful to check on approximations such as the delta method.

9.6.5 Dangers of the Bootstrap

All you ever learn using the bootstrap, without further modeling assumptions, are properties of $\widehat{F}_n$. Unless you have a way of saying how much and/or in what ways knowledge of $\widehat{F}_n$ can be transformed into knowledge of F, the bootstrap can only tell you about $\widehat{F}_n$, not about F [46].

9.6.6 The Number of Possible Bootstrap Samples

If we have a sample size of n there are only

$$\binom{2n-1}{n-1}$$

possible bootstrap samples. To see this imagine n boxes defined by $n-1$ lines

$$|\,| \;\cdots\; |\,|$$

The first bootstrap observation can be put one of the n boxes, the second into $n+1$ possible positions, the third $n+2, \ldots$, the nth into $2n-1$ positions.

1. The total is

$$n(n-1)\cdots(2n-1) = (2n-1)_{(n-1)} = \frac{(2n-1)!}{(n-1)!}$$

2. The balls can be ordered in $n!$ ways so that the total number of possible samples is

$$\frac{(2n-1)!}{(n-1)!n!} = \binom{2n-1}{n-1}$$

3. Thus it would be possible to enumerate all the possible samples.

   Recalling that (Stirling's Approximation)

$$r! \approx (2\pi r)^{-1/2} r^r e^{-r}$$

we have that

$$\binom{2n-1}{n-1} \approx \frac{[2\pi(2n-1)]^{-1/2}(2n-1)^{2n-1}e^{-(2n-1)}}{[2\pi n]^{1/2}n^n e^n [2\pi(n-1)]^{1/2}(n-1)^{n-1}}$$

$$= \left[\frac{2n-1}{2\pi n(n-1)}\right]^{1/2} \frac{\left\{n\left[2-\frac{1}{n}\right]\right\}^{2n-1}}{n^n\left\{n\left[1-\frac{1}{n}\right]\right\}^{n-1}}$$

$$= \sqrt{\frac{2 - \frac{1}{n}}{2\pi n(1 - \frac{1}{n})} \frac{\left[2 - \frac{1}{n}\right]^{2n-1}}{\left[1 - \frac{1}{n}\right]^{n-1}}}$$

$$\approx (\pi n)^{-1/2} 2^{2n-1}$$

Thus we have

n	5	10	15	20	30
Samples	10^2	10^5	10^8	10^{11}	10^{17}

One can also show that the original sample is the most probable of these to occur.

Chapter 10
Decision Theory

10.1 Introduction

- In this chapter we introduce some of the ideas and notation of decision theory.
- At one time it was thought that all statistical problems could be cast in the decision theoretic framework and statistics could thus be reduced to a study of optimization techniques.
- This subsided, partly due to the complexity of real-world problems and partly due to the realization that inference was more subtle than optimization.
- Nevertheless some knowledge of the basic concepts is useful for consolidation of ideas and as an introduction to Bayesian ideas.

10.1.1 Actions, Losses, and Risks

In the basic statistical model $(\mathcal{X}, f(x, \theta), \Theta)$ we consider an **action space**, $\mathcal{A}$, which represents all of the actions or decisions which the experimenter might consider regarding θ.

Examples of actions include

1. The action space might be the parameter space itself. In this case we have the **estimation** problem.
2. The action space might be deciding between two hypotheses H_0 and H_1. Here the action space is $\mathcal{A} = \{a_o, a_1\}$ and we have a **hypothesis testing** problem.
3. The action space might be the selection of a subset of the parameter space where we are confident that the subset contains the parameter. In this case we have an **interval estimation** problem.

© Springer International Publishing Switzerland 2014
C.A. Rohde, *Introductory Statistical Inference with the Likelihood Function*, DOI 10.1007/978-3-319-10461-4_10

Definition 10.1.1 (Loss function). Associated with each action and each value of the parameter is a **loss function**, L, such that if we take action a when θ is the true value of the parameter then we incur a loss $L(\theta, a)$, i.e., the loss function is a mapping:

$$L \, : \, \Theta \times \mathcal{A} \mapsto \mathbb{R}$$

- Choice of a loss function depends on the action and the consequences of making a wrong decision (choosing the wrong action).
- In certain problems conventional loss functions are typically chosen.

Example. In the estimation problem typical loss functions are

- **Squared error loss** $L(\theta, a) = (a - \theta)^2$
- **Absolute error loss** $L(\theta, a) = |a - \theta|$
- **0–1 loss**

$$L(\theta, a) = \begin{cases} 0 \ a = \theta \\ 1 \ a \neq \theta \end{cases}$$

Example. In the hypothesis testing problem we choose

$$L(\theta_0, a) = \begin{cases} c_0 \ a \neq \theta_0 \\ 0 \ a = \theta_0 \end{cases} \quad L(\theta_1, a) = \begin{cases} c_1 \ a \neq \theta_1 \\ 0 \ a = \theta_1 \end{cases}$$

Definition 10.1.2 (Decision space). Given a sample space $\mathcal{X}$ and an action space $\mathcal{A}$ the **decision space**, $\mathcal{D}$, is defined by

if $x \in \mathcal{X}$ occurs then we take action $a = d(x)$

Thus a decision function maps the sample space to the action space, $d \, : \, \mathcal{X} \mapsto \mathcal{A}$, and hence the decision space, $\mathcal{D}$, is a collection of functions mapping $\mathcal{X}$ to $\mathcal{A}$.

Definition 10.1.3. The **risk function**, R, is a function of $d \in \mathcal{D}$ and X defined by

$$R(\theta, d) = \mathbb{E}_\theta[L(\theta, d(X)]$$

The basic idea in decision theory is that the experimenter or decision maker should

1. Compare decision functions based on their risk function.
2. Choose that decision function which minimizes the risk.
3. It is essentially a frequentist concept since risks are averages over the sample space.
4. One central problem in decision theory is that there is usually no decision rule which uniformly (for all θ) minimizes the risk.
5. Therefore certain criteria are set up to reduce the number of decision rules and then search for a decision rule in this smaller collection.

10.2 Admissibility

Definition 10.2.1. If d and d' are two decision rules d is said to strictly dominate d' if

(i) $R(\theta, d) \leq R(\theta, d')$ for all θ
(ii) $R(\theta, d) < R(\theta, d')$ for at least one θ

Applying frequentist ideas we would prefer d to d'.

Definition 10.2.2. A decision rule is **inadmissible** if it is strictly dominated by another decision rule and admissable otherwise.

Finding admissable decision rules is not easy.

10.3 Bayes Risk and Bayes Rules

Definition 10.3.1 (Bayes risk). If π is a prior distribution for θ then the **Bayes risk** of the decision procedure δ for the prior π is

$$r(\pi, \delta) = \mathbb{E}_\pi \left\{ R(\theta, \delta) \right\}$$

The **Bayes decision rule** minimizes the Bayes risk.

Note that

$$r(\pi, \delta) = \int_\Theta \left\{ \int_\mathcal{X} L[\theta, \delta(x)] f(x; \theta) dm(x) \right\} \pi(\theta) d\lambda(\theta)$$

Under weak regularity conditions we can write

$$r(\pi, \delta) = \int_\Theta \left\{ \int_\mathcal{X} L[\theta, \delta(x)] f(x; \theta) d\lambda(x) \right\} \pi(\theta) d\lambda(\theta)$$

$$= \int_\mathcal{X} \left\{ \int_\Theta L(\theta, \delta(x)] f(x; \theta) \pi(\theta) d\lambda(\theta) \right\} d\lambda(x)$$

$$= \int_\mathcal{X} \left\{ \int_\Theta L[\theta, \delta(x)] \pi(\theta|x) d\lambda(\theta) \right\} f(x) d\lambda(x)$$

where

$$\pi(\theta|x) = \frac{f(x; \theta) \pi(\theta)}{f(x)} \quad \text{and} \quad f(x) = \int_\Theta f(x; \theta) \pi(\theta) d\lambda(\theta)$$

A Bayes decision rule is thus one in which we minimize the posterior risk

$$\int_\Theta L[\theta, \delta(x)]\pi(\theta|x)d\lambda(\theta)$$

1. Under weak conditions a Bayes rule with a proper prior is admissable and conversely every admissable decision rule, under weak conditions, is a Bayes rule with respect to some prior (possibly improper).
2. This result is what is known as a **complete class theorem** in which all admissable decision rules are characterized.
3. In frequentist statistics, the search for admissable rules involves a consideration of Bayes rules.
4. In Bayesian statistics the focus is on Bayes rules from the start.

10.4   Examples of Bayes Rules

Consider a random sample of size n from the normal distribution with parameters μ and σ^2 where σ^2 is known. Assume that the prior for μ is normal centered at μ_0 and variance σ_μ^2 (both assumed known).

We need to find the posterior distribution of μ. We can write

$$\mathbf{Y} = \mathbf{1}\mu + \mathbf{Z}_1$$

where $\mathbf{Z}_1$ is normal with mean vector $\mathbf{0}$ and variance covariance matrix $\sigma^2\mathbf{I}_n$. We can also write

$$\mu = \mu_0 + Z_2$$

where Z_2 is normal with mean 0 and variance σ_μ^2 and is independent of $\mathbf{Z}_1$.

It follows that

$$\begin{bmatrix} \mathbf{Y} \\ \mu \end{bmatrix} = \begin{bmatrix} \mathbf{1} \\ 1 \end{bmatrix} \mu_0 + \begin{bmatrix} \mathbf{I}_n & \mathbf{1} \\ \mathbf{0}^\top & 1 \end{bmatrix} \begin{bmatrix} \mathbf{Z}_1 \\ Z_2 \end{bmatrix}$$

and hence the joint distribution of $\mathbf{Y}$ and μ is normal with

$$\mathbb{E}\begin{bmatrix} \mathbf{Y} \\ \mu \end{bmatrix} = \begin{bmatrix} \mathbf{1} \\ 1 \end{bmatrix} \mu_0$$

and

$$\mathbb{V}\begin{bmatrix} \mathbf{Y} \\ \mu \end{bmatrix} = \begin{bmatrix} \sigma^2\mathbf{I}_n + \sigma_\mu^2\mathbf{1}\mathbf{1}^\top & \sigma_\mu^2\mathbf{1} \\ \sigma_\mu^2\mathbf{1}^\top & \sigma_\mu^2 \end{bmatrix}$$

- The conditional distribution of μ given $\mathbf{Y} = \mathbf{y}$ is thus normal (from theory on the multivariate normal).
- It follows that the Bayes estimator of μ is thus the conditional expected value of μ given $\mathbf{Y} = \mathbf{y}$ (using squared error loss).
- The formula for this expected value is

$$\mathbb{E}(\mu) + \mathbb{C}(\mu, \mathbf{Y})[\mathbb{V}(\mathbf{Y})^{-1}[\mathbf{y} - \mathbb{E}(\mathbf{Y})]$$

or

$$\mu_0 + \sigma_\mu^2 \mathbf{1}^\top \left[\sigma^2 \mathbf{I} + \sigma_\mu^2 \mathbf{1}\mathbf{1}^\top\right]^{-1} [\mathbf{y} - \mathbf{1}\mu_0]$$

For a matrix of the form

$$a\mathbf{I} + b\mathbf{1}\mathbf{1}^\top$$

The equation

$$[a\mathbf{I} + b\mathbf{1}\mathbf{1}^\top][c\mathbf{I} + d\mathbf{1}\mathbf{1}^\top] = ac\mathbf{I} + (bc + ad + nbd)\mathbf{1}\mathbf{1}^\top = \mathbf{I}$$

shows that

$$[a\mathbf{I} + b\mathbf{1}\mathbf{1}^\top]^{-1} = c\mathbf{I} + d\mathbf{1}\mathbf{1}^\top$$

where

$$c = \frac{1}{a} \;\; ; \;\; d = \frac{-b}{a(a + nb)}$$

In our case

$$a = \sigma^2 \;\; ; \;\; b = \sigma_\mu^2$$

It follows that

$$\sigma_\mu^2 \mathbf{1}^\top \left[\sigma^2 \mathbf{I} + \sigma_\mu^2 \mathbf{1}\mathbf{1}^\top\right]^{-1} = \sigma_\mu^2 \mathbf{1}^\top \left[\frac{1}{\sigma^2}\mathbf{I} - \frac{\sigma_\mu^2}{\sigma^2 + n\sigma_\mu^2}\right]$$

which reduces to

$$\frac{\sigma_\mu^2}{\sigma^2 + n\sigma_\mu^2}\mathbf{1}^\top$$

and hence the Bayes estimator is

$$\mu_0 + \frac{n\sigma_\mu^2}{\sigma^2 + n\sigma_\mu^2}(\overline{y} - \mu_0)$$

which can be written as

$$\frac{n\sigma_\mu^2\overline{y} + \sigma^2\mu_0}{\sigma^2 + n\sigma_\mu^2}$$

The Bayes estimator can be written in two equivalent forms

$$\frac{\frac{n\overline{y}}{\sigma^2} + \frac{\mu_0}{\sigma_\mu^2}}{\frac{n}{\sigma^2} + \frac{1}{\sigma_\mu^2}}$$

i.e., as a weighted combination of the usual estimator $\overline{y}$ and the prior mean μ_0 with weights equal to the variance of $\overline{y}$ and the variance of the prior distribution.

A second way to rewrite the Bayes estimator is as

$$\overline{y} - \frac{\sigma^2}{\sigma^2 + n\sigma_\mu^2}(\overline{y} - \mu_0)$$

i.e., the usual estimator is "shrunk" toward the prior mean. The amount of shrinkage depends on how far away the sample mean is from the prior mean, the sample size n, and the prior variance.

10.5   Stein's Result

In 1955 Charles Stein proved the remarkable result that the sample mean as an estimator of the mean of a multivariate normal distribution was inadmissible using squared error loss if the dimension of the parameter vector was greater than or equal to 3. This result lead to important insights into the nature of statistical procedures and the development of shrinkage estimators, etc.

The Stein estimator is

$$\delta^S(\mathbf{X}) = [1 - s(\mathbf{X})]\mathbf{X} = \left[1 - \frac{(p - 2)}{\sum_{j=1}^{p} X_j^2}\right]\mathbf{X}$$

where $\mathbf{X}$ is assumed multivariate normal with mean μ and variance covariance matrix $\mathbf{I}$.

The following argument is due to Dennis Lindley. Suppose now that we have the same assumptions as above, but we add the assumption that the μ_i are iid $N(0, \sigma^2)$, i.e.,

$$\boldsymbol{\mu} \text{ is } \text{MVN}(\mathbf{0}, \sigma^2\mathbf{I})$$

Then $\mathbf{X}$ and $\boldsymbol{\mu}$ are jointly multivariate normal with mean vectors given by

$$E(\mathbf{X}) = E[E(\mathbf{X}|\boldsymbol{\mu})] = E(\boldsymbol{\mu}) = \mathbf{0} \text{ and } E(\boldsymbol{\mu}) = \mathbf{0}$$

and variances and covariances given by

$$\begin{aligned}
\text{var}(\mathbf{X}) &= E[\text{var}(\mathbf{X}|\boldsymbol{\mu})] + \text{var}[E(\mathbf{X}|\boldsymbol{\mu})] \\
&= \mathbf{I} + \text{var}(\boldsymbol{\mu}) \\
&= \mathbf{I} + \sigma^2\mathbf{I} \\
\text{var}(\boldsymbol{\mu}) &= \sigma^2\mathbf{I} \\
\text{cov}(\mathbf{X}, \boldsymbol{\mu}) &= E(\mathbf{X}\boldsymbol{\mu}^\top) \\
&= E\{[E(\mathbf{X}|\boldsymbol{\mu}]\boldsymbol{\mu})^\top\} \\
&= E[\boldsymbol{\mu}\boldsymbol{\mu}^\top] \\
&= \sigma^2\mathbf{I}
\end{aligned}$$

It follows that the conditional distribution of $\boldsymbol{\mu}$ given $\mathbf{X}$ is multivariate normal with mean vector

$$\delta^B(\mathbf{X}) = \frac{\sigma^2}{1 + \sigma^2}\mathbf{X}$$

so that the Bayes estimator of $\boldsymbol{\mu}$ would be $\delta^B(\mathbf{X})$. We note that the Bayes estimator may be written as

$$\delta^B(\mathbf{X}) = \left(1 - \frac{1}{1 + \sigma^2}\right)\mathbf{X}$$

Now note that since the X_i are independent each normal with mean 0 and variance $1 + \sigma^2$ we have that

$$\frac{1}{1 + \sigma^2}\sum_{j=1}^{p}X_j^2 \sim \chi^2(p)$$

Thus a natural estimate of $1/(1 + \sigma^2)$ is, for $p \geq 3$,

$$\frac{p - 2}{\sum_{j=1}^{p}X_j^2} = s(\mathbf{X})$$

and we have another, simpler, derivation of the Stein estimator which shows that it is not as mysterious as first thought.

10.6   Exercises

1. The LINEX loss function for estimation is defined by

$$L(\theta, a) = \beta \left\{ e^{\alpha(a-\theta)} - \alpha(a - \theta) - 1 \right\} \quad \alpha \neq 0, \quad \beta > 0$$

(a) Plot the LINEX loss function for $b = 1$ and $\alpha = 0.2, 0.5, 1$ (use as horizontal axis $a - \theta$).

(b) Do the same for $b = 1$ and $\alpha = -0.2, -0.5, -1$ (use as horizontal axis $a - \theta$).

(c) Show that the posterior expected value of the LINEX loss function is

$$r(a, \pi) = \mathbb{E} \left\{ \beta \left[e^{\alpha(a-\theta)} - \alpha(a - \theta) - 1 \right] \right\}$$
$$= \beta \left\{ e^{\alpha a} M(-\alpha) - \alpha(a - \overline{\theta}) - 1 \right\}$$

where $\overline{\theta}$ is the mean of the posterior and $M(-\alpha)$ is the moment generating function of the posterior evaluated at $t = -\alpha$.

(d) Find the Bayes rule for (c).

(e) Find the Bayes rule when the posterior is a normal distribution with mean μ and variance σ^2.

Chapter 11
Sufficiency

11.1 Families of Distributions

We consider a set of observations **x** thought to be a realization of some random variable **X** whose probability distribution belongs to a set of distributions

$$\mathcal{F} = \{f(\cdot \, ; \, \theta) \, : \, \theta \in \Theta\}$$

The distributions in $\mathcal{F}$ are indexed by a parameter θ, i.e., the parameter θ determines which of the distributions is used to assign probabilities to **X**. The set Θ is called the parameter space and $\mathcal{F}$ is called the family of distributions. $\mathcal{F}$ along with **X** constitutes the probability model for the observed data.

Example 1. The binomial family in x is the observed number of successes in n Bernoulli trials and X is the random-variable with density in

$$\mathcal{F} = \binom{n}{x} \theta^x (1 - \theta)^{n-x} \quad x = 0, 1, 2, \ldots, n \, , \, \theta \in [0, 1]$$

Example 2. The Poisson family defined by

$$\mathbf{x} = (x_1, x_2, \ldots, x_n)$$
$$\mathbf{X} = (X_1, X_2, \ldots, X_n)$$
$$\mathcal{F} = \left\{ f_{\mathbf{X}}(\mathbf{x}; \theta) = \prod_{i=1}^{n} \frac{\theta^{x_i} e^{-\theta}}{x_i!} \, , \, 0 < \theta < \infty \, ; \, x_i = 0, 1, 2, \ldots \right\}$$

© Springer International Publishing Switzerland 2014
C.A. Rohde, *Introductory Statistical Inference with the Likelihood
Function*, DOI 10.1007/978-3-319-10461-4_11

Example 3. Let $\mathbf{X} = (\mathbf{X}_1, \mathbf{X}_2, \ldots, \mathbf{X}_n)$ be iid as f where $f\mathcal{F}$ is defined by

$$\mathcal{F} = \left\{ f_{\mathbf{X}} \; : \; f_{\mathbf{X}}(\mathbf{x}) = \prod_{i=1}^{n} f(x_i) \right\}$$

where f is any distribution on the nonnegative integers. This is a large family and cannot be indexed by a parameter.

11.1.1   Introduction to Sufficiency

Consider the number of coin tosses which are heads out of 5 tosses. We might use as the probability model $X \sim$ binomial$(5, \theta)$. To compare the evidence for θ_1 vs θ_2 given an observation of 4 heads, the Law of Likelihood suggests that we consider the ratio

$$\frac{f(4, \theta_1)}{f(4, \theta_2)} = \frac{\binom{5}{4}\theta_1^4(1 - \theta_1)}{\binom{5}{4}\theta_2^4(1 - \theta_2)}$$

of the two likelihoods. Note that in using the Law of Likelihood it is only the ratio of likelihoods that matters.

Thus we need only define the likelihood $L(\theta)$ up to a multiplicative constant. For example,

$$L(\theta) = \binom{5}{4}\theta^4(1 - \theta)$$

achieves its maximum at $\theta = \frac{4}{5}$ so that

$$\mathscr{L}(\theta) = \frac{\binom{5}{4}\theta^4(1 - \theta)}{\binom{5}{4}\left(\frac{4}{5}\right)^4 \left(1 - \frac{4}{5}\right)}$$

achieves its maximum of 1 at $\theta = \frac{4}{5}$ but is an equivalent version of the likelihood since

$$\frac{L(\theta_1)}{L(\theta_2)} = \frac{\mathscr{L}(\theta_1)}{\mathscr{L}(\theta_2)} = \frac{\theta_1^4(1 - \theta_1)}{\theta_2^4(1 - \theta_2)}$$

Suppose now that we are given the additional information that the result of the 5 tosses was (H, H, H, T, H). Then $\mathbf{X} = (\mathbf{X}_1, \mathbf{X}_2, \mathbf{X}_3, \mathbf{X}_4, \mathbf{X}_5)$ represents the results of 5 iid Bernoulli trials, i.e.,

$$f_{X_i} = \begin{cases} \theta & \text{if } x_i = 1 \\ 1 - \theta & \text{if } x_i = 0 \end{cases} = \theta^{x_i}(1 - \theta)^{1 - x_i}$$

and hence

$$f_{\mathbf{X}}(\mathbf{x}; \theta) = \prod_{i=1}^{5} f_{\mathbf{X}_i}(x_i; \theta) = \theta^{\sum_{i=1}^{5} x_i}(1 - \theta)^{5 - \sum_{i=1}^{5} x_i}$$

Thus if we observe $\mathbf{x} = (1, 1, 1, 0, 1)$ then $\sum_{i=1}^{5} x_i = 4$ and the likelihood ratio for comparing θ_1 to θ_2 is given by

$$\frac{L(\theta_1)}{L(\theta_2)} = \frac{\theta_1^4(1 - \theta_1)}{\theta_2^4(1 - \theta_2)}$$

Note that this likelihood ratio is exactly the same as if we are only told that the number of heads is 4.

It follows that knowing the order in which the observed results occurred does not provide any additional information about θ. Put another way, knowing the number of heads to be 4, i.e., $\sum_{i=1}^{5} x_i = 4$, the additional fact that $\mathbf{x} = (1, 1, 1, 0, 1)$ provides no additional information about θ.

For Bernoulli trials this is true in general since

$$P\left(\mathbf{X} = \mathbf{x}; \theta \middle| \sum_{i=1}^{n} x_i = s\right) = \frac{P(\mathbf{X} = \mathbf{x} \text{ and } \sum_{i=1}^{n} \mathbf{X}_i = s)}{P(\sum_{i=1}^{n} \mathbf{X}_i = s)}$$

$$= \frac{P(\sum_{i=1}^{n} X_i = s; \theta | \mathbf{X} = \mathbf{x})P(\mathbf{X} = \mathbf{x}; \theta)}{P(\sum_{i=1}^{n} \mathbf{X}_i = s)}$$

$$= \frac{\delta(s, \sum_{i=1}^{n} x_i)\theta^{\sum_{i=1}^{n} x_i}(1 - \theta)^{n - \sum_{i=1}^{n} x_i}}{\binom{n}{s}\theta^s(1 - \theta)^{n-s}}$$

$$= \begin{cases} \frac{\theta^s(1-\theta)^{n-s}}{\binom{n}{s}\theta^s(1-\theta)^{n-s}} & \text{if } s = \sum_{i=1}^{n} x_i \\ 0 & \text{otherwise} \end{cases}$$

$$= \begin{cases} \frac{1}{\binom{n}{s}} & \text{if } s = \sum_{i=1}^{n} x_i \\ 0 & \text{otherwise} \end{cases}$$

where

$$\delta(a, b) = \begin{cases} 1 \text{ if } a = b \\ 0 \text{ otherwise} \end{cases}$$

Thus if $\sum_{i=1}^{n} X_i = s$, $\mathbf{X}$ must be one of the $\binom{n}{s}$ sequences consisting of s 1's and $(n - s)$ 0's. Each of these sequences has the same probability which is independent of θ.

In this example each of these possible sequences has probability $\frac{1}{5}$. If, given $S = \sum_{i=1}^{5} X_i = 4$, we consider the Law of Likelihood for comparing θ_1 to θ_2 we find that

$$\frac{f_{\mathbf{X}|S=4}((1,1,1,0,1);\theta_1)}{f_{\mathbf{X}|S=4}((1,1,1,0,1);\theta_2)} = \frac{\frac{1}{5}}{\frac{1}{5}} = 1$$

i.e., if we know $S = 4$ knowledge of $\mathbf{x}$ provides no additional information about θ. Thus knowledge of S is sufficient and S is an example of a sufficient statistic.

Definition 11.1.1. Given random variables $\mathbf{X}$ and a family of probability distributions $\mathcal{F}$ for $\mathbf{X}$, a statistic $\mathbf{S}$ is sufficient for the family $\mathcal{F}$ if the conditional distribution of $\mathbf{X}$ given $\mathbf{S}$ is the same for every member of the family $\mathcal{F}$.

Definition 11.1.2. If $\mathcal{F}$ is indexed by a parameter θ we say that $\mathbf{S}$ is a sufficient statistic for θ if the conditional distribution of $\mathbf{X}$ given $\mathbf{S}$ is the same for all $\theta \in \Theta$. Thus $\mathbf{S}$ is a sufficient statistic for θ if and only if

$$P(\mathbf{X} \in A | \mathbf{S} = \mathbf{s})$$

is the same for all $\theta \in \Theta$.

Note. $\mathbf{X}$ itself is a sufficient statistic since for any set A

$$P(\mathbf{X} \in A | \mathbf{X} = \mathbf{x}) = \begin{cases} 1 & \mathbf{x} \in A \\ 0 & \text{otherwise} \end{cases}$$

Naturally we are interested in sufficient statistics which "reduce" the amount of data (i.e., have a smaller dimension).

11.1.2   Rationale for Sufficiency

The rationale for restricting attention to sufficient statistics runs as follows. Given $X = x$ and $t(X) = t$, if t is sufficient then the conditional distribution of X given $t(X) = t$ does not depend on θ. If we are given the value of $t(X)$, say t, then we can generate X' according to the conditional distribution, $f(x|t)$. It follows that X' has the same probability distribution as X and hence the inferences based on X' about θ should be the same. In this context **post-randomization** which does not depend on θ can provide no additional information about θ.

11.1.3 Factorization Criterion

It can be difficult to find conditional distributions. Fisher and Neyman produced the **factorization criterion**.

Theorem 11.1.1. *Let* $\mathbf{X}$ *have pdf* $f_{\mathbf{X}}(\mathbf{x} \; ; \; \boldsymbol{\theta})$ *for* $\boldsymbol{\theta} \in \boldsymbol{\Theta}$. *A statistic* $\mathbf{S} = \mathbf{s}(\mathbf{X})$ *is a sufficient statistic for* $\boldsymbol{\theta}$ *if and only if there exist functions* g *and* h *such that*

$$f_{\mathbf{X}}(\mathbf{x} \; ; \; \boldsymbol{\theta}) = g(s(\mathbf{x}) \; ; \; \boldsymbol{\theta})h(\mathbf{x})$$

where $h(\mathbf{x})$ *does not depend on* $\boldsymbol{\theta}$.

Example. Let $\mathbf{X} = (X_1, X_2, \ldots, X_n)$ where the $\mathbf{X}_i$ are iid $N(\theta, 1)$. Then

$$f_{\mathbf{X}}(\mathbf{x} \; ; \; \theta) = \prod_{i=1}^{n} \left(\frac{1}{\sqrt{2\pi}} \right) \exp \left\{ -\frac{(x_i - \theta)^2}{2} \right\}$$

$$= \left(\frac{1}{2\pi} \right)^{\frac{n}{2}} \exp \left\{ -\frac{\sum_{i=1}^{n}(x_i - \theta)^2}{2} \right\}$$

$$= \exp \left\{ -\frac{n(\bar{x} - \theta)^2}{2} \right\} \left[\left(\frac{1}{2\pi} \right)^{\frac{n}{2}} \exp \left\{ -\frac{\sum_{i=1}^{n}(x_i - \bar{x})^2}{2} \right\} \right]$$

It follows that $s(\mathbf{X}) = \bar{\mathbf{X}}$ is a sufficient statistic for θ.

Example. Let $\mathbf{X} = (X_1, X_2, \ldots, X_n)$ where the $\mathbf{X}_i$ are iid $N(\theta_1, \theta_2)$ where

$$-\infty < \theta_1 < +\infty \; ; \; 0 < \theta_2 < +\infty$$

Then

$$f_{\mathbf{X}}(\mathbf{x} \; ; \; \boldsymbol{\theta}) = \prod_{i=1}^{n} \left(\frac{1}{\sqrt{2\pi\theta_2}} \right) \exp \left\{ -\frac{(x_i - \theta_1)^2}{2\theta_2} \right\}$$

$$= \left(\frac{1}{2\pi\theta_2} \right)^{\frac{n}{2}} \exp \left\{ -\frac{\sum_{i=1}^{n}(x_i - \theta_1)^2}{2\theta_2} \right\}$$

$$= \left(\frac{1}{\theta_2} \right)^{\frac{n}{2}} \exp \left\{ -\frac{\sum_{i=1}^{n}(x_i - \bar{x})^2}{2\theta_2} - \frac{n(\bar{x} - \theta_1)^2}{2\theta_2} \right\} \left[\left(\frac{1}{2\pi} \right)^{\frac{n}{2}} \right]$$

and it follows that

$$\mathbf{s}(\mathbf{X}) = \left(\bar{X}, \sum_{i=1}^{n}(X_i - \bar{X})^2 \right)$$

is a sufficient statistic for $\boldsymbol{\theta} = (\theta_1, \theta_2)$.

More generally, if $\mathbf{X}$ has pdf $f_{\mathbf{X}}(\mathbf{x}) \in \mathcal{F}$, then a statistic $\mathbf{S} = \mathbf{s}(\mathbf{X})$ is a sufficient statistic for $\mathcal{F}$ if and only if

$$f_{\mathbf{X}}(\mathbf{x}) = g(\mathbf{s}(\mathbf{x}))h(\mathbf{x})$$

where $h(\mathbf{x})$ is the same for all $f \in \mathcal{F}$.

Example. Let $\mathbf{X} = (X_1, X_2, \dots, X_n)$ where the X_i are iid uniform on $0, \theta$. Then

$$f_{\mathbf{X}}(\mathbf{x}\,;\,\theta) = \begin{cases} \frac{1}{\theta^n} & 0 < x_1, x_2, \dots, x_n < \theta \\ 0 & \text{otherwise} \end{cases}$$

Here we must build in the dependence of the range of $\mathbf{X}$ into the functions g and h.

Let $y_1 \le y_2 \le \dots \le y_n$ denote the ordered values of $x_1, x_2, \dots, x_n$. The corresponding statistic is called the order statistic. Define

$$\mathbf{1}(a, b) = \begin{cases} 1 & \text{if } a \le b \\ 0 & \text{otherwise} \end{cases}$$

then

$$f_{\mathbf{X}}(\mathbf{x}\,;\,\theta) = \frac{1}{\theta^n}\mathbf{1}(y_n\,;\,\theta)\left[\prod_{i=1}^{n}\mathbf{1}(x_i\,;\,y_n)\right]$$

and hence $Y_n = \max(X_1, X_2, \dots, X_n)$ is a sufficient statistic for θ.

Note. It is often quite difficult to prove that a statistic is not a sufficient statistic using the factorization theorem. It may be that we are not clever enough in the use of the criterion.

Example. Given the family of distributions $\mathcal{F}$

$$\mathcal{F} = \left\{ f_{\mathbf{X}}\,:\, f_{\mathbf{X}}(\mathbf{x}) = \prod_{i=1}^{n} f(x_i)\,;\, f \text{ is a continuous pdf} \right\}$$

Let $\mathbf{Y}$ be the order statistic. Then

$$f_{\mathbf{X}}(\mathbf{x}) = \prod_{i=1}^{n} f(x_i) = \prod_{i=1}^{n} f(y_i)$$

for any $f \in \mathcal{F}$ so that $\mathbf{Y}$ is a sufficient statistic for $\mathcal{F}$.

11.1.4 Sketch of Proof of the Factorization Criterion

Let $s(\mathbf{X})$ be a sufficient statistic for θ. Then

$$f_{\mathbf{X}}(\mathbf{x} \; ; \; \theta) = P(\mathbf{X} = \mathbf{x} \; ; \; \theta)$$
$$= P(\mathbf{s}(\mathbf{X}) = \mathbf{s}(\mathbf{x}) \; ; \; \theta) P(\mathbf{X} = \mathbf{x} | \mathbf{s}(\mathbf{X}) = \mathbf{s}(\mathbf{x}))$$

The first term in the last expression is a function of θ and $\mathbf{s}(\mathbf{x})$ while the second does not involve θ since $\mathbf{s}(\mathbf{X})$ is a sufficient statistic for θ. Hence the factorization criteria is satisfied.

Conversely if $f_{\mathbf{X}}(\mathbf{x}) = g(\mathbf{s}(\mathbf{x}) \; ; \; \theta) h(\mathbf{x})$ then

$$f_{\mathbf{X}|\mathbf{s}(\mathbf{X})}(\mathbf{x}|\mathbf{s}(\mathbf{X}) = \mathbf{s}_0 \; ; \; \theta) = \frac{P(\mathbf{X} = \mathbf{x} \, , \, \mathbf{s}(\mathbf{x}) = \mathbf{s}_0 \; ; \; \theta)}{P(\mathbf{s}(\mathbf{X}) = \mathbf{s}_0 \; ; \; \theta)}$$
$$= \frac{\delta(\mathbf{s}(\mathbf{x}), \mathbf{s}_0) f_{\mathbf{X}}(\mathbf{x} \; ; \; \theta)}{P(\mathbf{s}(\mathbf{X}) = \mathbf{s}_0 \; ; \; \theta)}$$
$$= \frac{\delta(\mathbf{s}(\mathbf{x}), \mathbf{s}_0) g(\mathbf{s}_0 \; ; \; \theta) h(\mathbf{x})}{P(\mathbf{s}(\mathbf{X}) = \mathbf{s}_0 \; ; \; \theta)}$$

where

$$\delta(a, b) = \begin{cases} 1 & a = b \\ 0 & \text{otherwise} \end{cases}$$

If

$$A = \{\mathbf{x} \; : \; \mathbf{s}(\mathbf{x}) = \mathbf{s}_0\}$$

then

$$P(\mathbf{s}(\mathbf{X}) = \mathbf{s}_0 \; ; \; \theta) = \sum_{\mathbf{x}' \in A} f_{\mathbf{X}}(\mathbf{x}' \; ; \; \theta)$$
$$= \sum_{\mathbf{x}' \in A} g(\mathbf{s}_0 \; ; \; \theta) h(\mathbf{x}')$$
$$= g(\mathbf{s}_0 \; ; \; \theta) \sum_{\mathbf{x}' \in A} h(\mathbf{x}')$$

It follows that

$$P(\mathbf{X} = \mathbf{x} | \mathbf{s}(\mathbf{X}) = \mathbf{s}_0 \; ; \; \theta) = \frac{\delta(\mathbf{s}(\mathbf{x}), \mathbf{s}_0) g(\mathbf{s}_0 \; ; \; \theta) h(\mathbf{x})}{g(\mathbf{s}_0 \; ; \; \theta) \sum_{\mathbf{x}' \in A} h(\mathbf{x}')}$$
$$= \frac{\delta(\mathbf{s}(\mathbf{x}), \mathbf{s}_0) h(\mathbf{x})}{\sum_{\mathbf{x}' \in A} h(\mathbf{x}')}$$

which does not depend on θ so that $\mathbf{s}(\mathbf{X})$ is a sufficient statistic.

11.1.5   Properties of Sufficient Statistics

- If $s(\mathbf{X})$ is sufficient for a family $\mathcal{F}$, then $s(\mathbf{X})$ is sufficient for a subfamily of $\mathcal{F}$, but it may not be sufficient for a larger family.

  - If $X_1, X_2, \ldots, X_n$ are iid $N(\theta_1, \theta_2)$ then $(\bar{\mathbf{X}}, \sum_{i=1}^n (X_i - \bar{X})^2)$ is sufficient for (θ_1, θ_2) and for the case in which $X_1, X_2, \ldots, X_n$ are iid $N(\theta_1, 1)$.
  - If $X_1, X_2, \ldots, X_n$ are iid $N(\theta_1, 1)$ then $\bar{\mathbf{X}}$ is sufficient, but it is not sufficient when $X_1, X_2, \ldots, X_n$ are iid $N(\theta_1, \theta_2)$.

- If $t(\mathbf{X}) = u(s(\mathbf{X}))$ and $t(\mathbf{X})$ is sufficient then $s(\mathbf{X})$ is sufficient. This follows since to calculate $t(\mathbf{X})$ we need only know the value of $s(\mathbf{X})$ and not the value of $\mathbf{X}$ itself.

- Any one-to-one function of a sufficient statistic is also a sufficient statistic. For example, for n Bernoulli trials $X_1, X_2, \ldots, X_n$ the following are sufficient statistics:

  - $\mathbf{X}$
  - $\left(e^{X_1 + X_2}, \sum_{i=3}^n X_i\right)$
  - $S = \sum_{i=1}^n X_i$
  - $\frac{1}{S}$

  In this situation can we reduce the data further by considering a function of $S = \sum_{i=1}^n X_i$? For example,

$$h(S) = |S - \frac{1}{2}|$$

$$g(S) = \begin{cases} 1 \ S \geq \frac{n}{2} \\ 0 \ \text{otherwise} \end{cases}$$

The answer in this case is no. S is a minimal sufficient statistic as is $\frac{1}{S}$ and e^S.

11.1.6   Minimal Sufficient Statistics

The basic idea of a minimal sufficient statistic S is that the statistic is sufficient and the data cannot be reduced beyond S without losing sufficiency. More precisely:

Definition 11.1.3. A sufficient statistic S is a **minimal sufficient statistic** if it is a function of every other sufficient statistic. Thus S is a minimal sufficient statistic if

1. S is sufficient.
2. S can be calculated from any other sufficient statistic.

Finding minimal sufficient statistics involves the use of the **likelihood function**.

Definition 11.1.4. Let $\mathbf{X}$ have pdf $f_{\mathbf{X}}(\mathbf{x}\,;\,\boldsymbol{\theta})$. Given that $\mathbf{X} = \mathbf{x}$ is observed we call the function of $\boldsymbol{\theta}$,

$$L(\boldsymbol{\theta}\,;\,\mathbf{x}) = c(\mathbf{x})f_{\mathbf{X}}(\mathbf{x}\,;\,\boldsymbol{\theta}),$$

the likelihood function. Here $c(\mathbf{x})$ is any function of $\mathbf{x}$ which does not depend on θ.

By the Law of Likelihood, the comparison of two $\boldsymbol{\theta}$ values requires only the ratio of the likelihood at the two values. Consequently we call $f_{\mathbf{X}}(\mathbf{x}\,;\,\boldsymbol{\theta})$ or any constant multiple of $f_{\mathbf{X}}(\mathbf{x};\,\boldsymbol{\theta})$ the likelihood function of $\boldsymbol{\theta}$ for data $\mathbf{x}$. Note that the likelihood function is a statistic and is the minimal sufficient statistic for $\boldsymbol{\theta}$.

Example. If $X_1, X_2, \ldots, X_n$ are iid Poisson with parameter θ then for a fixed θ we have

$$f_{\mathbf{X}}(\mathbf{x}\,;\,\theta) = \frac{\theta^{\sum_i x_i}e^{-n\theta}}{\prod_i x_i!}$$

while for a fixed value of $\mathbf{X} = \mathbf{x}$ we have

$$L(\theta\,;\,\mathbf{x}) = \frac{\theta^{\sum_i x_i}e^{-n\theta}}{\prod_i x_i!}$$
$$= c(\mathbf{x})\theta^{\sum_i x_i}e^{-n\theta}$$

Theorem 11.1.2. *The likelihood function is the minimal sufficient statistic, i.e., we can determine the likelihood function from any other sufficient statistic.*

Example. Let $X_1, X_2, \ldots, X_n$ be iid Bernoulli trials. Then

$$f_{\mathbf{X}}(\mathbf{x}\,;\,\theta) = \theta^{\sum_i x_i}(1 - \theta)^{n - \sum_i x_i}$$

To determine the likelihood function we need only know $\sum_i x_i$. Conversely, if we know the likelihood function

$$L(\theta\,;\,\mathbf{x}) = c\theta^{\sum_i x_i}(1 - \theta)^{n - \sum_i x_i}$$

then we know $\sum_i x_i$.

By contrast, if $t(\mathbf{X}) = (t_1(\mathbf{X}), t_2(\mathbf{X}) = (X_1 + X_2, X_3 + \cdots + X_n)$ then $t(\mathbf{X})$ is sufficient and we can calculate the likelihood function from $t(\mathbf{X})$, but from the likelihood function we cannot calculate the values of $t_1(\mathbf{X})$ and $t_2(\mathbf{X})$ so that $t(\mathbf{X})$ is not a minimal sufficient statistic.

Theorem 11.1.3. *A statistic* $s(\mathbf{X})$ *is minimally sufficient if and only if, for any two points* $\mathbf{x}$ *and* $\mathbf{y}$ *in the sample space,*

$$s(\mathbf{x}) = s(\mathbf{y}) \iff f_{\mathbf{X}}(\mathbf{x} \,;\, \boldsymbol{\theta}) = c(\mathbf{x}, \mathbf{y}) f_{\mathbf{X}}(\mathbf{y} \,;\, \boldsymbol{\theta})$$

where $c(\mathbf{x}, \mathbf{y})$ *does not involve* $\boldsymbol{\theta}$. *In other words* $\mathbf{x}$ *and* $\mathbf{y}$ *generate the same likelihood function.*

Example. In n Bernoulli trials

$$f_{\mathbf{X}}(\mathbf{x} \,;\, \boldsymbol{\theta}) = c f_{\mathbf{X}}(\mathbf{y} \,;\, \boldsymbol{\theta})$$

means that the ratio

$$\frac{f_{\mathbf{X}}(\mathbf{x} \,;\, \boldsymbol{\theta})}{f_{\mathbf{X}}(\mathbf{y} \,;\, \boldsymbol{\theta})}$$

must not involve $\boldsymbol{\theta}$ or

$$\frac{\theta^{\sum_i x_i}(1-\theta)^{n-\sum_i x_i}}{\theta^{\sum_i y_i}(1-\theta)^{n-\sum_i y_i}} = \left(\frac{\theta}{1-\theta}\right)^{\sum_i x_i - \sum_i y_i}$$

must be free of $\boldsymbol{\theta}$, i.e., $\sum_i x_i$ must equal $\sum_i y_i$. Therefore $\sum_i X_i$ is the minimal sufficient statistic.

Example. If $X_1, X_2, \ldots, X_n$ are iid Gamma(r, λ) then

$$f_{\mathbf{X}}(\mathbf{x} \,;\, r, \lambda) = \frac{\lambda^{nr} \left(\prod_{i=1}^{n} x_i\right)^{r-1} \exp\left\{-\lambda \sum_{i=1}^{n} x_i\right\}}{[\Gamma(r)]^n}$$

Thus

$$\frac{f_{\mathbf{X}}(\mathbf{x} \,;\, r, \lambda)}{f_{\mathbf{X}}(\mathbf{y} \,;\, r, \lambda)} = c$$

is free of r and λ if and only if

$$\frac{\left(\prod_{i=1}^{n} x_i\right)^{r-1} \exp\left\{-\lambda \sum_{i=1}^{n} x_i\right\}}{\left(\prod_{i=1}^{n} y_i\right)^{r-1} \exp\left\{-\lambda \sum_{i=1}^{n} y_i\right\}} = c$$

i.e., if and only if $\prod_{i=1}^{n} x_i = \prod_{i=1}^{n} y_i$ and $\sum_{i=1}^{n} x_i = \sum_{i=1}^{n} y_i$. Thus

$$\left(\prod_{i=1}^{n} X_i \,,\, \sum_{i=1}^{n} X_i\right)$$

is the minimal sufficient statistic.

Example. If $X_1, X_2, \ldots, X_n$ are iid $N(\mu, \sigma^2)$ then

$$\frac{f_{\mathbf{X}}(\mathbf{x}\,;\mu,\sigma^2)}{f_{\mathbf{X}}(\mathbf{y}\,;\mu,\sigma^2)} = c$$

is free of μ and σ^2 if and only if

$$\left(\bar{x}, \sum_i (x_i - \bar{x})^2\right) = \left(\bar{y}, \sum_i (y_i - \bar{y})^2\right)$$

Therefore

$$\left(\bar{X}, \sum_i (X_i - \bar{X})^2\right)$$

is the minimally sufficient statistic as is

$$\left(\sum_i X_i, \sum_i X_i^2\right)$$

Example. If $X_1, X_2, \ldots, X_n$ are iid Cauchy then

$$f_{\mathbf{X}}(\mathbf{x}\,;\theta) = \left(\frac{1}{\pi}\right)^n \prod_{i=1}^n \frac{1}{1 + (x_i - \theta)^2}$$

Thus

$$\frac{f_{\mathbf{X}}(\mathbf{x}\,;\theta)}{f_{\mathbf{X}}(\mathbf{y}\,;\theta)} = c$$

is free of θ if and only if

$$\{x_j\,:\,j = 1, 2, \ldots, n\} = \{y_j\,:\,j = 1, 2, \ldots, n\}$$

It follows that the minimal sufficient statistic is the order statistic. Note that in this case the minimal sufficient statistic is n dimensional even though the parameter space is one dimensional. Recall also that the distribution of $\bar{X}$ for the Cauchy is the same as the distribution of each X_i.

11.2 Importance of Sufficient Statistics in Inference

11.2.1 Frequentist Statistics

Suppose that $t(X)$ is an estimator of θ with mean square error $MSE_t(\theta)$. Let $s(X)$ be a sufficient statistic for θ. Define a new estimator $\tilde{t}(S)$ by

$$\tilde{t}(S) = \mathbb{E}[t(X)|S]$$

Note that by sufficiency of S this conditional expectation does not depend on θ so it is an estimator of θ.

Theorem 11.2.1 (Rao-Blackwell). *The mean square error of $\tilde{t}(S)$ is no larger than the mean square error of t, i.e.,*

$$MSE_{\tilde{t}}(\theta) \leq MSE_t(\theta)$$

Proof.

$$
\begin{aligned}
MSE_t(\theta) &= \mathbb{E}[t(X) - \theta)]^2 \\
&= \mathbb{E}\left\{ [t(X) - \tilde{t}(S)] + [\tilde{t}(S) - \theta)] \right\}^2 \\
&= \mathbb{E}\left\{ [t(X) - \tilde{t}(S)]^2 \right\} + \mathbb{E}\left\{ [\tilde{t}(S) - \theta)]^2 \right\} \\
&\quad + 2\mathbb{E}\left\{ [t(X) - \tilde{t}(S)][\tilde{t}(S) - \theta)] \right\} \\
&= \mathbb{E}\left\{ [t(X) - \tilde{t}(S)]^2 \right\} + MSE_{\tilde{t}}(\theta)
\end{aligned}
$$

Since

$$\mathbb{E}\left\{ [t(X) - \tilde{t}(S)][\tilde{t}(S) - \theta)] \right\} = \mathbb{E}\left\{ [\tilde{t}(S) - \theta)]\mathbb{E}\left\{ [t(X) - \tilde{t}(S)]|S \right\} \right\} = 0$$

It follows that

$$MSE_{\tilde{t}}(\theta) \leq MSE_t(\theta)$$

If we consider testing problems then since the basis of tests is the likelihood ratio which clearly depends only on the sufficient statistic it is obvious that tests depend only on the sufficient statistic, all other parts of the data being irrelevant provided the model is true.

11.2.2 Bayesian Inference

If $s(X)$ is a sufficient statistic then by the factorization theorem

$$f(x; \theta) = g(s; \theta)h(x)$$

so that the posterior distribution of θ is

$$
\begin{aligned}
p(\theta|x) &= \frac{f(x;\theta)p(\theta)}{\int_\Theta f(x;\theta)p(\theta)dm(\theta)} \\
&= \frac{g(s;\theta)h(x)p(\theta)}{\int_\Theta g(s;\theta)h(x)p(\theta)dm(\theta)} \\
&= \frac{g(s;\theta)p(\theta)}{\int_\Theta g(s;\theta)p(\theta)dm(\theta)}
\end{aligned}
$$

Thus the posterior distribution of θ depends only on s so Bayesian statistics depends only on the value of the sufficient statistic.

11.2.3   Likelihood Inference

By the factorization theorem

$$ f(x;\theta) = g(s;\theta)h(x) $$

Thus the maximum of the likelihood over θ occurs when $g(s;\theta)$ is maximized so that the likelihood function satisfies

$$ \mathscr{L}(\theta;x) = \frac{f(x;\theta)}{f(x;\hat\theta)} = \frac{g(s;\theta)h(x)}{g(s;\hat\theta)h(x)} = \frac{g(s;\theta)}{g(s;\hat\theta)} $$

depends only on s so likelihood-based methods depend only on the value of the sufficient statistic assuming the model is true.

11.3   Alternative Proof of Factorization Theorem

If the density of X can be factored as

$$ f_X(x;\theta) = h(x|t)g(t;\theta) $$

where h does not depend on θ then t is a sufficient statistic for θ. To see this note that

$$ f(x,t;\theta) = h(x|t)g(t;\theta) = f_X(x;\theta) $$

It follows that

$$ f(t;\theta) = \int_A f(x,t;\theta) = \int_A h(x|t)g(t;\theta)d\mu(x) = g(t;\theta)\int_A h(x|t)d\mu(x) $$

where

$$A = \{x \; : \; g(x) = t\}$$

and hence

$$f(x; \theta|t) = \frac{f(x, t; \theta)}{f(t; \theta)} = \frac{h(x|t)}{\int_A h(x|t) d\mu(x)}$$

which is independent of θ so that t is sufficient for θ.

11.4   Exercises

1. If $X_1, X_2, \ldots, X_n$ are iid with a Beta(a,b) pdf find the minimal sufficient statistic for (a,b).
2. If $X_1, X_2, \ldots, X_n$ are iid with a uniform pdf over $\theta - 1/2, \theta + 1/2)$ pdf find the minimal sufficient statistic for θ.
3. If $X_1, X_2, \ldots, X_n$ are iid with a uniform pdf over $\theta - \rho, \theta + \rho)$ pdf find the minimal sufficient statistic for θ and rho.
4. If $Y_1, Y_2, \ldots, Y_n$ are independent $N(\beta_0 + \beta_1 x_i, \sigma^2)$ where the x_i are known find the minimal sufficient statistic for β_0, β_1 and σ^2.

Chapter 12
Conditionality

12.1 Ancillarity

Conditioning arguments are at the center of many disputes regarding the foundations of statistical inference. We present here only some simple arguments and examples.

Definition 12.1.1. A statistic A is **ancillary** (for θ) if its distribution does not depend on θ.

The basic idea in conditioning is that, since A provides no information on θ, we should use the conditional distribution, given A, for inference on θ. The idea originated with R.A. Fisher and has been discussed and disputed for decades. In some problems most statisticians condition on A, in other problems they do not.

In most problems the sample size is considered fixed, i.e., ancillary even though it may be determined by availability of funds or other considerations not related to the problem (θ) of interest. Similarly in regression type problems (linear models, generalized linear models, etc.) most statisticians condition on the covariates (design matrix). There seems to be no definite guidelines for when to condition and when not to condition.

Example. Cox introduced the following example. Consider two measuring devices. Device P produces measurements which are normal with mean θ and variance σ^2 and device I produces measurements which are normal with variance $k^2\sigma^2$ where k is much larger than 1. Which instrument is used is decided by the flip of a fair coin so that the precision of the measurement (i.e., what instrument is used) is ancillary.

Thus we would report the value of the measurement and the associated value of precision σ^2 or $k^2\sigma^2$ depending on the instrument **actually** used. However, if we do not condition, the true variance of X is

© Springer International Publishing Switzerland 2014
C.A. Rohde, *Introductory Statistical Inference with the Likelihood Function*, DOI 10.1007/978-3-319-10461-4_12

$$\mathbb{V}(X) = \mathbb{E}\left[\mathbb{V}(X|F)\right] + \mathbb{V}\left[\mathbb{E}(X|F)\right]$$
$$= \frac{\sigma^2}{2} + \frac{k^2\sigma^2}{2}$$

Note that

$$\sigma^2 < \sigma^2\left(\frac{1}{2} + \frac{k^2}{2}\right) < k^2\sigma^2$$

so that the reported standard error will be either too small or too large.

Example (Valliant, Dorfman and Royall). There is a population of size 1,000 from which we have selected a random sample of size 100 without replacement. The population mean is estimated by the sample mean which has variance estimated by

$$\mathbb{V}(\overline{Y}_s) = \left(1 - \frac{100}{1000}\right)\frac{s^2}{100} \quad \text{where} \quad s^2 = \frac{\sum_{i \in s}(y_i - \overline{y}_s)^2}{99}$$

and s denotes the set of items selected.

Before we drew the sample, we considered doing a complete census of all 1,000 objects, but we had another study of interest. To decide whether to do the complete census or a sample of size 100 and the other study we flipped a coin. If the result was a head we did the complete census; if the result was a tail we took the sample of size 100.

The variance of the sample mean is

$$\mathbb{V}(\overline{Y}_s) = \frac{1}{2}\mathbb{V}(\overline{Y}_s|n = 100) + \frac{1}{2}\mathbb{V}(\overline{Y}_s|n = 1000) = \frac{1}{2}\mathbb{V}(\overline{Y}_s|n = 100)$$

Using this an estimate of variability is clearly wrong, yet it is correct from a frequentist point of view. Note that the same variance would be required if we had done the complete census. In this case any confidence interval would consist of a set of points whereas we know the population mean exactly! Clearly there is need for conditioning in situations like this.

12.2   Problems with Conditioning

Examples in the previous section indicate that we should condition whenever there is an ancillary statistic. Unfortunately this is not always so easy. An excellent review article by Ghosh et al. [19] provides many examples and extensions. In particular there are examples given where there is no unique ancillary statistic.

Some authors have suggested that there are really two major types of ancillarity:

1. Experimental
2. Mathematical

Experimental ancillaries are those such as sample size, covariates, etc., i.e., situations where most statisticians routinely condition. Mathematical ancillaries are those that arise because of the specific nature of the statistical model.

Example (Continuous uniform). Let $X_1, X_2, \ldots, X_n$ be iid with pdf

$$f(x; \theta_1, \theta_2) = \begin{cases} \frac{1}{\Delta} & \theta_1 \leq x \leq \theta_2 \\ 0 & \text{elsewhere} \end{cases} \tag{12.1}$$

where $\Delta = \theta_2 - \theta_1$.

The joint density is given by

$$f(x_1, x_2, \ldots, x_n \, ; \, \theta_1, \theta_2) = \begin{cases} \frac{1}{\Delta^n} & \text{all } x_i \in [\theta_1, \theta_2] \\ 0 & \text{elsewhere} \end{cases} \tag{12.2}$$

It follows that the minimum and maximum of $X_1, X_2, \ldots, X_n$ are minimal sufficient statistics for θ_1 and θ_2.

The joint distribution of the minimum and maximum from a random sample with distribution function F and density function f is easily shown to be

$$f(y_1, y_n) = n(n-1)[F(y_n) - F(y_1)]^{n-2} f(y_1) f(y_n) \tag{12.3}$$

where Y_1 is the minimum of the X_i's and Y_n is the maximum

For the uniform distribution, we have that

$$F(y; \theta_1, \theta_2) = \frac{1}{\Delta} \int_{\theta_1}^{y} dx = \frac{y - \theta_1}{\Delta}$$

so that the joint pdf of Y_1 and Y_n is given by

$$f(y_1, y_n; \theta_1, \theta_2) = \frac{1}{\Delta^n} n(n-1)(y_n - y_1)^{n-2} \quad \theta_1 \leq y_1 \leq y_n \leq \theta_2$$

Let $\theta_1 = \theta - \rho$ and $\theta_2 = \theta + \rho$, then we have that $\Delta = 2\rho$ and hence the joint density is

$$f(y_1, y_n; \theta) = \frac{n(n-1)(y_n - y_1)^{n-2}}{\rho^n} \quad ; \quad \theta - \rho \leq y_1 \leq y_n \leq \theta + \rho$$

If we assume that ρ is known, then the likelihood function for θ is

$$\mathcal{L}(\theta) = 1 \; ; \; y_n - \rho \le \theta \le y_1 + \rho$$

For the special case where $\rho = 1/2$ it is easy to show that $[Y_1, Y_n]$ is a $100 \left(1 - \frac{1}{2^{n-1}}\right)$ confidence interval for θ.

Suppose now that

$$n = 5 \quad \text{and} \quad y_1 = 0.01, \; y_n = 0.99$$

Then the $100(1 - \frac{1}{16})\% = 93.75\%$ confidence interval for θ is .01 to .99. But since

$$y_1 \ge \theta - \frac{1}{2} \; ; \; y_n \le \theta + \frac{1}{2}$$

if and only if

$$0.51 = 0.01 + 0.5 \ge \theta \text{ and } 0.49 = 0.99 - 0.5 \le \theta$$

with certainty.

Thus with these observed values of y_1 and y_n we are certain that

$$0.49 \le \theta \le 0.51$$

and yet our 93.75 % confidence interval is

$$0.01 \le \theta \le 0.99$$

This is silly.

As Cox points out it is imperative to condition on the ancillary statistic in this example which is the range $R = Y_n - Y_1$.

Chapter 13
Statistical Principles

13.1 Introduction

A number of principles for evaluating the evidence (information) provided by data have been formulated:

- The **repeated sampling principle:** evidence (information) is evaluated using hypothetical repeated sampling.
- The **sufficiency principle:** evidence (information) should depend only on the value of a sufficient statistic.
- The **conditionality principle:** evidence (information) should depend only on the experiment actually performed.
- The **likelihood principle:** evidence (information) resulting from observations with proportional likelihoods should be the same.
- The **Bayesian coherency principle:** evidence (information) from data is used to obtain (beliefs) using Bayes theorem which requires consistent (coherent) betting behavior.
- **Birnbaum's confidence concept:** a concept of statistical evidence is not plausible unless it finds "strong evidence" for H_2 as against H_1 with small probability (α) when H_1 is true and with much larger probability $(1 - \beta)$ when H_2 is true.

We focus on the sufficiency, conditionality, and likelihood principles and their implications. The sufficiency and conditionality principles were shown to be "equivalent" to the likelihood principle by Birnbaum in 1962 which caused a major stir and revival of interest in the foundations of statistics. Recent work by Mayo [32] and Evans [14] has cast doubt on the force of Birnbaum's result. Another proof of the Likelihood Principle has been advanced by Gandenberger [18]. Nevertheless, the clarity with which Birnbaum presented the relevant concepts is still of great value.

© Springer International Publishing Switzerland 2014
C.A. Rohde, *Introductory Statistical Inference with the Likelihood Function*, DOI 10.1007/978-3-319-10461-4__13

The discussions are done only for a discrete sample space thus avoiding measure theoretic difficulties. However, references and comments will be made on the generalizations to other sample spaces.

13.1.1   Birnbaum's Formulation

Consider a random variable X with discrete sample space

$$\mathcal{X} = \{x_1, x_2, \ldots, x_k\}$$

and discrete parameter space

$$\Theta = \{\theta_1, \theta_2, \ldots, \theta_r\}$$

and model probabilities

$$f(x_i; \theta_j)$$

Represent the model probabilities as a matrix

θ	x_1	x_2	$\cdots$	x_k
θ_1	$f(x_1; \theta_1)$	$f(x_2; \theta_1)$	$\cdots$	$f(x_k; \theta_1)$
θ_2	$f(x_1; \theta_2)$	$f(x_2; \theta_2)$	$\cdots$	$f(x_k; \theta_2)$
$\vdots$	$\vdots$	$\vdots$	$\ddots$	$\vdots$
θ_r	$f(x_1; \theta_r)$	$f(x_2; \theta_r)$	$\cdots$	$f(x_k; \theta_r)$

Note that the row sums are 1. Elements in the columns are the (unscaled) likelihoods of θ for that value of x. In particular, note that if two elements in a column are equal than that value of x equally supports the θ values in the corresponding rows in the sense that the same probability is assigned to x by each of the θ values.

Regarding the discrete nature of the representation: "If we believe, as we must, that the real world is finite then this representation is universal." Moreover it allows careful discussion of the essentials of statistical principles without the troubles of the infinite. Actual applications of modern statistics in which computers play such an important role all computations (graphs, etc.) really are based on finite sample spaces and parameter spaces.

In Basu's words:

> I hold firmly to the view that this contingent and cognitive universe of ours is in reality only finite and, therefore, discrete. In this essay we steer clear of the logical quicksands of "infinity" and the "infinitesimal". Infinite and continuous models will be used in the sequel, but they are to be looked upon as mere approximations to the finite realities.

Now suppose that we have another random variable Y with distribution specified as follows:

θ	y_1	y_2	$\cdots$	y_n
θ_1	$g(y_1; \theta_1)$	$g(y_2; \theta_1)$	$\cdots$	$g(y_n; \theta_1)$
θ_2	$g(y_1; \theta_2)$	$g(y_2; \theta_2)$	$\cdots$	$g(y_n; \theta_2)$
$\vdots$	$\vdots$	$\vdots$	$\ddots$	$\vdots$
θ_r	$g(y_1; \theta_r)$	$g(y_2; \theta_r)$	$\cdots$	$g(y_n; \theta_r)$

i.e., we have the same parameter space but different sample spaces and a different density function. Again note that the row sums are 1.

Suppose that for some value of X, x_o, and some value of Y, y_o, we have that

$$f(x_o, \theta_i) = cg(y_o; \theta_i)$$

for $i = 1, 2, \ldots, r$ where $c > 0$

i.e., the likelihood functions for x_o and y_o are the same:

x_o	y_o
$f(x_o; \theta_1)$	$\frac{1}{c} f(y_o; \theta_1)$
$f(x_o; \theta_2)$	$\frac{1}{c} f(y_o; \theta_2)$
$\vdots$	$\vdots$
$f(x_o; \theta_r)$	$\frac{1}{c} f(y_o; \theta_r)$

The likelihood principle simply says that one cannot learn anymore about θ from x_o than one can from y_o or equivalently the evidence (information) provided by x_o is the same as that provided by y_o.

13.1.2   Framework and Notation

Consider a statistical model for random X

$$\mathcal{E} = (\mathcal{X}, f(x; \theta), \Theta)$$

We assume that X is discrete and that Θ is discrete as well so that

$$f(x; \theta) = P(X = x; \theta)$$

gives the probability of observing x when θ is the value of the parameter.

For a given observed value of X, say x, the pair $(\mathcal{E}, x)$ is an instance of **statistical evidence** which we write as

$$\text{Ev}(\mathcal{E}, x)$$

Note that we have not explicitly defined statistical evidence nor what we might use it for.

Definition 13.1.1. A statement that two statistical models E and E^* with the same parameter space and observed values x and x' represent equivalent (statistical) evidence is written as

$$\text{Ev}(\mathcal{E}, x) = \text{Ev}(\mathcal{E}^*, x')$$

13.1.3   Mathematical Equivalence

Definition 13.1.2 (Principle of mathematical equivalence). If two observations x and x' have the same probability for all parameter values then $\text{Ev}(\mathcal{E}_1, x)$ is equal to $\text{Ev}(\mathcal{E}_2, x')$, i.e.,

$$f(x; \theta) = f(x'; \theta) \ \text{ for all } \theta \in \Theta \implies \text{Ev}(\mathcal{E}_1, x) = \text{Ev}(\mathcal{E}_2, x')$$

The principle of mathematical equivalence simply states that relabelling of observations should not affect the evidence provided by the observations.

This was anticipated by Pratt [38] in his review of Lehman's book where he said:

A relabeling of the possible outcomes which does not affect the outcome actually observed surely should not change an inference or decision.

For example suppose that experiments 1 and 2 have probabilities given by

$$\mathcal{P}_1 = \begin{bmatrix} 0.9 & 0.1 \\ 0.3 & 0.7 \end{bmatrix} \quad \mathcal{P}_2 = \begin{bmatrix} 0.1 & 0.9 \\ 0.7 & 0.3 \end{bmatrix}$$

i.e., outcome 1 in experiment $\mathcal{E}_1$ has probability 0.9 when $\theta = 1$ and probability 0.3 when $\theta = 2$. Similarly outcome 2 in experiment $\mathcal{E}_2$ has probability 0.9 when $\theta = 1$ and probability 0.3 when $\theta = 2$.

Mathematical equivalence simply says that

$$\text{Ev}(\mathcal{E}_1, 1) = \text{Ev}(\mathcal{E}_2, 2)$$

13.1.4   Irrelevant Noise

Let x_s be a specified possible outcome of $\mathcal{E}$.

- Define a binary random variable Z, independent of X, such that

$$\mathbb{P}(Z = z) = \begin{cases} c & z = 1 \\ 1 - c & z = 0 \end{cases}$$

where $0 \leq c \leq 1$ and is known.
- Further define the random variable Y as a function of X and Z by

$$Y = \begin{cases} 1 \text{ if } x = x_s \text{ and } z = 1 \\ 0 \text{ otherwise} \end{cases}$$

Define the experiment $\mathcal{E}^*$ by

$$\mathcal{E}^* = (\mathcal{Y}, g_\theta, \Theta)$$

where

$$g_\theta(1) = g(1; \theta) = c\,f(x_s; \theta) \text{ and } g_\theta(0) = g(0; \theta) = 1 - c\,f(x_s; \theta)$$

Let Ev $(\mathcal{E}, x_s)$ denote the evidence about θ when $\mathcal{E}$ is performed and x_s is observed. Similarly let Ev $(\mathcal{E}^*, 1)$ denote the evidence when $\mathcal{E}^*$ arises from performance of $\mathcal{E}$ and $y = 1$ is observed.

Definition 13.1.3 (Principle of irrelevant noise).

$$Ev\,(\mathcal{E}, x_s) = Ev\,(\mathcal{E}^*, 1)$$

We call $\mathcal{E}^*$ the **stochastically censored** version of $\mathcal{E}$.

Suppose, for instance, an experiment has possible outcomes $a, b, c, d, \dots, x$. Suppose Meter 1 tells the outcome, while Meter 2 tells only whether the outcome was or was not d. If in fact the outcome is d, you would learn this from reading either meter and would want, therefore, to make the same inference or decision; yet the result of a significance test would ordinarily depend on which meter you were reading.

[38]

13.2   Likelihood Principle

Definition 13.2.1 (Likelihood Principle). If $\mathcal{E}$ and $\mathcal{E}^*$ are two experiments with common parameter space Θ and two outcomes $x_s \in \mathcal{X}$ and $y_s \in \mathcal{Y}$ are such that

$$f(x_s; \theta) = c\,f^*(y_s; \theta) \text{ for all } \theta \in \Theta$$

for some positive c then

$$\text{Ev}\,(\mathcal{E}, x_s) = \text{Ev}\,(\mathcal{E}^*, y_s)$$

13.3 Equivalence of Likelihood and Irrelevant Noise Plus Mathematical Equivalence

Theorem 13.3.1. *The likelihood principle and the irrelevant noise principle plus mathematical equivalence are equivalent.*

Let **L** stand for the likelihood principle, **IN** stand for the irrelevant noise principle, and **ME** stand for the mathematical equivalence principle. Then the statement of the theorem is

$$\textbf{L} \iff \textbf{IN} + \textbf{ME}$$

Proof.

$$\textbf{L} \implies \textbf{IN} + \textbf{ME}$$

Obviously

$$\textbf{L} \implies \textbf{ME}$$

In the setup of the irrelevant noise principle we have that

$$g(1; \theta) = c\, f(x_s; \theta) \quad \text{for all } \theta \in \Theta$$

Thus if the likelihood principle is assumed to be true

$$\text{Ev}\,(\mathcal{E}^*, 1) = \text{Ev}\,(\mathcal{E}, x_s)$$

which is simply the statement of the principle of irrelevant noise, i.e.,

$$\textbf{L} \implies \textbf{IN}$$

and hence the likelihood principle implies the principle of irrelevant noise and the principle of mathematical equivalence.

$$\textbf{IN} + \textbf{ME} \implies \textbf{L}$$

Suppose now that $(\mathcal{E}_1, x_s)$ and $(\mathcal{E}_2, y_s)$ are such that the parameter space is the same and

$$f_1(x_s; \theta) = c\, f_2(y_s; \theta) \quad \text{for all } \theta \in \Theta$$

for some positive c. We may assume $c \leq 1$ (if not just write $f_2(y_s; \theta) = \frac{1}{c} f(x_s; \theta)$ and now $\frac{1}{c} < 1$).

Now define $\mathcal{E}_1^*$ by taking $c_1 = 1$ and $x = x_s$, then

$$f_1^*(1; \theta) = f_1(x_s; \theta) \quad \text{for all } \theta \in \theta$$

Similarly define $\mathcal{E}_2^*$ by taking $c_2 = c$ and $y = y_s$, then

$$f_2^*(1; \theta) = c f_2(y_s; \theta) \quad \text{for all } \theta \in \theta$$

Note that $\mathcal{E}_1^*$ is the stochastically censored version of $\mathcal{E}_1$ and $\mathcal{E}_2^*$ is the stochastically censored version of $\mathcal{E}$.

Now note that

$$\begin{aligned}
f_1^*(1, \theta) &= f_1(x_s; \theta) \\
&= c\, f_2(y_s; \theta) \\
&= f_2^*(1; \theta)
\end{aligned}$$

for all $\theta \in \Theta$. Thus $(\mathcal{E}_1^*, 1)$ and $(\mathcal{E}_2^*, 1)$ are mathematically equivalent and hence

$$\text{Ev}\,(\mathcal{E}_1^*, 1) = \text{Ev}\,(\mathcal{E}_2^*, 1)$$

Thus we have, assuming the principle of irrelevant noise

$$\text{Ev}\,(\mathcal{E}_1, x_s) = \text{Ev}\,(\mathcal{E}_1^*, 1) = \text{Ev}\,(\mathcal{E}_2^*, 1) = \text{Ev}\,(\mathcal{E}_2, y_s)$$

i.e.,

$$\text{Ev}\,(\mathcal{E}_1, x_s) = \text{Ev}\,(\mathcal{E}_2, y_s)$$

i.e.,

$$\mathbf{IN + ME} \implies \mathbf{L}$$

Pratt again anticipated this result:

In the meter reading example: A direct continuation of this argument shows an inference or decision should depend on the probability under the possible hypotheses of the outcome observed only (and this only up to multiplication by a constant). The use of probabilities of other outcomes also, as in the Neyman-Pearson formulation, inevitably leads to inconsistencies.

[38] $\square$

13.4   Sufficiency, Conditionality, and Likelihood Principles

In the context of a statistical model we recall that

Definition 13.4.1. A statistic s is **sufficient** if f can be written as

$$f(x; \theta) = g[s(x); \theta] p[x|s(x)]$$

where

- $g[s(x); \theta]$ is the pdf of $s(X)$ at x,
- the pdf of X given $s(X) = s(x)$, $p(x|s)$, does not depend on θ.

Let (E', s) denote the instance of statistical evidence determined by the statistical model for the experiment defined by

$$E' = (\mathcal{S}, \Theta, g)$$

where $\mathcal{S} = \{s : \ s = s(x), \ x \in \mathcal{X}\}$ and g is the pdf of s.

Definition 13.4.2 (Sufficiency principle). The sufficiency principle **S** states that if s is a sufficient statistic then

$$\mathrm{Ev}(\mathcal{E}, x) = \mathrm{Ev}(\mathcal{E}', s(x))$$

In short the sufficiency principle says that whatever the evidence in $(\mathcal{E}, x)$ is, it is equivalent to the evidence provided by $(\mathcal{E}', s(x))$ The sufficiency principle simply states that post-randomization does not influence the amount of evidence provided by an experiment.

In the context of a statistical model an ancillary statistic is defined by

Definition 13.4.3. A statistic h is said to be an **ancillary statistic** if f can be written as

$$f(x; \theta) = p[h(x)] g[x; \theta|h(x)]$$

where

- $g[x; \theta|h(x)]$ is the conditional pdf of X given $h(X)$ and
- the pdf of h, $p(h) = P[h(X) = h]$ does not depend on θ.

In the presence of an ancillary statistic the instance of statistical evidence (E, x) can be represented as follows:

- Let (E_h, x) denote the model of statistical evidence determined by the statistical model

$$E_h = (\mathcal{X}_h, \Theta, g_h) \ \text{ where } \ \mathcal{X}_h = \{x : \ h(x) = h\}$$

- The statistical model $E = (\mathcal{X}, \Theta, f)$ can then be thought of as a mixture model with components E_h having probabilities given by g_h.

Definition 13.4.4 (Conditionality principle). The conditionality principle **C:** states that if h is an ancillary statistic then

$$\mathrm{Ev}(E, x) = \mathrm{Ev}(E_h, x) \quad \text{where} \quad h = h(x)$$

In short, the conditionality principle says that whatever the evidence in (E, x) is, it is equivalent to the evidence in (E_h, x) if h is ancillary. The conditionality principle simple states that a pre-randomization (which does not depend on θ) should have no impact on the evidence provided by the experiment.

Recall the likelihood principle:

Definition 13.4.5 (Likelihood principle). The likelihood principle **L** states that if

$$f(x; \theta) = cf^*(x^*; \theta) \quad \text{for some } c > 0 \text{ and all } \theta \in \Theta$$

then

$$\mathrm{Ev}(E, x) = \mathrm{Ev}(E^*, x^*)$$

In short, the likelihood principle states that whatever the evidence is in two experiments with the same likelihood it is equivalent.

13.5 Fundamental Result

Theorem 13.5.1 (Birnbaum, 1962). *The conditionality principle and the sufficiency principle imply the likelihood principle and conversely.*

If **L** denotes the likelihood principle, **C** denotes the conditionality principle, and **S** denotes the sufficiency principle Birnbaum's result states that

$$\mathbf{L} \iff \mathbf{S} \text{ and } \mathbf{C}$$

As previously mentioned there are now doubts about Birnbaum's proof which we present here. Consequently one either believes the likelihood principle or not. Since it is "equivalent" to other sensible procedures it must be accorded some prominence.

proof. Let E and E' denote two statistical models having a common parameter space Θ, i.e.,

$$E = (\mathcal{X}, \Theta, f_\theta) \quad \text{and} \quad E' = (\mathcal{Y}, \Theta, g_\theta)$$

Let $x \in \mathcal{X}$ and $y \in \mathcal{Y}$ determine the same likelihood function, i.e.,

$$f_\theta(x) = f(x; \theta) = cg_\theta(y) = cg(y; \theta)$$

for some $c > 0$ and all $\theta \in \Theta$.

We will show that

$$\mathrm{Ev}(E, x) = \mathrm{Ev}(E', y)$$

using the conditionality and sufficiency principles.

Define a mixture model E^* by the statistic h where

$$h = 1 \implies E \text{ is observed}$$
$$h = 2 \implies E' \text{ is observed}$$

and

$$P(H = h) = \begin{cases} k & h = 1 \\ 1 - k & h = 2 \end{cases}$$

where

$$k = \frac{1}{(1 + c)}$$

Note that the distribution of $h(X)$ does not depend on θ so that $h(X)$ is ancillary.

If z represents an outcome of E^* and $h_\theta(z) = h(z; \theta)$ is the pdf we have

$$h(x, \theta) = kf(x; \theta)$$
$$= \frac{1}{1+c} f(x; \theta)$$
$$= \frac{c}{1+c} g(y; \theta)$$
$$= (1 - k)g(y; \theta)$$
$$= h(y; \theta)$$

Hence by the sufficiency principle **S** we have that

$$\mathrm{Ev}(E^*, x) = \mathrm{Ev}(E^*, y)$$

By the conditionality principle **C** we have

$$\mathrm{Ev}(E^*, x) = \mathrm{Ev}(E, x) \text{ and } \mathrm{Ev}(E^*, y) = \mathrm{Ev}(E', y)$$

It follows that

$$\text{Ev}(E, x) = \text{Ev}(E^*, x) = \text{Ev}(E^*, y) = \text{Ev}(E', y)$$

$\square$

13.6 Stopping Rules

Consider a model in which observations are taken one at a time. Let $X_1, X_2, \ldots$ be a sequence of random variables in a sequential experiment. Assume that the joint density of $\mathbf{X}^{(j)} = X_1, X_2, \ldots, X_j)$, $f(\mathbf{x}^{(j)}; \theta)$ exists for all j.

Definition 13.6.1. A **stopping rule** is a sequence

$$\underline{\tau} = (\tau_0, \tau_1, \ldots)$$

where τ_m is a function of $\mathbf{x}^{(m)}$ for $m \geq 1$ and

$$\tau_0 = \{1\}, \quad \tau_m = \{0, 1\} \ m \geq 1$$

Thus $\tau_m(\mathbf{x}^{(m)} = 1$ means we stop after observing the mth X and $\tau_m(\mathbf{x}^{(m)} = 0$ means we take another observation.

Definition 13.6.2. The **stopping time** N is the random sample size in the sequential experiment. It depends on τ and the data. The stopping time is proper if

$$\mathbb{P}(N < \infty; \theta) = 1 \ \text{ for all } \theta$$

We consider only proper stopping times.

Example. Let $X_1, X_2, \ldots$ be iid each $N(0, 1)$. Consider the stopping rule defined by

$$\tau_0 = 1 \ ; \quad \tau_m = \begin{cases} 1 & \bar{x}_m \geq km^{-1/2} \\ 0 & \text{otherwise} \end{cases}$$

i.e., we sample until the sample mean exceeds k times the standard error. The Law of the iterated logarithm shows that this is a proper stopping rule, *but* the expected time until we stop is infinite!

It follows that the joint density at the point where stopping occurs is

$$g_\theta(x_1, x_2, \ldots, x_n; \theta) = \left\{ \prod_{j=0}^{n-1} [1 - \tau_j(\mathbf{x}^{(j)})] \right\} \tau_n(\mathbf{x}^{(n)}) \ f(\mathbf{x}^{(n)}; \theta)$$

Definition 13.6.3 (SR). The **stopping rule** principle simply states that the evidence about θ depends only of $f(\mathbf{x}^{(n)}; \theta)$ and not on the stopping rule.

If the likelihood principle is true then since the likelihood functions for these two experiments are the same it follows that the likelihood principle implies that the stopping rule principle is true.

The implications of the stopping rule principle are profound in that any stopping rule which does not depend on the parameter value is irrelevant at the analysis stage.

13.6.1   Comments

In classical statistics one has to be very careful about stopping rules. Suppose in the second example of the previous section if one analyzed the results as if the sample size was fixed then one could be sure to reject the null hypothesis $\mu = 0$ even though it is true. This is called sampling to a foregone conclusion.

13.6.2   Jeffreys/Lindley Paradox

Suppose that $X_1, X_2, \ldots, X_n$ are independent normal with mean θ and variance 1. Then

$$f(\mathbf{x}; \theta) = (2\pi)^{-n/2} \exp\left\{ -\frac{\sum_{i=1}^{n}(x_i - \theta)^2}{2} \right\}$$

Assume that we have a prior of the form

$$\pi(\theta) = \begin{cases} \lambda & \theta = 0 \\ (1 - \lambda)(2\pi\rho^2)^{-1/2} \exp\left\{ -\frac{\theta^2}{2\rho^2} \right\} & \theta \neq 0 \end{cases}$$

Then it can be shown that the posterior probability that $\theta = 0$ is over 50% for an observed value of $\bar{x}$ equal to kn^{-1} and suitable values of n, ρ, k and λ. That is, even though we have observed a value of the sample mean 3 standard errors from 0 (which a frequentist would say constituted evidence against $\theta = 0$) we have a posterior probability of over 50% that $\theta = 0$, hardly evidence against $\theta = 0$.

If the stopping rule principle is adopted the intentions of the experimenter are not relevant.

Savage put it best:

> I learned the stopping rule principle from Professor Barnard, in conversations in the summer of 1952. Frankly, I then thought it a scandal that anyone in the profession could advance an idea so patently wrong, even as today I can scarcely believe that some people resist an idea so patently right.

Example. Berger-Wolpert [3] Consider an experiment with two treatment groups T_1 and T_2 and a control group C with results as follows: If one compares T_1 and

	Treatment		
Result	C	T_1	T_2
Success	8	12	2
Failure	12	8	8

C, one finds that there is no significant difference. If one compares the pooled data from C and T_2 with T_1 there is a significant difference.

If, in a report, the experimenter says that T_2 was thought to be not different from the control (and hence pooling is justified), how can we know for sure that this was the case and it was not manipulating the data to gain significance? We can't. The likelihood principle says that we needn't be concerned about the experimenters intentions.

13.6.3 Randomization

Consider an experiment involving n pairs of subjects matched in some way so as to compare a treatment $T = 1$ vs a control $C = 0$. Let the pairs be denoted

$$\{(S_1^0, S_1^1), (S_2^0, S_2^1), \ldots, (S_n^0, S_n^1)\}$$

i.e., $((S_j^0, S_j^1)$ denotes the jth pair of subjects in which one of the subjects, S_j^0 gets the control, and the other subject, S_j^1, gets the treatment.

Randomization is often used to decide which of the subjects gets the treatment. Let $(r_1, r_2, \ldots, r_n)$ denote the realized result of the randomization, i.e.,

$$P(R_i = 0) = P(R_i = 1) = \frac{1}{2}$$

The experimental result will be $(x_1, x_2, \ldots, x_n)$ where

$$x_i = \begin{cases} 0 \text{ if control is better} \\ 1 \text{ if treatment is better} \end{cases}$$

The randomization analysis uses the test statistic

$$X = \sum_{i=1}^{n} x_i$$

and rejects if X is too large the p-value is

$$P(X \geq x = \sum_{i=1}^{n} x_i) = \sum_{j=x}^{n} \binom{n}{j} 2^{-n}$$

Note that the p-value is based solely on the probabilities assigned by the randomization procedure. Once, however, the randomization is applied the conditionality principle applies and these probabilities are irrelevant!

A much more sensible solution is to define θ as the proportion of the population where the treatment is superior to the control,

Then the joint density of the randomization probabilities $\mathbf{R}$ and $\mathbf{X}$ is given by

$$f(\mathbf{r}, \mathbf{x}; \theta) = 2^{-n} \theta^x (1 - \theta)^{n-x}$$

where $x = \sum_{i=1}^{n} x_i$. We may then base inference on the likelihood function

$$\mathscr{L}(\theta, x) = \frac{\theta^x (1 - \theta)^{n-x}}{\hat{\theta}^x (1 - \hat{\theta})^{n-x}}$$

where $\hat{\theta} = x/n$.

13.6.4   Permutation or Randomization Tests

Consider two samples

$$X_1, X_2, \ldots, X_m \text{ and } Y_1, Y_2, \ldots, Y_n$$

where the X_i's are assumed to be iid. as F_X and the Y_i's are assumed to be iid. as F_Y. Of interest is the null hypothesis $F_X = F_Y$ vs the alternative hypothesis that $F_X \neq F_Y$. In this form a test was introduced by R.A. Fisher called the **Fisher Randomization Test**. Another name for this test is the **permutation test**.

Suppose that there is a test statistic T for which large values indicate that the null hypothesis is not true. If $N = m + n$ then under the null hypothesis all $N!$ permutations of the data are equally likely. If we compute the test statistic for each of the permutations then the **permutation distribution** of T is defined as

$$\mathbb{P}_0(T_j) = \frac{1}{N!} \text{ for } j = 1, 2, \ldots, N!$$

The p-value for the **permutation test** is given by

$$\mathbb{P}_0(T > t_{obs}) = \frac{1}{N!} \sum_{j=1}^{N!} \mathbf{1}(T_j > t_{obs})$$

where $\mathbf{1}(A)$ is the indicator function of the set A.

The permutation test is very attractive since it makes very few assumptions (none in fact about the form of the distribution). There exist packages which calculate the exact p-values for a variety of problems.

However, the Fisher Randomization Test, along with other permutation test, has doubtful scientific validity as the following example due to D.V.Lindley shows:

13.6.4.1 Lindley's Example on Permutation Tests

Two scientists decide to conduct an experiment to compare a treatment T and a control C. Four experimental units will be used, two units for the control and two for the treatment.

There are thus six possible designs. Experimenter A selects one of the six possible designs at random. Experimenter B does not like either of the designs (T, T, C, C) or (C, C, T, T) and decides to select his design at random from the remaining four designs. As it turned out experimenter A, as the result of selecting a design at random, chose to use the design (T, C, T, C) while experimenter B happened to also randomly choose (T, C, T, C) as his design.

The designs and the results needed for the randomization test are given below:

	Design	Differences
	$TTCC$	$+4$
	$TCTC$	$+2$
	$TCCT$	0
	$CTTC$	0
	$CTCT$	-2
	$CCTT$	-4
	Results	5,4,3,2

where the differences are treatment minus control.

Assuming that large values of the difference indicate superiority of the treatment the p-value for experimenter A is

$$\text{p-value}_A = \mathbb{P}_0(D = +2) + \mathbb{P}_0(D = +4) = \frac{1}{6} + \frac{1}{6} = \frac{1}{3}$$

since the observed value was $D = +2$.

The p-value for experimenter B is

$$\text{p-value}_B = \mathbb{P}_0(D = +2) = \frac{1}{4}$$

Thus we have two experimenters who did exactly the same experiment with exactly the same result and yet they have two entirely different p-values. As Lindley comments:

Randomization analysis is surely not logical.

Chapter 14
Bayesian Inference

14.1 Frequentist vs Bayesian

In the frequentist approach to parametric statistical inference:

1. Probability models are based on the relative frequency interpretation of probabilities.
2. Parameters of the resulting probability models are assumed to be fixed, unknown constants.
3. Observations on random variables with a probability model depending on the parameters are used to construct statistics. These are used to make inferential statements about the parameters.
4. Inferences are evaluated and interpreted on the basis of the sampling distribution of the statistics used for the inference. Thus an interval which claims to be a 95 % confidence interval for θ has the property that it contains θ 95 % of the time in repeated use.
5. In all cases inferences are evaluated on the basis of **data not observed**.

Bayesian statistics, on the other hand:

1. Allows probabilities to be degrees of belief.
2. Probability statements can be made about parameters and represent degrees of belief about a parameter.
3. From observations with a given probability model and a prior distribution we determine the probability distribution of the parameter given the observed data using Bayes theorem.
4. Any inferential statements are then based on this distribution.
5. Since inferences depend on the prior the degrees of belief and hence inferences can differ for a given set of observations.

© Springer International Publishing Switzerland 2014
C.A. Rohde, *Introductory Statistical Inference with the Likelihood Function*, DOI 10.1007/978-3-319-10461-4_14

14.2   The Bayesian Model for Inference

The basic parametric statistical model is

$$(\mathcal{X}, f(x; \theta), \Theta)$$

We observe X which has sample space $\mathcal{X}$. The probability density for $X = x$ is $f(x; \theta)$; θ is a parameter(s) having values in the parameter space Θ.

In the Bayesian approach

1. $f(x; \theta)$ is interpreted as the conditional probability density of x given θ.
2. We interpret $f(x; \theta)$ as $f(x|\theta)$ implicitly replacing the ; by a | indicating conditioning on θ.
3. A **prior** density, $p(\theta)$, of θ which describes our beliefs about θ before the data is observed, is assumed.
4. Bayes theorem is then used to obtain the **posterior** distribution, $\mathbf{P}(\theta|x)$ of θ given the data x, i.e.,

$$\mathbf{P}(\theta|x) = \frac{f(x; \theta)p(\theta)}{f(x)}$$

1. Where

$$f(x) = \int_{\Theta} f(x; \theta)p(\theta)\mu(d\theta)$$

is a normalizing constant (the marginal distribution of x).

The posterior result may also be written as

$$\mathbf{P}(\theta|x) \propto \mathscr{L}(\theta; x)g(\theta)$$

where $\mathscr{L}(\theta; x)$ is the likelihood of θ having observed x. The posterior represents what we believe about θ after we have observed the data. It represents an updating of our beliefs about θ having observed the data.

14.3   Why Bayesian? Exchangeability

If $X_1, X_2, \ldots, X_n$ are independent and identically distributed (iid) then for any $(x_1, x_2, \ldots, x_n)$ the joint density $f(x_1, x_2, \ldots, x_n)$ can be written as

$$f(x_1, x_2, \ldots, x_n) = \prod_{i=1}^{n} f(x_i)$$

where $f(x)$ is the density function of any X at x.

A **permutation** of $\mathbf{x} = (x_1, x_2, \ldots, x_n)$, $\pi(\mathbf{x})$, is any rearrangement of $\mathbf{x}$. For example, $(x_{i_1}, x_{i_2}, \ldots, x_{i_n})$. There are $n!$ such permutations.

Definition 14.3.1. If

$$f(\pi(\mathbf{x})) = f(\mathbf{x})$$

for every permutation and every $\mathbf{x}$ the random variables $X_1, X_2, \ldots, X_n$ are said to be **exchangeable**.

Clearly if $X_1, X_2, \ldots, X_n$ are iid then they are exchangeable.

Theorem 14.3.1. *If $X_1, X_2, \ldots, X_n$ are iid given θ then they are exchangeable*

Proof. For any $x_1, x_2, \ldots, x_n$ we have

$$f(x_1, x_2, \ldots, x_n) = \int_\Theta f(x_1, x_2, \ldots, x_n | \theta) g(\theta) d\mu(\theta)$$

$$= \int_\Theta \prod_{i=1}^n f(x_i | \theta) g(\theta) d\mu(\theta)$$

$$= \int_\Theta \prod_{j=1}^n f(x_{i_j} | \theta) g(\theta) d\mu(\theta)$$

$$= \int_\Theta f(x_{i_1}, x_{i_2}, \ldots, x_{i_n} | \theta) g(\theta) d\mu(\theta)$$

$$= f(x_{i_1}, x_{i_2}, \ldots, x_{i_n})$$

A famous theorem due to de Finetti provides a partial converse to the fact that conditionally iid random variables are exchangeable. $\qquad \square$

Theorem 14.3.2 (de Finetti). *If $X_1, X_2, \ldots$ is a sequence of random variables which are exchangeable for every n then there is a distribution g such that*

$$f(x_1, x_2, \ldots, x_n) = \int_\Theta \prod_{i=1}^n f(x_i | \theta) g(\theta) d\mu(\theta)$$

i.e., $X_1, X_2, \ldots, X_n$ can be viewed as conditionally independent given θ where θ has distribution defined by g

Jose Bernardo, a leading proponent of the use of Bayesian statistics, states:

It is important to realize that if the observations are conditionally independent, -as it is implicitly assumed when they are considered to be a random sample from some model-, then they are necessarily exchangeable. The representation theorem, -a pure probability theory result- proves that if observations are judged to be *exchangeable*, then they must indeed be a random sample from some model *and* there *must exist* a prior probability distribution over the parameter of the model, hence requiring a *Bayesian* approach.

Note however that the representation theorem is an existence theorem: it generally does not specify the model, and it never specifies the required prior distribution. The additional assumptions which are usually necessary to specify a particular model are described in particular representation theorems. An additional effort is necessary to assess a prior distribution for the parameter of the model.

The key point is that exchangeability implies the existence of a prior and provides a powerful justification for the use of Bayesian methods to describe beliefs.

Other justifications for the use of Bayesian methods are based on the concept of utilities and decision making and rely on the concept of coherence:

1. One important point in using Bayesian methods is that the choice of prior need not reflect true prior knowledge about the parameter.
2. This is the basis for the **objective Bayes** approach. The prior in this case represents that function of the parameter which has minimal impact on the posterior.
3. It need not be a proper probability distribution, but the posterior is required to be a proper probability distribution.

In fact some Bayesians are even more forthright:

The posterior density is a probability density on the parameter (space), which does not mean that the parameter need be a genuine random variable. This density is used as an inferential tool, not as a truthful representation.

[31]

Let X be binomial with parameters n and θ where we assume that n is known. That is

$$f(x; \theta) = \binom{n}{x} \theta^x (1 - \theta)^{n-x}$$

for $x = 0, 1, \ldots, n$. Suppose we represent prior information by a distribution of the form

$$g(\theta; \alpha, \beta) = \frac{\theta^{\alpha-1}(1 - \theta)^{\beta-1}}{\mathbf{B}(\alpha, \beta)}$$

where α and β are both positive.

This prior is a Beta distribution with parameters α and β and

$$\mathbf{B}(\alpha, \beta) = \int_0^1 t^{\alpha-1}(1 - t)^{\beta-1} dt$$

It is known that $\mathbf{B}(\alpha, \beta)$ is given by

$$\mathbf{B}(\alpha, \beta) = \frac{\Gamma(\alpha)\Gamma(\beta)}{\Gamma(\alpha + \beta)}$$

where

$$\Gamma(\delta) = \int_0^\infty t^{\delta-1}e^{-t}dt$$

for $\delta > 0$ is the Gamma function.

With this choice of prior we have that

$$f(x) = \int_\Theta f(x;\theta)g(\theta;\alpha,\beta)d\theta$$

$$= \int_0^1 \binom{n}{x}\theta^x(1-\theta)^{n-x}\frac{\theta^{\alpha-1}(1-\theta)^{\beta-1}}{\mathbf{B}(\alpha,\beta)}d\theta$$

$$= \frac{\binom{n}{x}}{\mathbf{B}(\alpha,\beta)}\int_0^1 \theta^{x+\alpha-1}(1-\theta)^{n-x+\beta-1}d\theta$$

$$= \frac{\binom{n}{x}\mathbf{B}(x+\alpha-1,n-x+\beta-1)}{\mathbf{B}(\alpha,\beta)}$$

Thus the posterior density of θ is given by

$$g(\theta|x) = \frac{\theta^{x+\alpha-1}(1-\theta)^{n-x+\beta-1}}{\mathbf{B}(x+\alpha,n-x+\beta)}$$

i.e., a beta distribution with parameters $x+\alpha$ and $n-x+\beta$. Note that the posterior distribution depends on the parameters α and β

It is known that the Beta distribution with parameters α' and β' has expected value given by

$$\frac{\alpha'}{(\alpha'+\beta')}$$

Thus the expected value of the posterior is given by

$$\frac{(x+\alpha)}{(n+\alpha+\beta)}$$

which is a natural Bayes estimate of θ,

Note that this estimate is not the same as the conventional estimate x/n. In fact

$$\frac{x+\alpha}{n+\alpha+\beta} = (1-w_n)\frac{x}{n} + w_n\frac{\alpha}{\alpha+\beta}$$

where

$$w_n = \frac{\alpha + \beta}{n + \alpha + \beta}$$

i.e., the posterior mean is a weighted combination of the prior mean and the usual estimate.

This may also be written as

$$\frac{x + \alpha}{n + \alpha + \beta} = \frac{x}{n} - w_n \left(\frac{x}{n} - \frac{\alpha}{\alpha + \beta} \right)$$

which shows that the usual estimate is "shrunk" toward the prior mean. Note that the shrinkage factor, w_n, approaches 0 for large sample sizes.

Suppose that we have observed $x_1, x_2, \ldots, x_n$ assumed to be realized values of independent random variables which are Poisson with parameter λ. Then the density given λ is

$$f(x_1, x_2, \ldots, x_n; \lambda) = \prod_{i=1}^{n} \frac{\lambda^{x_i} e^{-\lambda}}{x_i!} = \frac{\lambda^{n\bar{x}} e^{-n\lambda}}{\prod_{i=1}^{n} x_i!}$$

Assume a prior for λ of the form

$$p(\lambda) = \frac{\lambda^{\alpha-1} e^{-\lambda/\beta}}{\Gamma(\alpha)\beta^{\alpha}}$$

i.e., a Gamma distribution with parameters $\alpha > 0$ and $\beta > 0$

Then the posterior of λ is proportional to

$$\lambda^{n\bar{x}+\alpha-1} e^{-\lambda(n+1/\beta)}$$

and hence the posterior is Gamma with parameters

$$a = n\bar{x} + \alpha \ \text{ and } \ b = \frac{1}{n + \frac{1}{\beta}}$$

One natural (Bayes) estimate of λ is the mean of the posterior given by

$$ab = \frac{n\bar{x} + \alpha}{n + \frac{1}{\beta}}$$

Note that the posterior mean can be written as

$$(1 - w_n)\bar{x} + w_n \alpha \beta$$

where

$$w_n = \frac{1}{1 + n\beta}$$

Thus the posterior mean is a linear combination of the prior mean and the maximum likelihood estimate. This can also be written as

$$\bar{x} - w_n \left(\bar{x} - \alpha\beta\right)$$

which again shows the shrinkage of the usual estimate to the prior mean. Again note that for large n the posterior mean is very nearly equal to the maximum likelihood estimate.

Another estimate is the mode of the posterior which, in this case, is given by

$$\frac{\bar{x} + \frac{\alpha - 1}{n}}{1 + \frac{1}{n\beta}}$$

For large n this is very nearly equal to the maximum likelihood estimate (this result is true quite generally).

Suppose that $\mathbf{Y}$ obeys a general linear model, i.e., $\mathbf{Y}$ is normal with

$$\mathbb{E}(\mathbf{Y}) = \mathbf{X}\boldsymbol{\beta} \ \text{ and } \ \mathbb{V}(\mathbf{Y}) = \mathbf{I}\sigma^2$$

Suppose further that the prior distribution for $\boldsymbol{\beta}$ is also normal with mean and variance-covariance matrix given by

$$\mathbb{E}(\boldsymbol{\beta}) = \boldsymbol{\beta}_0 \ \text{ and } \ \mathbb{V}(\boldsymbol{\beta}) = \mathbf{V}$$

The joint distribution of $\mathbf{Y}$ and $\boldsymbol{\beta}$ is thus also normal with

$$\mathbb{E}\left(\begin{bmatrix} \mathbf{Y} \\ \boldsymbol{\beta} \end{bmatrix}\right) = \begin{bmatrix} \mathbf{X} \\ \mathbf{I} \end{bmatrix} \boldsymbol{\beta}$$

and

$$\mathbb{V}\left(\begin{bmatrix} \mathbf{Y} \\ \boldsymbol{\beta} \end{bmatrix}\right) = \begin{bmatrix} \mathbf{I}\sigma^2 + \mathbf{X}\mathbf{V}\mathbf{X}^\top & \mathbf{X}\mathbf{V} \\ \mathbf{V}\mathbf{X}^\top & \mathbf{V} \end{bmatrix}$$

It then follows that the posterior distribution of $\boldsymbol{\beta}$ given $\mathbf{Y} = \mathbf{y}$ is normal with

$$\mathbb{E}(\boldsymbol{\beta}) = \boldsymbol{\beta}_0 + \mathbf{V}\mathbf{X}^\top \left[\mathbf{I}\sigma^2 + \mathbf{X}\mathbf{V}\mathbf{X}^\top\right]^{-1} \mathbf{X}\mathbf{V}(\mathbf{y} - \mathbf{X}\boldsymbol{\beta}_0)$$

and

$$\mathbb{V}(\beta) = \left[\mathbf{I} + \mathbf{XVX}^\top\right]^{-1}$$

Lots of complex, but routine, matrix algebra shows that the mean of the posterior distribution of β can be written as

$$\left[(\mathbf{X}^\top \mathbf{X})\sigma^{-2} + \mathbf{V}^{-1}\right]^{-1}\left\{\sigma^{-2}\mathbf{X}^\top \mathbf{Xb} + \mathbf{V}^{-1}\beta_0\right\}$$

where $\mathbf{b}$ is the least squares estimate

$$\mathbf{b} = (\mathbf{X}^\top \mathbf{X})^{-1}\mathbf{X}^\top \mathbf{y}$$

i.e., the mean of the posterior is a weighted linear combination of the prior mean β_0 and the maximum likelihood estimate $\mathbf{b}$.

Examples 1–3 have priors which are **conjugate**.

If a prior and a posterior belong to the same family of distributions they are said to be conjugate.

14.4   Stable Estimation

Intuitively, with large amounts of data, the impact of the prior should be small.

More formally, if the likelihood $\mathscr{L}(\theta|x)$ is highly concentrated over a region $\Theta_s \subset \Theta$, then the posterior will satisfy

$$\pi(\theta|x) \approx \frac{\mathscr{L}(\theta; x)}{\int_{\Theta_s} \mathscr{L}(\theta; x)d\mu(\theta)} \quad \theta \in \Theta_s$$

Thus the prior has essentially no impact on the posterior and we have robustness to prior misspecification.

This is called **stable estimation**.

14.5   Bayesian Consistency

If the posterior converges to a distribution which is concentrated at the true value of the parameter θ_0 we have Bayesian consistency.

Under weak regularity conditions most commonly used models with sensible priors lead to a posterior which is consistent.

14.6 Relation to Maximum Likelihood

1. Suppose that $X_1, X_2, \ldots, X_n$ are iid with pdf $f(x; \theta)$ where

$$\boldsymbol{\theta} = (\theta_1, \theta_2, \ldots, \theta_p)$$

2. Assume that the prior $\pi(\boldsymbol{\theta})$ and $f(\mathbf{x}; \boldsymbol{\theta})$ are positive and twice differentiable near the maximum likelihood estimate of $\boldsymbol{\theta}$, $\widehat{\boldsymbol{\theta}}$.
3. Then under suitable regularity conditions (similar to those for maximum likelihood estimation) we have the Bernstein-von Mises result as stated in Berger (1987).

The posterior density of $\boldsymbol{\theta}$

$$\pi_n(\boldsymbol{\theta}|\mathbf{x}) = \frac{f(\mathbf{x}; \boldsymbol{\theta})\pi(\boldsymbol{\theta})}{f(\mathbf{x})}$$

can be approximated for large n in the following four ways:

(i) π_n is approximately MVN $(\boldsymbol{\mu}^*(\mathbf{x}), \mathbb{V}(\mathbf{x}))$ where $\boldsymbol{\mu}^*(\mathbf{x})$ and $\mathbb{V}^*(\mathbf{x})$ are the posterior mean and posterior covariance matrix.

(ii) π_n is approximately MVN $\left(\widehat{\boldsymbol{\theta}}^*; [\mathcal{I}^\pi(\mathbf{x})]^{-1}\right)$ where $\widehat{\boldsymbol{\theta}}^*$ is the generalized maximum likelihood estimate for $\boldsymbol{\theta}$, i.e., the maximum likelihood estimator for $\boldsymbol{\theta}$ is the model with likelihood

$$\mathscr{L}^*(\boldsymbol{\theta}, \mathbf{x}) = f(\mathbf{x}; \boldsymbol{\theta})\pi(\boldsymbol{\theta})$$

and $\mathcal{I}^\pi(\mathbf{x})$ is the $p \times p$ matrix with (i, j) element given by

$$\mathcal{I}_{ij}^\pi(\mathbf{x}) = -\left[\frac{\partial^2 \ln[f(\mathbf{x}; \boldsymbol{\theta})\pi(\boldsymbol{\theta})]}{\partial\theta_i\partial\theta_j}\right]_{\boldsymbol{\theta}=\widehat{\boldsymbol{\theta}}^*}$$

(iii) π_n is approximately MVN $\left(\widehat{\boldsymbol{\theta}}; [\widehat{\mathcal{I}}(\mathbf{x})]^{-1}\right)$ where $\widehat{\boldsymbol{\theta}}$ is the maximum likelihood estimate for $\boldsymbol{\theta}$ and $\widehat{\mathcal{I}}(\mathbf{x})$ is the $p \times p$ observed Fisher information matrix with (i, j) element given by

$$\widehat{\mathcal{I}}_{ij}(\mathbf{x}) = -\left[\frac{\partial^2 \ln[f(\mathbf{x}; \boldsymbol{\theta})]}{\partial\theta_i\partial\theta_j}\right]_{\boldsymbol{\theta}=\widehat{\boldsymbol{\theta}}} = -\sum_{k=1}^n \left[\frac{\partial^2 \ln[f(x_k; \boldsymbol{\theta})]}{\partial\theta_i\partial\theta_j}\right]_{\boldsymbol{\theta}=\widehat{\boldsymbol{\theta}}}$$

(iv) π_n is approximately MVN $\left(\widehat{\boldsymbol{\theta}}; [\mathcal{I}(\widehat{\boldsymbol{\theta}})]^{-1}\right)$ where $\widehat{\boldsymbol{\theta}}$ is the maximum likelihood estimate for $\boldsymbol{\theta}$ and $\mathcal{I}(\boldsymbol{\theta})$ is the $p \times p$ expected Fisher information matrix with (i, j) element given by

$$\mathcal{I}_{ij}(\boldsymbol{\theta}) = -n\mathbb{E}_{\boldsymbol{\theta}}\left[\frac{\partial^2\,\ln[f(X_1;\boldsymbol{\theta})]}{\partial\theta_i\partial\theta_j}\right]$$

In general the approximations are ordered (i)–(iv) with (i) better than (ii), (ii) better than (iii), and (iii) better than (iv).

If the prior is "uninformative" then the result gives "objective" posterior approximations.

It follows that large sample posterior intervals are approximately

$$\widehat{\theta}_n \pm z_{1-\alpha/2}\sqrt{\frac{1}{n\,i(\widehat{\theta})}}$$

It also follows that large sample posterior intervals for $g(\theta)$ are given by

$$g(\widehat{\theta}_n) \pm z_{1-\alpha/2}\sqrt{\frac{|g^{(1)}(\widehat{\theta}_n)|}{n\,i(\widehat{\theta})}}$$

Remember Efron's statement that estimate plus or minus two standard errors has good credentials in any theory of statistical inference.

14.7 Priors

Many scientists and statisticians often say that they would use Bayesian methods if they could find or justify use of a particular prior. What they are arguing about is the choice of prior not the basic methodology, i.e., there is an acceptance of the treatment of parameters as random. Exchangeability ensures that there is a prior.

Much has been written on the choice of priors and much more will surely be written.

Example. Consider a room which we are told is square and between 10 and 20 feet on a side. If θ_1 is the parameter representing the length of a side, pleading ignorance leads to a prior of the form

$$p(\theta_1) = \begin{cases} \frac{1}{10} & \text{if } 10 \leq \theta_1 \leq 20 \\ 0 & \text{elsewhere} \end{cases}$$

If θ_2 is the parameter representing the area of the room then again pleading ignorance leads to a prior of the form

$$p(\theta_2) = \begin{cases} \frac{1}{400} & \text{if } 100 \leq \theta_2 \leq 400 \\ 0 & \text{elsewhere} \end{cases}$$

Note that the probability that the length of the side is between 10 and 15 feet is $\frac{1}{2}$ which corresponds to an area between 100 and 225 square feet.

The probability assigned to this area under the ignorance model for the area is

$$\int_{100}^{225} \frac{1}{400} d\theta_2 = \left.\frac{\theta_2}{400}\right|_{100}^{225} = \frac{225 - 100}{400} = \frac{125}{400} = \frac{5}{8}$$

Thus, the two ignorance assignments are not compatible.

Reference: Bayesianism: Its Scope and Limits, Elliott Sobel

Many view the above example as a key counterexample to the use of Bayesian statistics. If it were, interest in Bayesian statistics would have waned decades ago.

What has happened is the search for priors which are **transformation invariant** and yet, in some sense, do not convey "much" prior information, i.e., the prior is dominated by the likelihood, even for small samples.

14.7.1 Different Types of Priors

Basically there are four approaches:

1. A formal mathematical approach which uses **conjugate priors**
2. An ad hoc approach which uses **vague, flat,** or **uniform priors** to represent "ignorance"
3. A formal approach using **reference priors** which are designed to "let the data speak for themselves"
4. A formal approach which elicits information to determine a truly **subjective prior**

14.7.1.1 Conjugate Priors

If, in a given problem, there is a prior which, when combined with the likelihood, yields a posterior which is in the same family as the prior, then the prior is said to be a **conjugate prior**. It is tacitly assumed that a case can be made that this prior represents prior beliefs about the parameter.

Conjugate priors have the great advantage that closed forms can be obtained for the posterior and hence inferences are computationally simple.

Conjugate priors are not often available, but they are in one special family of distributions called **the exponential family**.

For example:

(i) If the likelihood is binomial then the beta distribution is a conjugate prior.
(ii) If the likelihood is Poisson then the Gamma distribution is a conjugate prior.
(iii) If the likelihood is normal then the normal is a conjugate prior.

Thus many of the simplest inference problems have conjugate priors and hence closed form expressions for the posterior distributions can be found.

More generally linear combinations of conjugate priors can be used to find priors. There are compendiums of conjugate priors available, e.g, Fink [15]

14.7.2 Vague Priors

Vague priors, also called flat or non-informative priors, are priors which are such that they are constant over the range of parameter values for which the likelihood is moderate in size.

Thus the posterior is essentially the likelihood normalized so as to integrate or sum to 1.

Whenever the prior is of this type it is usually not a density. There is, for example, no constant density that integrates to 1 over the interval $[0, \infty)$.

Thus one always needs to check that the posterior is in fact a density function when flat priors are used. Such a posterior is called **proper**.

Vague priors are supposed to represent **ignorance**, i.e., any parameter value is considered to be equally likely a priori. However this means that while we are ignorant about θ we are not ignorant about $g(\theta)$ since its density will not be uniform. (The Jacobian of the transformation form θ to $g(\theta)$ is not, in general, a constant.)

Thus vague priors are not **transformation invariant**. Reread the slides on the problem of ignorance.

14.7.2.1 Jeffrey's Priors

Jeffrey's priors are a class of default priors which are translation invariant.

These priors, when applicable, choose the prior

$$p(\theta) \propto \sqrt{i(\theta)}$$

where $i(\theta)$ is Fisher's information. For the multiple parameter case these priors are of the form

$$p(\boldsymbol{\theta}) \propto \sqrt{\det(i(\boldsymbol{\theta})}$$

i.e., to the determinant of Fisher's information matrix for a sample of size 1.

Example. For the Bernoulli we know that Fisher's information is $i(\theta) = 1/[\theta(1 - \theta)]$ so that the Jeffrey's prior is given by

$$i(\theta) = \frac{1}{\theta^{1/2}(1 - \theta)^{1/2}}$$

and hence the posterior for a binomial using Jeffrey's prior is given by

$$p(\theta|x) \propto \theta^{x-\frac{1}{2}}(1-\theta)^{n-x-\frac{1}{2}}$$

i.e., a beta distribution with parameter $a = x + 1/2$ and $b = n - x + 1/2$.

Example. For the normal with known variance, Jeffrey's prior is given by

$$p(\theta) = 1$$

which is an improper prior. For the normal with unknown mean and variance Jeffrey's prior is given by

$$g(\theta, \sigma^2) = \frac{1}{\sigma}$$

which is also an improper prior. In both cases the posterior is a proper prior.

Jeffrey's priors are not flat, but they are transformation invariant and are widely used.

14.7.2.2 Reference Priors

In the last three decades much work has been done on developing a class of prior distributions, called **reference priors**, which "let the data speak for themselves." Essentially these priors maximize the distance between the prior and the posterior, using distance specified by the Kullback-Leibler divergence.

"Intuitively, a reference prior for θ is one which maximizes what is **not known** about θ, **relative** to what could possibly be learnt from the result of a particular experiment. More formally a reference prior for θ is defined to be one which maximizes, within some class of candidate priors, the **missing information** about the quantity of interest θ, defined as a limiting form of the amount of information about its value which data from the assumed model could possibly provide."

The amount of missing information is defined in terms of the Kullback-Leibler divergence. Determination of these priors is quite technical, but often they turn out to be Jeffrey's prior.

"Reference priors are not descriptions of personal beliefs; they are proposed as formal **consensus** priors to be used as standards for scientific communication."

The quotations above are from papers by Bernardo. His website has excellent papers on objective Bayes procedures.

Here is a short summary of reference priors for common statistical problems:

Likelihood	Prior	Posterior
Binomial	Beta(1/2,1/2)	Beta(x+1/2,n-x+1/2)
Poisson	$\lambda^{-1/2}$	Gamma(x+1/2,1)
Normal (known σ^2)	Constant	Normal($\bar{x}, \sigma^2/n$)
Normal (unknown σ^2)	σ^{-1}	Student's t

A complete list of reference priors appears in [56].

14.7.2.3   Subjective Priors

One important method of obtaining priors is to convene a group of experts in the field under study and have them assess a prior distribution. Much has been written about this under the name **prior elicitation**.

Chapter 15
Bayesian Statistics: Computation

15.1 Computation

- By Bayes theorem the posterior density of θ is given by

$$p(\theta|x) = \frac{f(x;\theta)p(\theta)}{f(x)}$$

where

$$f(x) = \int_{\Theta} f(x;\theta)p(\theta)dm(\theta)$$

- The calculation of the posterior thus requires calculation of an integral of the likelihood weighted by the prior.
- Usually this integral can only be determined in closed form for conjugate priors.
- For many years Bayesian analysis was reduced to using conjugate priors (resulting in only a few practical applications)
- Or in relying on large sample approximations using large sample maximum likelihood results.
- The introduction of fast reliable computing has changed all of that.

15.1.1 *Monte Carlo Integration*

Suppose that we want to evaluate

$$\mathbf{I} = \int h(x)f(x)dx = \mathbb{E}_f[h(X)]$$

© Springer International Publishing Switzerland 2014
C.A. Rohde, *Introductory Statistical Inference with the Likelihood Function*, DOI 10.1007/978-3-319-10461-4_15

where f is a density function. Given random sample $X_1, X_2, \ldots, X_n$, where n is large then the law of large numbers tells us that

$$\frac{1}{n} \sum_{i=1}^{h} (X_i) \xrightarrow{p} \mathbb{E}[h(X)]$$

Thus

$$\frac{1}{n} \sum_{i=1}^{n} h(x_i)$$

is an estimate of the integral **I**. The variance of this estimate is estimated by

$$s_I^2 = \frac{1}{n-1} \sum_{i=1}^{n} (y_i - \overline{y})^2$$

where $y_i = h(x_i)$. It follows that the standard error of the approximation to the integral is estimated by

$$\sqrt{\frac{s^2}{n}}$$

Sampling from any density function is relatively easy since we can generate uniform $[0,1]$ random variables and use the fact that if Y has distribution function F then $F^{-1}(Y)$ is uniform $[0,1]$.

15.1.2 Importance Sampling

If we know how to draw samples from f there is no problem in approximating

$$\int h(x) f(x) dx$$

If, however, we do not know how to draw samples from f basic Monte Carlo sampling will not be feasible. If we know how to sample from g we can write

$$\mathbf{I} = \int h(x) f(x) dx = \int \frac{h(x) f(x)}{g(x)} g(x) dx = \mathbb{E}_g(Y)$$

where

$$Y = \frac{h(X) f(X)}{g(X)}$$

Since we can simulate from g, we obtain $X_1 = x_1, X_2 = x_2, \ldots, X_n = x_n$ from g and approximate $\mathbf{I}$ by

$$\frac{1}{n}\sum_{i=1}^{n} y_i = \frac{1}{n}\sum_{i=1}^{n} \frac{h(x_i)f(x_i)}{g(x_i)}$$

This is called **importance sampling**. It works well provided the tails of the density g are thicker than the tails of the density f but is otherwise similar to f.

15.1.3   Markov Chain Monte Carlo

The basic problem of evaluating

$$\mathbf{I} = \int h(x)f(x)dx$$

can also be solved by constructing a Markov chain $X_1, X_2, \ldots$ whose stationary distribution has density f. Then by a law of large numbers for Markov chains,

$$\frac{1}{n}\sum_{i=1}^{n} h(X_i) \ \xrightarrow{p} \ \mathbb{E}_f[h(X)]$$

Hence we can obtain a sample from $f(\boldsymbol{x})$ and use this sample to approximate f and hence the posterior.

There are a variety of different algorithms to perform markov chain monte carlo (MCMC). One important one is **Gibbs Sampling**.

15.1.4   The Gibbs Sampler

The Gibbs sampler is a method that generates observations from a marginal density f without having to calculate f. To understand Gibbs sampling it is necessary to understand a little about **stochastic processes**. I have included in the appendix a short section on stochastic processes.

Suppose that $\mathbf{y}$ is k dimensional. Let $\mathbf{y}^{(0)}$ be an initial starting value and define

$$f_i(y_i|\mathbf{y}_{-i})$$

to be the conditional density of $\mathbf{Y}_i$ given the rest of the Y_i's, i.e., $\mathbf{y}_{-i}$ is the $k-1$ dimensional vector obtained by eliminating the ith coordinate of $\mathbf{y}$. At the end of the jth step we have calculated

$$\mathbf{y}^{(j)} = (y_1^{(j)}, y_2^{(j)}, \ldots, y_k^{(j)})$$

We then generate the next random observation as follows:

1. Generate a random observation $y_1^{(j+1)}$ from

$$f_1(y_1 | Y_2 = y_2^{(j)}, Y_3 = y_3^{(j)}, \ldots, Y_k = y_k^{(j)})$$

2. Generate a random observation $y_2^{(j+1)}$ from

$$f_2(y_2 | Y_1 = y_1^{(j+1)}, Y_3 = y_3^{(j)}, \ldots, Y_k = y_k^{(j)})$$

3. Generate a random observation $y_3^{(j+1)}$ from

$$f_3(y_3 | Y_1 = y_1^{(j+1)}, Y_2 = y_2^{(j+1)}, \ldots, Y_k = y_k^{(j)})$$

....

(k) Generate a random observation $y_k^{(j+1)}$ from

$$f_k(y_k | Y_1 = y_1^{(j+1)}, Y_2 = y_2^{(j+1)}, \ldots, Y_{k-1} = y_{k-1}^{(j+1)})$$

Then

$$\mathbf{y}^{(j+1)} = (y_1^{(j+1)}, y_2^{(j+1)}, \ldots, y_k^{(j+1)})$$

The sequence

$$\mathbf{y}^{(0)}, \mathbf{y}^{(1)}, \ldots, \mathbf{y}^{(j)}, \mathbf{y}^{(j+1)}, \ldots$$

is a realization of a Markov chain, under suitable conditions, for j large the distribution of $\mathbf{y}^{(j)}$ will converge to the stationary distribution which can be shown to be $f(\mathbf{y})$.

Hence we have a random observation from $f(\mathbf{y})$. We repeat this process a large number N of times and then have a (large) random sample from f which can be used to estimate f or some other function of f.

15.1.5   Software

Fortunately there is now much software available to obtain posterior densities using MCMC. The most widely used of these is **WinBUGS** which is short for Bayesian analysis using Gibbs Sampling implemented for Windows. It appears to be no longer supported by its developers, but there are excellent alternatives, namely JAGS (Just Another Gibbs Sampler), MCMCPack in R, STAN, etc. Even SAS now has an excellent PROC for doing Bayesian analysis. The excellent texts by Albert and Huff, in addition to providing introductions to Bayesian statistics, provide R code for doing many of the basic analyses. The text by Marin and Robert [31] also should be mentioned as should ABC (Approximate Bayesian Computation).

Chapter 16
Bayesian Inference: Miscellaneous

16.1 Bayesian Updating

Suppose you have obtained a posterior distribution for θ based on data y_1. At a later date you are given data y_2 whose distribution depends on the same parameter and is independent of the previous data. Then we have that

$$
\begin{aligned}
p(\theta|y_1, y_2) &= \frac{f(y_1, y_2; \theta)g(\theta)}{\int_\Theta f(y_1, y_2; \theta)g(\theta)d\theta} \\[2mm]
&= \frac{f(y_2; \theta)f(y_1; \theta)g(\theta)}{\int_\Theta f(y_2; \theta)f(y_1; \theta)g(\theta)d\theta} \\[2mm]
&= \frac{f(y_2; \theta)\frac{f(y_1; \theta)g(\theta)}{f(y_1)}}{\int_\Theta f(y_2; \theta)\frac{f(y_1; \theta)g(\theta)}{f(y_1)}d\theta} \\[2mm]
&= \frac{f(y_2; \theta)p(\theta|y_1)}{\int_\Theta f(y_2; \theta)p(\theta|y_1)d\theta}
\end{aligned}
$$

i.e., "yesterday's posterior becomes today's prior."

This feature of Bayesian inference is very compatible with the way in which science operates, incorporating information in a logical and orderly way.

16.2 Bayesian Prediction

Suppose that we have observed $X_1 = x_1, X_2 = x_2, \ldots, X_n = x_n$ where the X_i are iid as $f(x; \theta)$. Suppose that interest focuses on the **prediction** of X_{n+1}, the next (or a later value of X).

© Springer International Publishing Switzerland 2014
C.A. Rohde, *Introductory Statistical Inference with the Likelihood Function*, DOI 10.1007/978-3-319-10461-4_16

We note that

$$f(x_{n+1}|x_1, x_2, \ldots, x_n) = \frac{f(x_1, x_2, \ldots, x_n, x_{n+1})}{f(x_1, x_2, \ldots, x_n)}$$

$$= \frac{\int_\Theta f(x_1, x_2, \ldots, x_n, x_{n+1}, \theta) p(\theta) d\theta}{f(x_1, x_2, \ldots, x_n)}$$

$$= \frac{\int_\Theta f(x_1, x_2, \ldots, x_n; \theta) p(\theta) f(x_{n+1}; \theta) d\theta}{f(x_1, x_2, \ldots, x_n)}$$

$$= \int_\Theta p(\theta|x_1, x_2, \ldots, x_n) f(x_{n+1}; \theta) d\theta$$

Example. We have $X_1, X_2, \ldots, X_n$ as iid normal with mean θ and known variance σ^2 and we want to predict X_{n+1}, the next value of X. We know that the posterior of μ is

$$p(\mu|\mathbf{x}) = [(2\pi\sigma_*^2)]^{-1/2} \exp\left\{-\frac{(\mu - \mu_*)^2}{2\sigma_*^2}\right\}$$

where

$$\mu_* = \frac{1}{\frac{n}{\sigma^2} + \frac{1}{\sigma_o^2}} \left(\frac{n\overline{x}}{\sigma^2} + \frac{\mu_o}{\sigma_o^2}\right) \quad \text{and} \quad \sigma_*^2 = \frac{1}{\frac{n}{\sigma^2} + \frac{1}{\sigma_o^2}}$$

and μ_0, σ_0^2 are the mean and variance of the conjugate prior for μ.

It follows that the predictive density for x_{n+1} is

$$p(x_{n+1}(x|\mathbf{x}) = \int_{-\infty}^{\infty} p(\mu|\mathbf{x}) f(x_{n+1}; \mu) d\mu$$

or

$$\int_{-\infty}^{\infty} (2\pi\sigma_*^2)^{-1/2} \exp\left\{-\frac{(\mu - \mu_*)^2}{2\sigma_*^2}\right\} (2\pi\sigma^2)^{-1/2} \exp\left\{-\frac{(x_{n+1} - \mu)^2}{2\sigma^2}\right\} d\mu$$

which reduces to

$$K \int_{-\infty}^{\infty} \exp\left\{-\frac{\mu^2}{2}\left(\frac{1}{\sigma_*^2} + \frac{1}{\sigma^2}\right) + \mu\left(\frac{\mu_*}{\sigma_*^2} + \frac{x_{n+1}}{\sigma}\right)\right\} d\mu$$

where

$$K = \frac{\exp\left\{-\frac{\mu_*^2}{2\sigma_*^2} - \frac{x_{n+1}^2}{2\sigma^2}\right\}}{\sqrt{2\pi\sigma_*^2}\sqrt{2\pi\sigma^2}}$$

Now note that

$$\int_{-\infty}^{\infty} \frac{\exp\left\{-\frac{(\mu-a)^2}{2b^2}\right\}}{\sqrt{2\pi b^2}} = 1$$

implies that

$$\int_{-\infty}^{\infty} \exp\left\{-\frac{\mu^2}{2b^2} + \frac{\mu}{b^2}\right\} d\mu = \sqrt{(2\pi b^2}\exp\left\{\frac{a^2}{2b^2}\right\}$$

so that to evaluate the integral we only need to identify a and b.
    Note that

$$b^2 = \frac{1}{\frac{1}{\sigma_*^2} + \frac{1}{\sigma^2}} = \frac{\sigma_*^2\sigma^2}{\sigma_*^2 + \sigma^2}$$

and that

$$\frac{a}{b^2} = \left(\frac{\mu_*}{\sigma_*^2} + \frac{x_{n+1}}{\sigma}\right)$$

so that

$$a = \left(\frac{\mu_*}{\sigma_*^2} + \frac{x_{n+1}}{\sigma}\right)b^2$$

and hence

$$\frac{a^2}{2b^2} = \frac{1}{2}\left(\frac{\mu_*}{\sigma_*^2} + \frac{x_{n+1}}{\sigma^2}\right)^2 b^2$$

It follows that $p(x_{n+1}|\mathbf{x})$ is given by

$$\left\{\frac{\exp\left\{-\frac{\mu_*^2}{2\sigma_*^2} - \frac{x_{n+1}^2}{2\sigma^2}\right\}}{\sqrt{2\pi\sigma_*^2}\sqrt{2\pi\sigma^2}}\right\}$$

$$\times$$

$$\left\{\frac{\sqrt{2\pi\sigma_*^2}\sqrt{2\pi\sigma^2}}{\sqrt{\sigma_*^2 + \sigma^2}}\exp\left\{\frac{1}{2}\left(\frac{\mu_*}{\sigma_*^2} + \frac{x_{n+1}}{\sigma^2}\right)^2 b^2\right\}\right\}$$

or

$$\frac{1}{\sqrt{2\pi(\sigma_*^2 + \sigma^2)}} \exp\left\{ -\frac{\mu_*^2}{2\sigma_*^2} - \frac{x_{n+1}^2}{2\sigma^2} \right\}$$

$$\times$$

$$\exp\left\{ \frac{\mu_*^2\sigma^2}{2\sigma_*^2(\sigma_*^2 + \sigma^2)} + \frac{x_{n+1}^2\sigma_*^2}{2\sigma^2(\sigma_*^2 + \sigma^2)} - \frac{\mu_* x_{n+1}}{(\sigma_*^2 + \sigma^2)} \right\}$$

which reduces to

$$\frac{1}{\sqrt{2\pi(\sigma_*^2 + \sigma^2)}} \exp\left\{ -\frac{(x_{n+1} - \mu_*)^2}{2(\sigma_*^2 + \sigma^2)} \right\}$$

i.e., normal with mean μ_* and variance $\sigma_*^2 + \sigma^2$.

For the same problem we can note that

$$X_{n+1} = \mu + Z_{n+1}$$

where $Z_{n+1} \stackrel{d}{\sim} N(0, \sigma^2)$ is independent of $X_1, X_2, \ldots, X_n$ so that

$$\widehat{X}_{n+1} = \widehat{\mu} + Z_{n+1} \stackrel{d}{\sim} N(\mu, \sigma^2/n + \sigma^2)$$

A totally ad hoc but reasonable predictor.

16.3   Stopping Rules in Bayesian Inference

Recall that $t(x)$ is a sufficient statistic for θ if

$$f(x; \theta) = h(x)g(t(x); \theta)$$

where $h(x)$ does not depend on θ. As previously noted, with prior $p(\theta)$, the posterior of θ is

$$p(\theta|x) = \frac{f(x; \theta)p(\theta)}{\int_\Theta f(x; \theta)p(\theta)d\theta}$$

$$= \frac{g(t(x); \theta)h(x)p(\theta)}{\int_\Theta g(t(x); \theta)h(x)p(\theta)d\theta}$$

$$= \frac{g(t(x); \theta)p(\theta)}{\int_\Theta g(t(x); \theta)p(\theta)d\theta}$$

i.e., the posterior depends only on the sufficient statistic, $t(x)$.

In many applications the sufficient statistic can be written as

$$t(x) = [a(x), s(x)]$$

where the density of $a(x)$ does not depend on θ.

Definition 16.3.1. A statistic $a(x)$ is said to be **ancillary** if the distribution of $a(x)$ does not depend on θ.

In the case of an ancillary statistic we have

$$g(t(x); \theta) = g(s(x); \theta|a(x))g(a(x); \theta)$$
$$= g(s(x); \theta|a(x))g(a(x))$$

It follows that

$$p(\theta|x) = \frac{g(s(x); \theta|a(x))g(a(x))p(\theta)}{\int_\Theta g(s(x); \theta|a(x))g(a(x))p(\theta)d\theta}$$
$$= \frac{g(s(x); \theta|a(x))p(\theta)}{\int_\Theta g(s(x); \theta|a(x))p(\theta)d\theta}$$

Thus in Bayesian inference, in the presence of an ancillary statistic, we may use the distribution of the sufficient statistic conditional on the ancillary statistic as the basic "likelihood."

Consider the Bernoulli trial model in which

$$f(x_1, x_2, \ldots, x_n) = \prod_{i=1}^{n} f(x_i; \theta) = \theta^{s_n}(1 - \theta)^{n - s_n}$$

where $s_n = x_1 + x_2 + \ldots + x_n$ is the sufficient statistic.

It is clear that (n, s_n) is a sufficient (minimal). If we write

$$g(n, s_n; \theta) = g(s_n; \theta|n)g(n|\theta)$$

where $g(n|\theta)$ does not depend on θ then we may base inference on

$$g(s_n; \theta|n) = \binom{n}{s_n} \theta^{s_n}(1 - \theta)^{n - s_n}$$

the binomial density.

If in the same problem we write

$$g(n, s_n; \theta) = g(n; \theta|s_n)g(s_n; \theta)$$

and we assume that for all $s_n \geq 1$, $g(s_n; \theta)$ does not depend on θ then s_n is ancillary and inference can be based on

$$g(n; \theta | s_n)$$

which is a negative binomial distribution, i.e.,

$$g(n : \theta | s_n) = \binom{n-1}{s_n - 1} \theta^{s_n} (1 - \theta)^{n - s_n}$$

Note that the posterior distributions for each of these situations are the same

$$p(\theta | s_n) \propto \theta^{s_n} (1 - \theta)^{n - s_n} p(\theta)$$

This is a result of the likelihood principle in Bayesian inference.

Principle 16.3.1 (Likelihood Principle). Whenever two likelihood functions are proportional, i.e.,

$$g_1(x_1; \theta) \propto g_2(x_2; \theta) \quad \text{for all} \quad \theta,$$

then the posterior densities for θ are identical.

As the example shows, while it is obvious that the sample size n is usually fixed in advance of the experiment, inferences can be the same under different rules for the termination of the experiment. This has important practical considerations. In particular can we consider n as being fixed if

- "Stop when you have obtained a significant result."
- "Stop when you run out of money."

What we know is that, provided the rule which leads to the final n does not depend on θ, Bayesian inferences should be the same.

Definition 16.3.2 (Stopping Rule). A stopping rule h, for sequential sampling from a sequence $x_1 \in \mathcal{X}_1, x_2 \in \mathcal{X}_2, \ldots$ is a sequence of functions

$$h_n : \mathcal{X}_1 \times \mathcal{X}_2 \times \cdots \times \mathcal{X}_n \mapsto [0, 1]$$

such that

- If $x_{(n)} = (x_1, x_2, \ldots, x_n)$ is observed stop with probability $h(x_{(n)})$
- Otherwise observe x_{n+1}
- A stopping rule is **proper** if the distribution $p_h(n)$ guarantees that the sample size is finite
- A stopping rule is deterministic if $h(x_{(n)}) \in \{0, 1\}$; otherwise it is said to be a randomized stopping rule

In the general case it is necessary to consider the data resulting from a sequential experiment as consisting of **both** n, as chosen by the rule, h, and the observed values $x_{(n)} = x_1, x_2, \ldots, x_n$. Thus the probability model is of the form $f(n, x_{(n)}; \theta | h)$, i.e., we must condition on h.

Suppose we ignore the sampling rule h and analyze the data as if the observed sample size was fixed in advance, i.e., we assume that

$$f(n, x_{(n)}; \theta | h) = f(x_{(n)}; \theta)$$

What are the consequences of such an assumption?

Example. Consider Bernoulli trials with parameter θ and a stopping rule h defined by

$$h_1(1) = 1 \; ; \; h_1(0) = 0 \; ; \; h_2(x_1, x_2) = 1 \quad \text{for all } x_1, x_2$$

i.e., if the first trial is a success we stop; if it is a failure we observe x_2 and stop.

This is clearly a **biased** sampling rule since it seems to be in favor of larger values of θ.

Note, however, that

$$
\begin{aligned}
f(n = 1, x_1 = 1; \theta | h) &= f(x_1; \theta | n = 1, h) \mathbb{P}(n = 1; \theta | h) \\
&= f(x_1 = 1; \theta) \\
&= \theta
\end{aligned}
$$

and for $x = 0, 1$

$$
\begin{aligned}
f(n = 2, x_1 = 0, x_2 = x; \theta | h) &= f(x_1, x_2 = x; \theta | n = 2, h) \mathbb{P}(n = 2; \theta | h) \\
&= f(x_1 = 0; \theta | n = 2, h) f(x_2 = x; \theta | x_1 = 0, n = 2, h) \mathbb{P}(n = 2; \theta | h) \\
&= f(x_2 = x; \theta | x_1 = 0) f(x_1 = 0; \theta) \\
&= (1 - \theta) \theta^x (1 - \theta)^{1 - x}
\end{aligned}
$$

It follows that for all $(n, x_{(n)})$ we have that

$$f(n, x_{(n)}; \theta | h) = f(x_{(n)}; \theta)$$

and hence the posteriors will be the same and thus Bayesian inferences will be the same.

Theorem 16.3.1. *For any stopping rule, h, as defined in the previous definition we have that*

$$f(n, x_{(n)}; \theta | h) \propto f(x_{(n)}; \theta) \quad \theta \in \Theta$$

where $f(x_{(n)}; \theta)$ is the fixed sample size parametric model for $x_{(n)}$. That is, stopping rules as defined are likelihood non-informative, and posterior inferences will not depend on the stopping rule.

Suppose that $x_1, x_2, \ldots, x_n$ are iid as normal with mean θ and variance 1. Also suppose that an investigator wants to "prove" that θ is not 0 by sampling until the p-value is less than α. That is sample until $\bar{x}$ exceeds $k(\alpha)/\sqrt{n}$, e.g., $k(0.05) = 1.96$.

Thus the stopping rule is

$$h_n(x_{(n)}) = \begin{cases} 1 \text{ if } |\bar{x}_n| > k(\alpha)/\sqrt{n} \\ 0 \text{ if } |\bar{x}_n| \le k(\alpha)/\sqrt{n} \end{cases}$$

This can be shown by the Law of the Iterated Logarithm when $\theta = 0$ to be a proper stopping rule and hence is likelihood non-informative.

Does this mean that a Bayesian can be tricked by such an investigator? After all the posterior with vague prior is $N(\bar{x}, 1/n)$ so that a $1 - \alpha$ credible interval is

$$\bar{x} \pm k(\alpha)/\sqrt{n}$$

Thus the credible interval **does not contain the true value** $\theta = 0$!

A solution is provided when we realize that $\theta = 0$ is a special value of the parameter (as is any point null hypothesis). If we assign a positive prior probability π to $\theta = 0$ and a normal conjugate prior with large variance to the rest of the parameter, i.e., use a prior of the form

$$p(\theta) = \pi \mathbf{1}_{\theta=0}(\theta) + (1 - \pi)\mathbf{1}_{\theta \ne 0}(\theta)N(\theta, 0, \sigma_0^2)$$

The resulting posterior consists of a spike at $\theta = 0$ given by

$$\pi^* = \left\{ 1 + \frac{1 - \pi}{\pi}\left(1 + n\sigma_0^2\right)^{-1/2} \exp\left[\frac{1}{2}(\sqrt{n}\bar{x})^2(1 + n\sigma_0^2)^{-1}\right] \right\}^{-1}$$

Suppose now that α is very small so that $k(\alpha)$ is large. In this case n is likely to be large and when we stop we have $\bar{x} \approx k(\alpha)/\sqrt{n}$ and in this case

$$\pi^* \approx \left\{ 1 + \frac{1 - \pi}{\pi}\left(1 + n\sigma_0^2\right)^{-1/2} \exp\left[\frac{1}{2}k^2(\alpha)\right] \right\}^{-1} \approx 1$$

Thus, even though a frequentist argument would say that $\theta \ne 0$ a careful Bayesian argument shows that the posterior probability that $\theta = 0$ is close to one! This is another variant of the Jeffrey's Lindley paradox and shows, once again, the basic incompatibility of frequentist and Bayesian inferences.

16.4   Nuisance Parameters

Suppose that the parameter θ can be written as $\theta = (\phi, \lambda)$ where ϕ is of interest and λ is called a **nuisance parameter**.

1. Classical statistics has no general theory regarding inference in the presence of nuisance parameters. A variety of ad hoc techniques is used, e.g., pivots and marginalization.
2. Bayesian inference on the other hand has a logical surefire way to deal with nuisance parameters: simply assign them a prior and integrate them out.

Thus first calculate

$$p(\theta|x) = \frac{f(x; \theta)p(\theta)}{f(x)}$$

and then

$$p(\phi|x) = \int p(\theta|x)d\lambda = \int p(phi, \lambda|x)d\lambda$$

where

$$f(x) = \int f(x; \phi, \lambda)p(\phi, \lambda)d\phi d\lambda$$

Alternatively we might calculate the **integrated likelihood** for ϕ as

$$f(x; \phi) = \int f(x; \phi.\lambda)p(\lambda|\phi)d\lambda$$

and use this likelihood to calculate the posterior for ϕ as

$$p(\phi|x) = \frac{f(x; \phi)p(\phi)}{f(x)}$$

In any case the elimination of nuisance parameters is straightforward *but* depends heavily on the prior; reference priors are the best choice.

16.5   Summing Up

No inferential argument in statistics has anything going for it unless a sensible Bayesian interpretation can be found for it.

D. Basu

Chapter 17
Pure Likelihood Methods

17.1 Introduction

As we have seen in previous chapters use of the likelihood is important in frequentist methods and in Bayesian methods. In this chapter we explore the use of the likelihood function in another context, that of providing a self-contained method of statistical inference. Richard Royall in his book, Statistical Evidence: A Likelihood Paradigm, carefully developed the foundation for this method building on the work of Ian Hacking and Anthony Edwards. Royall lists three questions of interest to statisticians and scientists after having observed some data

1. What do I do?
2. What do I believe?
3. What evidence do I now have?

In the context of the usual parametric statistical model where we have an observed value x_{obs} of random X having sample space $\mathcal{X}$, parameter space Θ, and probability density function $f(x_{obs}; \theta)$ at the observed value, x_{obs} of X the first question is a decision theoretic problem re the actions to be taken on the basis of the model and the observed data and the second concerns what do I believe about θ given the observed data and presumably some prior knowledge about θ. The third question concerns characterizing what evidence the data has provided us about θ and requires no actions or beliefs. It is simply a question of "what do the data say" (about θ).

We have already stated the Law of Likelihood:

Axiom 17.1.1. *(Law of Likelihood).* *For two parameter values, θ_1 and θ_0, in the model $\mathcal{X}, f(x; \theta), \Theta$), the magnitude of the likelihood ratio*

$$L(\theta_1, \theta_0; x_{obs}) = \frac{f(x_{obs}; \theta_1)}{f(x_{obs}; \theta_0)}$$

© Springer International Publishing Switzerland 2014
C.A. Rohde, *Introductory Statistical Inference with the Likelihood Function*, DOI 10.1007/978-3-319-10461-4_17

measures the statistical evidence for θ_1 vs θ_0. If the ratio is greater than 1 we have statistical evidence for θ_1 vs θ_0 while if less than 1 we have statistical evidence for θ_0 vs θ_1.

I have used the term statistical evidence so as to not conflict with the use of the word evidence in other contexts, e.g., in P-values. We say the statistical evidence for θ_1 vs θ_0 is of strength $k > 1$ if $L(\theta_1, \theta_0; \boldsymbol{x}_{obs}) > k$.

17.2   Misleading Statistical Evidence

Since we are dealing with probability models it is possible to observe a value, $\boldsymbol{x}_{obs}$, for which $L(\theta_1, \theta_0; \boldsymbol{x}_{obs}) > k$, and yet θ_0 is true. This is called **misleading evidence**. The following is called the **universal bound** and shows that the probability of misleading evidence can be kept small by choice of k.

Theorem 17.2.1. *The probability of misleading evidence is bounded by $1/k$, i.e.,*

$$\mathbb{P}_{\theta_0}\left\{\frac{f(\boldsymbol{X};\theta_1)}{f(\boldsymbol{X};\theta_0)} \geq k\right\} \leq \frac{1}{k}$$

Proof. Let M be the set

$$M = \left\{\boldsymbol{x} \; : \; \frac{f(\boldsymbol{X};\theta_1)}{f(\boldsymbol{X};\theta_0)} \geq k\right\}$$

Then

$$\int_M f(\boldsymbol{x};\theta_0)d\mu(\boldsymbol{x}) \leq \int_M \frac{1}{k}f(\boldsymbol{x};\theta_1)d\mu(\boldsymbol{x})$$

$$\leq \frac{1}{k}\int_{\mathcal{X}} f(\boldsymbol{x};\theta_1)d\mu(\boldsymbol{x})$$

$$= \frac{1}{k}$$

In fact a much stronger result is true. Consider a sequence of observations

$$\mathbf{X}_n = (X_1, X_2, \ldots, X_n)$$

such that if A is true then $\mathbf{X}_n \sim f_n$ and when B is true $\mathbf{X}_n \sim g_n$. The likelihood ratio

$$\frac{g_n(\mathbf{x}_n)}{f_n(\mathbf{x}_n)} = z_n$$

is the LR in favor of B after n observations. Then we have the following theorem.

Theorem 17.2.2. *If A is true then*

$$P_A(Z_n \geq k \ for \ some \ n = 1, 2, \ldots) \leq \frac{1}{k}$$

Robbins [41]

In many circumstances the universal bound is far too conservative. Consider the situation where we have $X_1, X_2, \ldots, X_n$ where the X_i are iid as $N(\mu, \sigma^2)$ where, for simplicity, σ^2 is assumed known. The joint density is given by

$$f(\mathbf{y}; \mu) = \prod_{i=1}^{n} (2\pi\sigma^2)^{-\frac{1}{2}} \exp\left\{ -\frac{(y_i - \mu)^2}{2\sigma^2} \right\}$$

After some algebraic simplification the likelihood ratio for comparing μ_1 vs μ_0 is given by

$$\exp\left\{ \left(\bar{x} - \frac{\mu_0 + \mu_1}{2} \right) \frac{n(\mu_1 - \mu_0)}{\sigma^2} \right\}$$

It follows that the likelihood ratio exceeds k if and only if

$$\frac{n(\mu_1 - \mu_0)}{\sigma^2} \left(\bar{x} - \frac{\mu_1 + \mu_0}{2} \right) \geq \ln(k)$$

Thus, without loss of generality, if $\mu_1 - \mu_0 > 0$, the likelihood ratio exceeds k if and only if

$$\bar{x} \geq \frac{\mu_1 + \mu_0}{2} + \frac{\sigma^2}{n(\mu_1 - \mu_0)} \ln(k)$$

Thus the probability of misleading statistical evidence when $H_0 = \mu_0$ is assumed true is given by

$$
\begin{aligned}
\text{PMLEV}_1 &= P_{\mu=\mu_0} \left\{ \frac{f(\mathbf{X}; \mu_1)}{f(\mathbf{X}; \mu_0)} \geq k \right\} \\
&= P_{\mu=\mu_0} \left\{ \overline{X} \geq \frac{\mu_1 + \mu_0}{2} + \frac{\sigma^2}{n\mu_1 - \mu_0} \ln(k) \right\} \\
&= P_{\mu=\mu_0} \left\{ \frac{\sqrt{n}(\overline{X} - \mu_0)}{\sigma} \geq \frac{\sqrt{n}(\mu_1 - \mu_0)}{2\sigma} + \frac{\sigma \ln(k)}{\sqrt{n}(\mu_1 - \mu_0)} \right\} \\
&= P\left(Z \geq \frac{\sqrt{n}c}{2} + \frac{\ln(k_2)}{\sqrt{n}c} \right)
\end{aligned}
$$

$$= \Phi\left(-\frac{c\sqrt{n}}{2} - \frac{\ln(k)}{c\sqrt{n}}\right)$$

where $\Phi(z)$ is the standard normal distribution function evaluated at z and

$$c = \frac{|\mu_1 - \mu_0|}{\sigma}$$

If $\mu_1 - \mu_0 < 0$ similar calculations show that the probability of misleading evidence when μ_0 is assumed true is given by the same expression. It follows that the probability of misleading evidence when $H_0 = \mu_0$ is true is

$$\text{PMLEV} = \Phi\left(-\frac{c\sqrt{n}}{2} - \frac{\ln(k_2)}{c\sqrt{n}}\right)$$

where

$$c = \frac{|\mu_2 - \mu_1|}{\sigma}$$

and Φ is the standard normal distribution function. The function

$$B(c, k, n) = \Phi\left(-\frac{c\sqrt{n}}{2} - \frac{\ln(k)}{c\sqrt{n}}\right)$$

has been called the **bump function** by Royall.

Also note that c is often called the **effect size** in the social science literature and represents the difference between μ_0 and μ_1 in standard deviation units. The following are rules of thumb for judging the magnitude of the effect size:

- $c \le 0.1$ trivial
- $0.1 < c \le 0.6$ small
- $0.6 < c \le 1.2$ moderate
- $c \ge 1.2$ large

Note that the derivative with respect to c of the bump function is

$$\phi\left(-\frac{c\sqrt{n}}{2} - \frac{\ln(k)}{c\sqrt{n}}\right)\left(-\frac{\sqrt{n}}{2} + \frac{\ln(k)}{c^2\sqrt{n}}\right)$$

which vanishes when

$$\frac{\sqrt{n}}{2} = \frac{\ln(k)}{c^2\sqrt{n}}$$

i.e., when

$$c = \sqrt{\frac{2\ln(k)}{n}} = c^*$$

The second derivative with respect to c is

$$\phi\left(-\frac{c\sqrt{n}}{2} - \frac{\ln(k)}{c\sqrt{n}}\right)\left(-\frac{\sqrt{n}}{2} + \frac{\ln(k)}{c^2\sqrt{n}}\right)^2 \phi\left(-\frac{c\sqrt{n}}{2} - \frac{\ln(k)}{c\sqrt{n}}\right)$$
$$+ \left(-\frac{2\ln(k)}{c^3\sqrt{n}}\right)$$

which is negative when $c = c^*$ so that the bump function has a maximum at $c = c^*$ given by

$$B(c^*, k, n) = \Phi\left(-\frac{c^*\sqrt{n}}{2} - \frac{\ln(k)}{c^*\sqrt{n}}\right) = \Phi(-\sqrt{2\ln(k)})$$

It is well known that

$$\frac{t}{1+t^2}\phi(t) \le \Phi(-t) \le \frac{1}{t}\phi(t)$$

so that

$$\Phi(-\sqrt{2\ln(k)}) \le \frac{1}{\sqrt{2\ln(k)}}\phi(\sqrt{2\ln(k)})$$

$$= \frac{1}{2\sqrt{\pi\ln(k)}}\exp\left\{-(\sqrt{2\ln(k)})^2/2\right\}$$

$$= \frac{1}{2\sqrt{\pi\ln(k)}}\exp\left\{-\ln(k)\right\}$$

$$= \frac{1}{k2\sqrt{\pi\ln(k)}}$$

which is considerably less than the universal bound of $1/k$.

17.2.1 Weak Statistical Evidence

Again, since we are dealing with probability models, it is possible to observe a value, x_{obs}, for which

$$\frac{1}{k} < L(\theta_1, \theta_0; x_{obs}) < k$$

This is called **weak statistical evidence**. We have weak evidence in the example of normally distributed observations if and only if

$$-\ln(k) \leq \left(\bar{x} - \frac{\mu_1 + \mu_0}{2}\right) \frac{n(\mu_1 - \mu_0)}{\sigma^2} \leq \ln(k)$$

If $\mu_1 - \mu_0 > 0$ the condition for weak statistical evidence is that $\bar{x}$ must lie between

$$\frac{\mu_1 + \mu_0}{2} - \frac{\sigma^2}{n(\mu_1 - \mu_0)} \ln(k)$$

and

$$\frac{\mu_1 + \mu_0}{2} + \frac{\sigma^2}{n(\mu_1 - \mu_0)} \ln(k)$$

If we define

$$g_n(\mu_0, \mu_1, k) = \frac{\mu_1 + \mu_0}{2} + \frac{\sigma^2}{n(\mu_1 - \mu_0)} \ln(k)$$

then the condition for weak evidence becomes

$$g_n(\mu_0, \mu_1, 1/k) \leq \bar{x} \leq g_n(\mu_0, \mu_1, k)$$

and the probability of weak evidence is given by

$$\Pr\left\{g_n(\mu_0, \mu_1, 1/k) \leq \bar{X} \leq g_n(\mu_0, \mu_1, k)\right\}$$

which is easily evaluated under H_0 and H_1 since $\bar{X}$ has an $N\left(\mu, \frac{\sigma^2}{n}\right)$ distribution.
Now we note that

$$\frac{\sqrt{n}}{\sigma}[g_n(\mu_0, \mu_1, k) - \mu_0] = \frac{c\sqrt{n}}{2} + \frac{\ln(k)}{c\sqrt{n}}$$

It follows that the probability of weak evidence, $P_{\mu = \mu_0}(\text{WEV})$, is given by

$$\Phi\left(\frac{c\sqrt{n}}{2} + \frac{\ln(k)}{c\sqrt{n}}\right) - \Phi\left(\frac{c\sqrt{n}}{2} - \frac{\ln(k)}{c\sqrt{n}}\right)$$

Similarly

$$\frac{\sqrt{n}}{\sigma}[g_n(\mu_0, \mu_1, k) - \mu_2] = \frac{-c\sqrt{n}}{2} + \frac{\ln(k)}{c\sqrt{n}}$$

It follows that the probability of weak evidence $P_{\mu=\mu_1}(\text{WEV})$ is given by

$$\Phi\left(\frac{c\sqrt{n}}{2} + \frac{\ln(k)}{c\sqrt{n}}\right) - \Phi\left(\frac{c\sqrt{n}}{2} - \frac{\ln(k)}{c\sqrt{n}}\right)$$

If we define

$$W(x,y) = \Phi\left(\frac{c\sqrt{n}}{2} + \frac{\ln(k_1)}{c\sqrt{n}}\right) - \Phi\left(\frac{c\sqrt{n}}{2} - \frac{\ln(k_2)}{c\sqrt{n}}\right)$$

then the two probabilities are given by

$$W_1 = P_1(\text{WEV}) = W(k_2, k_1)$$
$$\text{and}$$
$$W_2 = P_2(\text{WEV}) = W(k_1, k_2)$$

There is nothing that requires the same level of statistical evidence be the same for μ_1 vs μ_0 as for μ_0 vs μ_1. That is we say we have statistical evidence for μ_1 vs μ_0 of level k_1 if $L(\theta_1, \theta_0; x_{obs}) > k_1$ and statistical evidence for μ_0 vs μ_1 of level k_0 if $L(\theta_0, \theta_1; x_{obs}) > k_0$.

We then have the following summary of results for the normal distribution example.

- When H_0 is true the probability of misleading evidence for H_1 at level k_1 defined by $(L_1/L_0 \geq k_1)$ is

$$M_0 = \Phi\left(-\frac{c\sqrt{n}}{2} - \frac{\ln(k_2)}{c\sqrt{n}}\right)$$

- When H_0 is true the probability of weak evidence is

$$W_0 = P_{\mu=\mu_0}\left(\frac{1}{k_0} \leq \frac{L_1}{L_0} \leq k_1\right)$$
$$= \Phi\left(\frac{c\sqrt{n}}{2} + \frac{\ln(k_1)}{c\sqrt{n}}\right) - \Phi\left(\frac{c\sqrt{n}}{2} - \frac{\ln(k_0)}{c\sqrt{n}}\right)$$

- When H_1 is true the probability of misleading evidence for H_0 at level k_0 defined by $(L_0/L_1 \geq k_0$ is

$$M_1 = \Phi\left(-\frac{c\sqrt{n}}{2} - \frac{\ln(k_1)}{c\sqrt{n}}\right)$$

- When H_1 is true the probability of weak evidence is

$$W_1 = P_{\mu=\mu_1} \left(\frac{1}{k_0} \leq \frac{L_2}{L_1} \leq k_1 \right)$$

$$= \Phi \left(\frac{c\sqrt{n}}{2} + \frac{\ln(k_0)}{c\sqrt{n}} \right) - \Phi \left(\frac{c\sqrt{n}}{2} - \frac{\ln(k_1)}{c\sqrt{n}} \right)$$

17.2.2 Sample Size

There is no doubt that one of the questions most asked of a statistician is

How many observations do I need?

Actually the usual question is how many subjects do I need to get a statistically significant result that is publishable? This question is easily answered, so let us consider refining the question.

Suppose that we will observe $X_1, X_2, \ldots, X_n$ assumed independent and identically distributed as normal with mean μ and variance σ^2 assumed known (usually based on past work with similar instruments, and so on). Of interest is a (null) hypothesis $H_0 : \mu = \mu_0$ and an alternative $H_1 : \mu = \mu_1$ where without loss of generality we assume that $\mu_1 > \mu_0$. It is assumed that μ_1 represents a value of μ which is of scientific importance,i.e., if μ_1 is true then a result of scientific or practical importance has been discovered.

The Neyman–Pearson theory has been used for decades to determine sample size is the default method. It is required in submitting grants to NIH, NSF, FDA, etc., as well as in reporting the results of published studies and dissertations. The Neyman–Pearson approach to sample size selection is as follows:

1. Choose a value α for the significance level (usually $\alpha = 0.05$).
2. Choose a value $1 - \beta$ for the power (usually $\beta = 0.20$ so that the power is 0.8).
3. Select the sample size n so that

$$P(\text{Type I error}) = P(\text{reject } H_0 | H_0 \text{ true}) = \alpha$$
$$1 - P(\text{Type II error}) = P(\text{reject } H_0 | H_1 \text{ true}) = 1 - \beta$$

In the case of a normal distribution with known variance we have that

$$P(\text{Type I error}) = P(\overline{X} \geq C | \mu = \mu_0)$$

$$= P \left(\frac{\sqrt{n}(\overline{X} - \mu_0)}{\sigma} \geq \frac{\sqrt{n}(C - \mu_1)}{\sigma} \bigg| \mu = \mu_0 \right)$$

$$= 1 - \Phi \left(\frac{C - \mu_1}{\sigma} \right)$$

and it follows that

$$C = \mu_0 + z_{1-\alpha/2}\frac{\sigma}{\sqrt{n}} = \mu_0 + 1.645\frac{\sigma}{\sqrt{n}} \text{ if } \alpha = 0.05$$

and

$$\text{Power} = P(\overline{X} \geq C | \mu = \mu_1)$$

$$= P\left(\overline{X} \geq \mu_0 + z_{1-\alpha/2}\frac{\sigma}{\sqrt{n}} \middle| \mu = \mu_1\right)$$

$$= P\left(\frac{\sqrt{n}(\overline{X} - \mu_1)}{\sigma} \geq z_{1-\alpha/2} - (\mu_1 - \mu_0)\frac{\sqrt{n}}{\sigma} \middle| \mu = \mu_1\right)$$

$$= 1 - \Phi\left(z_{1-\alpha/2} - (\mu_1 - \mu_0)\frac{\sqrt{n}}{\sigma}\right)$$

$$= 1 - \Phi(z_{1-\alpha/2} - c\sqrt{n})$$

In order to have power $1 - \beta$ we must have

$$\Phi\left(z_{1-\alpha/2} - (\mu_1 - \mu_0)\frac{\sqrt{n}}{\sigma}\right) = \beta$$

i.e.,

$$z_{1-\alpha/2} - (\mu_1 - \mu_0)\frac{\sqrt{n}}{\sigma} = z_\beta$$

or

$$z_{1-\alpha/2} - z_\beta = (\mu_1 - \mu_0)\frac{\sqrt{n}}{\sigma}$$

and it follows that

$$n = \frac{(z_{1-\alpha/2} + z_{1-\beta})^2}{c^2}$$

where

$$c = \frac{\mu_1 - \mu_0}{\sigma}$$

This is the prototype of sample size formulas.

The Neyman-Pearson approach is inadequate when we want to quantify statistical evidence for H_1 vs H_0 we now consider the selection of sample size necessary to quantify statistical evidence. Recall that there are four probabilities involved:

1. The probability of misleading statistical evidence for H_1 when H_0 is true
2. The probability of misleading statistical evidence for H_0 when H_1 is true
3. The probability of weak statistical evidence when H_0 is true
4. The probability of weak evidence when H_1 is true

The analogue to the Type I error probability is the probability of finding misleading evidence for H_1 when H_0 is true. For the normal distribution we have the correspondence for $\alpha = 0.05$ and M_0 given by

$$\alpha = 0.05 \quad M_0 = \Phi\left(-\frac{c\sqrt{n}}{2} - \frac{\ln(8)}{c\sqrt{n}}\right)$$

and if we take $c = 0.5$, a moderate effect size, we have the correspondence

$$\alpha = 0.05 \quad M_0 = \Phi\left(-\frac{\sqrt{n}}{4} - \frac{4\ln(8)}{\sqrt{n}}\right)$$

For the analogue to the Type II error we must be more careful. The probability of failing to find evidence supporting H_1 when H_0 is true is composed of two parts:

1. The probability of misleading evidence in favor of H_0 when H_1 is true
2. The probability of weak evidence when H_1 is true

For the normal distribution we have the correspondence

$$\beta = P(\text{Type II error}) = \Phi\left(z_{1-\alpha/2} - (\mu_2 - \mu_1)\frac{\sqrt{n}}{\sigma}\right)$$

$$M_1 + W_1 = \Phi\left(-\frac{c\sqrt{n}}{2} - \frac{\ln(k_1)}{c\sqrt{n}}\right) + \Phi\left(\frac{c\sqrt{n}}{2} + \frac{\ln(k_1)}{c\sqrt{n}}\right) - \Phi\left(\frac{c\sqrt{n}}{2} - \frac{\ln(k_2)}{c\sqrt{n}}\right)$$

$$= 1 - \Phi\left(\frac{c\sqrt{n}}{2} - \frac{\ln(k_2)}{c\sqrt{n}}\right)$$

$$= \Phi\left(\frac{-c\sqrt{n}}{2} + \frac{\ln(k_2)}{c\sqrt{n}}\right)$$

and if $\beta = 0.2$, $c = 0.5$ and $k_2 = 8$ we have

$$\beta = 0.2 \; ; \; M_2 + W_2 = \Phi\left(-\frac{\sqrt{n}}{4} + \frac{2\ln(8)}{\sqrt{n}}\right)$$

For the Neyman Pearson sample size formula for $\alpha = 0.05$, $\beta = 0.20$ and $c = 0.5$ we get a sample size of

$$n = \frac{(1645 + 0.84)^2}{0.5^2} = 25$$

For this sample size we find that $M_1 + W_1$ is equal to

$$M_1 + W_1 = \Phi\left(-\frac{\sqrt{25}}{4} + \frac{2\ln(8)}{\sqrt{25}}\right) = \Phi(-0.418) = 0.34$$

Thus the conventional sample size formula does not lead to a small probability of finding weak evidence.

Exercises in Royall's book show that the this is true in general, i.e., conventional sample size formulas do not guarantee finding strong evidence.

17.3 Birnbaum's Confidence Concept

Recall Birnbaum's confidence concept which he advocated after becoming skeptical of the likelihood principle.

A concept of statistical evidence is not plausible unless it finds "strong evidence" for H_2 as against H_1 with small probability (α) when H_1 is true and with much larger probability ($1 - \beta$) when H_2 is true.

What the results in the sample size section show is that it is possible in certain cases to satisfy the confidence concept with sufficient observations.

17.4 Combining Evidence

Suppose that we have two independent estimators, t_1 and t_2 of a parameter θ where t_1 is normal with expected value θ and variance v_1 and t_2 is normal with expected value θ and variance v_2. Assume that v_1 and v_2 are known.

The joint density of t_1 and t_2 is

$$f(t_1, t_2; \theta) = \frac{1}{2\pi\sqrt{v_1 v_2}} \exp\left\{-\frac{(t_1 - \theta)^2}{2v_1} - \frac{(t_2 - \theta)^2}{2v_2}\right\}$$

which has logarithm

$$-\ln[2\pi\sqrt{v_1 v_2}] - \frac{(t_1 - \theta)^2}{2v_1} - \frac{(t_2 - \theta)^2}{2v_2}$$

The derivative with respect to θ is thus

$$\frac{(t_1 - \theta)}{v_1} - \frac{t_2 - \theta}{v_2}$$

and hence the maximum likelihood estimate of θ is

$$\widehat{\theta} = \frac{\frac{t_1}{v_1} + \frac{t_2}{v_2}}{\frac{1}{v_1} + \frac{1}{v_2}}$$

At this value of θ the joint density is

$$f(t_1, t_2; \widehat{\theta}) = \frac{1}{2\pi\sqrt{v_1 v_2}} \exp\left\{-\frac{(t_1 - \widehat{\theta})^2}{2v_1} - \frac{(t_2 - \widehat{\theta})^2}{2v_2}\right\}$$

and hence the likelihood for θ is

$$\mathscr{L}(\theta; t_1, t_2) = \frac{f(t_1, t_2; \theta)}{f(t_1, t_2; \widehat{\theta})} = \frac{\frac{1}{2\pi\sqrt{v_1 v_2}} \exp\left\{-\frac{(t_1 - \theta)^2}{2v_1} - \frac{(t_2 - \theta)^2}{2v_2}\right\}}{\frac{1}{2\pi\sqrt{v_1 v_2}} \exp\left\{-\frac{(t_1 - \widehat{\theta})^2}{2v_1} - \frac{(t_2 - \widehat{\theta})^2}{2v_2}\right\}}$$

or

$$\mathscr{L}(\theta; t_1, t_2) = \exp\left\{\frac{t_1\theta}{v_1} + \frac{t_2\theta}{v_2} - \frac{\theta^2}{2v_1} - \frac{\theta^2}{2v_2} - \frac{t_1\widehat{\theta}}{v_1} - \frac{t_2\widehat{\theta}}{v_2} + \frac{\widehat{\theta}^2}{2v_1} + \frac{\widehat{\theta}^2}{2v_2}\right\}$$

$$= \exp\left\{\theta\left(\frac{t_1}{v_1} + \frac{t_2}{v_2}\right) - \frac{\theta^2}{2}\left(\frac{1}{v_1} + \frac{1}{v_2}\right) - \widehat{\theta}\left(\frac{t_1}{v_1} + \frac{t_2}{v_2}\right)\right.$$
$$\left. + \frac{\widehat{\theta}^2}{2}\left(\frac{1}{v_1} + \frac{1}{v_2}\right)\right\}$$

$$= \exp\left\{\theta\widehat{\theta}\left(\frac{1}{v_1} + \frac{1}{v_2}\right) - \frac{\theta^2}{2}\left(\frac{1}{v_1} + \frac{1}{v_2}\right) - \frac{\widehat{\theta}^2}{2}\left(\frac{1}{v_1} + \frac{1}{v_2}\right)\right\}$$

$$= \exp\left\{-\frac{1}{2}\left(\frac{1}{v_1} + \frac{1}{v_2}\right)\left(\theta^2 - 2\theta\widehat{\theta} + \widehat{\theta}^2\right)\right\}$$

$$= \exp\left\{-\left(\frac{1}{v_1} + \frac{1}{v_2}\right)\frac{(\theta - \widehat{\theta})^2}{2}\right\}$$

$$= \exp\left\{\frac{(\theta - \widehat{\theta})^2}{2v}\right\}$$

where

$$v = \frac{1}{\frac{1}{v_1} + \frac{1}{v_2}}$$

which is a normal likelihood centered at $\widehat{\theta}$ and curvature v.

This is a likelihood version of the standard result that to combine unbiased uncorrelated estimators weight inversely as their variance and divide the result by the sum of the weights.

In general note that if we have x_1 observations from $f(x; \theta)$ and independent observations x_2 from $f(x; \theta)$ then the evidence for θ_1 vs θ_0 based on (x_1, x_2) is

$$\frac{f(x_1, x_2; \theta_1)}{f(x_1, x_2; \theta_0)} = \left[\frac{f(x_1; \theta_1)}{f(x_1; \theta_0)}\right] \left[\frac{f(x_2; \theta_1)}{f(x_2; \theta_0)}\right]$$

i.e., evidence is multiplicative.

17.5 Exercises

1. Suppose that $X_1, X_2, \ldots, X_n$ are iid, each Poisson with parameter λ. Let $k = 8$, $n = 1, 10, 25$. Draw graphs of the probability of misleading evidence for $\lambda_1 = 2$ vs $\lambda_0 = 1$.
2. Repeat Exercise 1 for the binomial with $n = 10, 25, 100, 1000$ and $p = 0.6$ vs $p = 0.5$.

Chapter 18
Pure Likelihood Methods and Nuisance Parameters

18.1 Nuisance Parameters

18.1.1 Introduction

In most, if not all, statistical problems we have not one parameter but many. However, we are often interested in inference or statements on just one of the parameters. Suppose then that the parameter of interest is θ and that the remaining parameters, called nuisance parameters, are denoted by γ.

The elimination of nuisance parameters so as to focus on the parameter of interest is a complex problem in statistics with no universal solution. In fact, in some cases, there may be no way to overcome the problem without additional related data.

Recall that a statistical model is a collection (family) of probability distributions. The family is parametric if it can be indexed by a k-dimensional parameter vector Δ where $\Delta \in R^k$. In most applications the elements of Δ consist of two types:

- Parameters of primary interest denoted by θ
- Parameters not of primary interest denoted by γ and called nuisance parameters

The most important case occurs when

$$\Delta = (\theta, \gamma)$$

and $\theta \in \Theta \subseteq R^p, \gamma \in \Gamma \subseteq R^{k-p}$

The parameters θ and γ are said to be

variation independent if $\Delta = \Theta \times \Gamma$

Example. Let X be normal with mean μ and variance σ^2. Then μ and σ^2 are variation independent and we might have

© Springer International Publishing Switzerland 2014
C.A. Rohde, *Introductory Statistical Inference with the Likelihood Function*, DOI 10.1007/978-3-319-10461-4_18

$$\theta = \mu, \gamma = \sigma^2 \quad \text{or} \quad \theta = \sigma^2, \gamma = \mu$$

Example. Again let X be normal with mean μ and variance σ^2 with σ^2 known. We might have $\theta = |\mu|$ and $\gamma = \text{sign}(\mu)$.

Suppose now that we have n observations $y_1, y_2, \ldots, y_n$ which are observed values of independent random variables $Y_1, Y_2, \ldots, Y_n$. The joint density is then

$$f_y(y; \delta) = \prod_{i=1}^{n} f_{Y_i}(y_i; \delta_i)$$

There are two important situations

(1) $\delta_i = (\theta, \gamma)$
(2) $\delta_i = (\theta, \gamma_i)$

In the first case the number of nuisance parameters is independent of the sample size while in the second case the number of nuisance parameters increases with the number of observations.

18.1.2   Neyman-Scott Problem

Suppose that $Y_1, Y_2, \ldots, Y_n$ are independent with normal distributions where

$$E(Y_i) = E\left(\begin{bmatrix} Y_{i1} \\ Y_{i2} \end{bmatrix}\right) = \begin{bmatrix} \mu_{i1} \\ \mu_{i2} \end{bmatrix}$$
$$\text{and}$$
$$\text{var}(Y_i) = \text{var}\left(\begin{bmatrix} Y_{i1} \\ Y_{i2} \end{bmatrix}\right) = \begin{bmatrix} \sigma^2 & 0 \\ 0 & \sigma^2 \end{bmatrix}$$

and that

$$\theta = \sigma^2 \; ; \; \gamma = (\mu_1, \mu_2, \ldots, \mu_n)$$

The joint density, $f(y; \sigma^2, \mu_1, \mu_2, \ldots, \mu_n)$, is given by

$$\prod_{i=1}^{n}(2\pi\sigma^2)^{-1} \exp\left\{-\frac{1}{2\sigma^2}(y_{i1} - \mu_i)^2 - \frac{1}{2\sigma^2}(y_{i2} - \mu_i)^2\right\}$$

Clearly the maximum likelihood estimate of μ_i is $\overline{y}_i$ which yields a maximized likelihood with respect to γ of

$$(2\pi\sigma^2)^{-1} \exp\left\{-\frac{1}{2\sigma^2} \sum_{i=1}^{n} S_i^2\right\}$$

where

$$S_i^2 = \sum_{j=1}^{2} (y_{ij} - \overline{y}_i)^2$$

The log likelihood is given by

$$-n\ln(2\pi\sigma^2) - \frac{1}{2\sigma^2} \sum_{i=1}^{2} S_i^2$$

which has the first derivative

$$-\frac{n}{\sigma^2} - \frac{1}{2\sigma^4} \sum_{i=1}^{n} S_i^2$$

It follows that the maximum likelihood estimate of σ^2 is given by

$$\widehat{\sigma^2} = \frac{1}{2n} \sum_{i=1}^{n} S_i^2$$

Recall that

$$\frac{S_i^2}{\sigma^2} \sim \text{chi-square}(1)$$

so that

$$E(S_i^2) = \sigma^2 \quad \text{and} \quad \text{var}(S_i^2) = 2\sigma^4$$

It follows that

$$E(\widehat{\sigma}^2) = \frac{\sigma^2}{2} \quad \text{and} \quad \text{var}(\widehat{\sigma}^2) = \frac{\sigma^4}{2n}$$

and hence

$$\widehat{\sigma}^2 \xrightarrow{p} \frac{\sigma^2}{2}$$

i.e., $\widehat{\sigma}^2$ is not a consistent estimator for σ^2.

18.2   Elimination Methods

Assume that the basic model consists of a sample space $\mathcal{X}$ and a family of distributions P indexed by two parameters $\theta \in \Theta$ and $\gamma \in \Gamma$, which may be vector valued.

We also assume, for simplicity, that the full parameter space Δ is equal to $\Theta \times \Gamma$, i.e., θ and γ are variation independent.

The following is a partial list (with overlap) of techniques which have been used to eliminate the parameters in Γ. In general some information about θ is lost when any of these approaches are used:

- Replace the model $(\mathcal{X}, P_{(\theta, \gamma)})$ by a new model $(\mathcal{T}, Q_\theta)$ where, as the notation indicates, the family Q is indexed by θ alone. **Marginal** and **conditional** likelihoods fit into this category.
- Replace the parameter γ by an estimate $\widetilde{\gamma}$ and use the model $(\mathcal{X}, P_{(\theta, \widetilde{\gamma})})$. **Profile** and **estimated** likelihoods are examples of this type of approach as are the usual methods of inference in generalized linear models and other types of regression models.
- Use a **pivot** or other argument to obtain a statistic whose distribution is free of the nuisance parameter. Inference on θ is then based on this statistic.
- Restrict attention to a class of inference procedures such as unbiased estimators, unbiased tests, fixed size confidence intervals, etc., whose repeated sampling properties are free of the nuisance parameter.
- Eliminate the nuisance parameter from the risk function (or estimating equations) by maximization (minimization) and choose the decision rule for θ based on this new risk function (estimating equation).
- Choose a prior for γ, integrate out (marginalize) over γ, and base inference on the remaining likelihood which is called the **integrated likelihood**.
- Use an indirect method to obtain a statistics whose distribution depends only on θ.

18.3   Evidence in the Presence of Nuisance Parameters

From the perspective of this chapter, i.e., "what do the data say?" about θ, The likelihood ratio

$$\frac{L(\theta_2; x)}{L(\theta_1; x)}$$

measures the statistical evidence for θ_2 vs θ_1. Thus the basic methodology is to "look at the likelihood function." The problem is that when the dimension of $\Theta = p > 1$ it is hard to visualize and understand the likelihood function.

Example. In a $N(\mu, \sigma^2)$ problem we may be interested in μ alone. We want to know "What do the data say" about μ? In this analysis σ^2 is a **nuisance parameter**.
   The likelihood ratio for comparing μ_2 to μ_1 is, after simplification,

$$\exp\left\{ \frac{n(\mu_2 - \mu_1)}{\sigma^2} \left[\bar{x} - \frac{\mu_2 + \mu_1}{2}\right]\right\}$$

and the presence of σ^2 shows that the evidence is dependent on the value of σ^2.

Example. In the two-binomial problem where the model for $P_{(\theta_1, \theta_2)}$ $(X = x, Y = y)$ is

$$\binom{n_1}{x} \theta_1^x (1 - \theta_1)^{n_1 - x} \binom{n_2}{y} \theta_2^y (1 - \theta_2)^{n_2 - y}$$

we may ask "what do the data say" about

$$\theta_1, \quad \text{or} \quad \theta_2,$$
$$\frac{\theta_1}{\theta_2} \text{ (the relative risk)}$$
$$\frac{\theta_1(1-\theta_1)}{\theta_2/(1-\theta_2)} \text{ (the odds ratio)}$$

It would be possible to do a contour plot of $L(\theta_1, \theta_2; x)$ which would completely represent the evidence about θ_1, θ_2. But we would like to break the problem down into components and look at them one at a time.

   Suppose then that the parameter is (θ, γ) where θ is of interest and γ is the nuisance parameter. The question is then: "What do the data say" about θ?

- That is, we want to look at the evidence about θ_2 vs θ_1.
- Which is better supported and by how much?
- The problem is that the likelihood ratio

$$\frac{L(\theta_2, \gamma_0; x)}{L(\theta_1, \gamma_0; x)}$$

measures the support for θ_2 vs θ_1 when $\gamma = \gamma_0$. In general this depends on the specific value of γ_0.

18.3.1   Orthogonal Parameters

Sometimes the ratio is free of γ, i.e., suppose the likelihood function factors as

$$L(\theta, \gamma; x) = L_1(\theta; x) L_2(\gamma; x)$$

In this case

$$\frac{L(\theta_2, \gamma; x)}{L(\theta_1, \gamma; x)} = \frac{L_1(\theta_2; x)L_2(\gamma; x)}{L_1(\theta_1; x)L_2(\gamma; x)} = \frac{L_1(\theta_2; x)}{L_1(\theta_1; x)}$$

so that $L_1(\theta; x)$ may be used as a likelihood for θ. In such a case we say that θ and γ are **orthogonal parameters**.

Example. In the case of two independent binomials the likelihood for θ_1 and θ_2 is

$$\theta_1^x (1 - \theta_1)^{n_1 - x} \theta_2^y (1 - \theta_2)^{n_2 - y} = L_1(\theta_1)L(\theta_2)$$

and hence

$$L_1(\theta_1; x) = \theta_1^x (1 - \theta_1)^{n_1 - x} \text{ is the likelihood function for } \theta_1$$
$$L(\theta_2; y) = \theta_2^y (1 - \theta_2)^{n_2 - y} \text{ is the likelihood function for } \theta_2$$

Example. Suppose that X and Y are independent Poisson with means λ_1, λ_2 and that we are interested in

$$\theta = \frac{\lambda_1}{\lambda_1 + \lambda_2}$$

The joint density of X and Y is given by

$$f_{X,Y}(x, y) = \frac{\lambda_1^x \lambda_2^y e^{-\lambda_1} e^{-\lambda_2}}{x! y!} \quad x, y = 0, 1, 2, \ldots$$

where $0 < \lambda_1 < \infty$ and $0 < \lambda_2 < \infty$. We can reparametrize as

$$\theta = \frac{\lambda_1}{\lambda_1 + \lambda_2} , \quad \gamma = \lambda_1 + \lambda_2$$

Thus

$$\lambda_1 = \theta\gamma \quad \lambda_2 = \gamma - \lambda_1 = \gamma(1 - \theta)$$

The joint density of X and Y in terms of the new parameters is

$$f_{X,Y}(x, y) = \frac{(\theta\gamma)^x e^{-\theta\gamma} [\gamma(1 - \theta)]^y e^{-\theta(1-\gamma)}}{x! y!}$$

$$= \frac{\theta^x (1 - \theta)^y \gamma^{x+y} e^{-\gamma}}{x! y!}$$

It follows that

$$L_1(\theta; x, y) \propto \theta^x (1 - \theta)^y \text{ and } L_2(\gamma; x, y) \propto \gamma^{x+y} e^{-\gamma}$$

More generally if X_i, Y_i are independent observations from the above model then

$$L(\lambda_1, \lambda_2) \propto \lambda_1^{\sum_i x_i} e^{-n\lambda_1} \lambda_2^{\sum_i y_i} e^{-n\lambda_2}$$
$$L(\theta, \gamma) \propto \theta^{\sum_i x_i} (1 - \theta)^{\sum_i y_i} \gamma^{\sum_i x_i + \sum_i y_i} e^{-n\gamma}$$

so that

$$L_1(\theta) \propto \theta^{\sum_i x_i} (1 - \theta)^{\sum_i y_i}$$
$$\text{and}$$
$$L_2(\gamma) \propto \gamma^{\sum_i x_i + \sum_i y_i} e^{-n\gamma}$$

What if we reparametrize differently? For example, let $\lambda_2 = \gamma$ be the nuisance parameter. Then

$$(\lambda_1, \lambda_2) \mapsto (\theta, \gamma) \quad \text{and} \quad \theta = \frac{\lambda_1}{\lambda_1 + \lambda_2}, \quad \gamma = \lambda_2$$

and hence

$$\lambda_1 = \frac{\theta}{1 - \theta} \gamma, \quad \lambda_2 = \gamma$$

In this case

$$L(\theta, \gamma; x, y) \propto \left(\frac{\theta}{1 - \theta} \right)^x \gamma^{x+y} e^{-\gamma} e^{-\frac{\theta\gamma}{1-\theta}}$$

and the parameters are not orthogonal:

- The point is that it is not obvious whether an orthogonal reparametrization exists, i.e., does there exist $\gamma(\lambda_1, \lambda_2)$ such that $(\lambda_1, \lambda_2) \mapsto (\theta, \gamma)$ is 1–1 and $L(\theta, \gamma)$ factors?
- And even when there is an orthogonal reparametrization it might be hard to find.

18.3.2 Orthogonal Reparametrizations

If there exists an orthogonal reparametrization, $L(\theta)$ is unique. That is, even if there is more than one way to reparametrize in terms of θ and an orthogonal nuisance parameter γ, the likelihood for θ is unique.

One very important special case when orthogonalization is possible is when X has a p-dimensional normal distribution, i.e.,

$$X \overset{d}{\sim} \text{MVN}(\boldsymbol{\mu}, \boldsymbol{\Sigma})$$

where Σ is fixed and known but not necessarily diagonal and

$$\boldsymbol{\mu} = (\boldsymbol{\mu}_1, \boldsymbol{\mu}_2)$$

where $\boldsymbol{\mu}_1$ is q dimensional and $\boldsymbol{\mu}_2$ is $p - q$ dimensional. This model can be reparametrized in terms of a mean vector $\boldsymbol{\theta} = (\boldsymbol{\theta}_1, \theta 2)$, where $\boldsymbol{\theta}_1$ equals $\boldsymbol{\mu}_1$ and is orthogonal to $\boldsymbol{\theta}_2$. Moreover this orthogonal likelihood is the one obtained from the marginal distribution of $\boldsymbol{X}_1$.

Define $\boldsymbol{\theta} = \boldsymbol{A}\boldsymbol{\mu}$, where

$$\boldsymbol{A} = \begin{bmatrix} \boldsymbol{I} & \boldsymbol{0} \\ -\boldsymbol{\Sigma}_{21}\boldsymbol{\Sigma}_{11}^{-1} & \boldsymbol{I} \end{bmatrix}$$

The likelihood for $\boldsymbol{\mu}$ is proportional to

$$\exp\left\{-\frac{1}{2}(\boldsymbol{y} - \boldsymbol{\mu})^{\top}\boldsymbol{\Sigma}^{-1}(\boldsymbol{y} - \boldsymbol{\mu})\right\}$$

so the likelihood for $\boldsymbol{\theta} = \boldsymbol{A}^{-1}\boldsymbol{\mu}$ is

$$\exp\left\{-\frac{1}{2}(\boldsymbol{y} - \boldsymbol{A}^{-1}\boldsymbol{\theta})^{\top}\boldsymbol{\Sigma}^{-1}(\boldsymbol{y} - \boldsymbol{A}^{-1}\boldsymbol{\theta})\right\}$$

which may be rewritten as

$$\exp\left\{-\frac{1}{2}(\boldsymbol{A}\boldsymbol{y} - \boldsymbol{\theta})^{\top}[\boldsymbol{A}\boldsymbol{\Sigma}\boldsymbol{A}^{\top}]^{-1}(\boldsymbol{A}\boldsymbol{y} - \boldsymbol{\theta})\right\}$$

Now note that

$$\boldsymbol{A}\boldsymbol{y} - \boldsymbol{\theta} = \begin{bmatrix} \boldsymbol{I} & \boldsymbol{0} \\ -\boldsymbol{\Sigma}_{21}\boldsymbol{\Sigma}_{11}^{-1} & \boldsymbol{I} \end{bmatrix}\begin{bmatrix} \boldsymbol{y}_1 \\ \boldsymbol{y}_2 \end{bmatrix} - \begin{bmatrix} \boldsymbol{\theta}_1 \\ \boldsymbol{\theta}_2 \end{bmatrix} = \begin{bmatrix} \boldsymbol{y}_1 \\ \boldsymbol{y}_2^* \end{bmatrix}$$

and that

$$\boldsymbol{A}\boldsymbol{\Sigma}\boldsymbol{A}^{\top} = \begin{bmatrix} \boldsymbol{I} & \boldsymbol{0} \\ -\boldsymbol{\Sigma}_{21}\boldsymbol{\Sigma}_{11}^{-1} & \boldsymbol{I} \end{bmatrix}\begin{bmatrix} \boldsymbol{\Sigma}_{11} & \boldsymbol{\Sigma}_{12} \\ \boldsymbol{\Sigma}_{21} & \boldsymbol{\Sigma}_{22} \end{bmatrix}\begin{bmatrix} \boldsymbol{I} & -\boldsymbol{\Sigma}_{11}^{-1}\boldsymbol{\Sigma}_{12} \\ \boldsymbol{0} & \boldsymbol{I} \end{bmatrix}$$

$$= \begin{bmatrix} \boldsymbol{\Sigma}_{11} & \boldsymbol{0} \\ \boldsymbol{0} & \boldsymbol{\Sigma}_{22} - \boldsymbol{\Sigma}_{21}\boldsymbol{\Sigma}_{11}^{-1}\boldsymbol{\Sigma}_{12} \end{bmatrix}$$

It follows that the likelihood for $\boldsymbol{\theta}$ is proportional to

$$\exp\left\{-\frac{1}{2}(\boldsymbol{y}_1 - \boldsymbol{\theta}_1)^{\top}\boldsymbol{\Sigma}_{11}^{-1}(\boldsymbol{y}_1 - \boldsymbol{\theta}_1)\right\}\exp\left\{-\frac{1}{2}(\boldsymbol{y}_2^* - \boldsymbol{\theta}_2)^{\top}[\boldsymbol{\Sigma}_{22}^{-1} - \boldsymbol{\Sigma}_{21}\boldsymbol{\Sigma}_{11}^{-1}\boldsymbol{\Sigma}_{12}]^{-1}(\boldsymbol{y}_2^* - \boldsymbol{\theta}_2)\right\}$$

It is clear that the orthogonal likelihood for $\theta_1 = \mu_1$ is the first term which is simply the likelihood for μ_1 based on the marginal distribution of y_1.

This result generalizes directly: for any linear function $\theta = \ell^\top \mu$ of interest. Reparametrize in terms of

$$\theta = L\mu \quad \text{where} \quad L = \begin{bmatrix} \ell^\top \\ L_1 \end{bmatrix} \quad \text{is non-singular}$$

The distribution of $Y^* = LY$ is MVN$(\theta, L\Sigma L^\top)$ and the above result applies so that the likelihood function for $\ell^\top \mu$ is that from the marginal distribution of $\ell^\top Y$, i.e., from a N $(\ell^\top \mu, \ell^\top \Sigma \ell)$ distribution.

We can't always orthogonalize, however. For example, In an N (μ, σ^2) model where we are interested in $\theta = \mu$, there is no $\gamma(\mu, \sigma^2)$ such that

$$(\mu, \sigma^2) \mapsto (\theta, \gamma) \quad \text{is 1-1 and } \theta, \gamma \text{ are orthogonal}$$

18.4 Varieties of Likelihood

In problems involving nuisance parameters various kinds of likelihoods have been introduced. These include:

True Likelihoods:

1. Marginal likelihood
2. Conditional likelihood

True likelihoods are characterized by the fact that they are based on the distribution of a statistic S which is **observable** and whose distribution depends only on the parameter of interest.

Pseudo-likelihoods:

1. Estimated likelihood (also called sliced likelihood)
2. Profile likelihood (also called concentrated likelihood)
3. Modified or adjusted profile likelihood
4. Partial likelihood
5. Composite likelihood
6. Quasi-likelihood
7. Canonical likelihood
8. Penalized likelihood
9. Empirical likelihood
10. Approximate likelihood
11. Pivotal likelihood
12. Predictive likelihood

13. h likelihood
14. Induced likelihood
15. Indirect likelihood
16. Many others

The pseudo-likelihoods are derived from the full likelihood of the observations and are not, in general, observable.

Example. The profile likelihood for μ in a normal (μ, σ^2) model is obtained by maximizing

$$(2\pi\sigma^2)^{-n/2} \exp\left\{-\frac{1}{2\sigma^2} \sum_{i=1}^{n} (x_i - \mu)^2\right\}$$

with respect to σ^2 for fixed μ. It is easy to show that

$$\tilde{\sigma}^2(\mu) = \frac{1}{n} \sum_{i=1}^{n} (x_i - \mu)^2$$

Hence the profile likelihood for μ is proportional to

$$\left[\sum_{i=1}^{n} (x_i - \mu)^2\right]^{-n/2}$$

This is maximized when $\mu = \overline{x}$ so that the profile likelihood is given by

$$\left[\frac{\sum_{i=1}^{n} (x_i - \overline{x})^2}{\sum_{i=1}^{n} (x_i - \mu)^2}\right]^{n/2}$$

since

$$\sum_{i=1}^{n} (x_i - \mu)^2 = \sum_{i=1}^{n} (x_i - \overline{x})^2 + n(\mu - \overline{x})^2$$

the profile likelihood is given by

$$\left\{\frac{1}{1 + \frac{t^2(\mu)}{n-1}}\right\}^{n/2}$$

where

$$t^2(\mu) = \frac{n(\mu - \overline{x})^2}{s^2}$$

is the square of the Student's t statistic.

18.5 Information Loss

A major concern in reducing the experiment to another experiment, based on a statistic, is the amount of information lost in the reduction.

If nuisance parameters γ are present we suppose that there are statistics U and V such that

$$f(x; \theta, \gamma) = f_V(v; \theta, \gamma) f_{U|V}(u; v, \theta, \gamma) f_{X|U,V}(x; u, v, \theta, \gamma)$$

If x is a one to one function of (u, v) then V is **partially sufficient** for θ if

$$f_{U|V}(u; v, \theta, \gamma) = f_{U|V}(u; \gamma, v)$$

i.e., the distribution of U given V does not depend on θ.

If x is in a one-to-one correspondence with (u, v) and V is degenerate then U is **partially ancillary** for θ if

$$f_{U|V}(u; v, \theta, \gamma) = f_U(u; \gamma)$$

i.e., the distribution of U V does not depend on θ.

In both these cases data reduction can take place. We must assume, however, that the amount of information in the ignored factor of the likelihood provides little or no information about the parameter of interest. Unfortunately, all attempts to formalize a concept of lack of information have been lacking in generality. Jorgenson

18.6 Marginal Likelihood

In some circumstances we can find a statistic S that has a distribution which depends on θ but does not depend on γ. In this case $f_S(s, \theta)$ is a true likelihood and is called the **marginal likelihood** of θ. In general if S, V is a sufficient statistic for (θ, γ) and we have that

$$f_{U,V}(u, v; \theta, \gamma) = f_V(v; \theta) f_{U|V}(u; v, \theta, \gamma)$$

The function

$$f_V(v; \theta)$$

is the basis for the marginal likelihood of θ. This implies that there is little information about θ contained in the second factor.

Example. If $Y_1, Y_2, \ldots, Y_n$ are iid $N(\mu, \sigma^2)$, then the distribution of

$$S^2 = \sum_{i=1}^{n} (Y_i - \bar{Y})^2$$

does not depend on μ, so its distribution may be used as a marginal likelihood. More precisely, the distribution of $U = S^2/\sigma^2$ is chi-square with $n - 1$ degrees of freedom, i.e.,

$$f_U(u) = \frac{u^{\frac{n-1}{2}-1} \exp\left\{-\frac{u}{2}\right\}}{2^{\frac{n-1}{2}} \Gamma\left(\frac{n-1}{2}\right)}$$

It follows that the distribution of

$$V = S^2 = \sigma^2 U$$

is given by

$$f_V(v, \sigma^2) = \frac{v^{\frac{n-1}{2}-1} \exp\left\{-\frac{v}{2\sigma^2}\right\}}{2^{\frac{n-1}{2}} \Gamma\left(\frac{n-1}{2}\right) (\sigma^2)^{\frac{n-1}{2}}}$$

which defines the marginal likelihood for σ^2.

18.7   Conditional Likelihood

In some circumstances we can find a statistic S such that the distribution of Y given S depends on θ but does not depend on γ, the nuisance parameter. In this case $f_{Y|S}(y, \theta)$ is a true likelihood and is called the **conditional likelihood** of θ.

More generally, if S is a statistic such that

$$f(x; \theta, \gamma) = f_U(u; \theta, \gamma) f_{X|U}(x; \theta, u)$$

then the likelihood based on $f_{X|U}(x; \theta, u)$ is called a conditional likelihood. In this case the factor $f_U(u; \theta, \gamma)$ should not contain much information about θ. Note that in general the maximum of this likelihood is not the same as the overall maximum likelihood estimate.

Example. Let X and Y be independent binomial, n_1, p_1 and n_2, p_2, respectively. Interest focuses on the odds ratio

$$\theta = \frac{\frac{p_2}{1-p_2}}{\frac{p_1}{1-p_1}}$$

Consider the conditional distribution of Y given $S = X + Y$:

$$
\begin{aligned}
f_{Y|S}(y|s) &= \frac{P(Y = y, S = s)}{P(S = s)} \\
&= \frac{P(Y = y, X = s - y)}{P(S = s)} \\
&= \frac{\binom{n_1}{s-y}\binom{n_2}{y}p_1^{s-y}(1-p_1)^{n_1-s+y}p_2^y(1-p_2)^{n_2-y}}{\sum_z \binom{n_1}{s-z}\binom{n_2}{z}p_1^{s-z}(1-p_1)^{n_1-s+z}p_2^z(1-p_2)^{n_2-z}} \\
&= \frac{\binom{n_1}{s-y}\binom{n_2}{y}\theta^y}{\sum_z \binom{n_1}{s-z}\binom{n_2}{z}\theta^z}
\end{aligned}
$$

This distribution is known as the non-central hypergeometric distribution with parameters n_1, n_2, s, and non-centrality parameter θ. It forms the basis of Fisher's exact test in frequentist statistics. Note that the maximum of this likelihood is not the maximum likelihood estimate obtained by maximizing the full likelihood.

Note that both marginal and conditional likelihoods are true likelihoods. They arise, however, mainly in exponential families and in group families of distributions.

18.7.1 Estimated Likelihoods

Since we can't always orthogonalize or find marginal or conditional likelihoods how do we eliminate nuisance parameters?

One simple idea would be to estimate the nuisance parameters and consider the likelihood function for θ with the nuisance parameters replaced by the estimate, i.e., use

$$
L_e(\theta) = L(\theta, \widehat{\gamma})
$$

which is called the **estimated likelihood**.

Usually the estimate is chosen to be a consistent estimator of γ, e.g., the maximum likelihood estimate.

Consider the probability of misleading evidence at

$$
\theta = \theta_0 + \frac{c}{\sqrt{ni_{\theta\theta}}}
$$

We have that

$$
P_{\theta_0}\left[\frac{L_e(\theta)}{L_e(\theta_0)}\right] \to \Phi\left(-(1 - \rho_{\theta\gamma}^2)^{\frac{1}{2}}\left[\frac{c}{2} + \frac{\ln(k)}{c}\right]\right)
$$

where

$$\begin{bmatrix} i_{\theta\theta} & i_{\theta\gamma} \\ i_{\gamma\theta} & i_{\gamma\gamma} \end{bmatrix} \quad \text{is the information matrix}$$

and

$$\rho_{\theta\gamma}^2 = \frac{i_{\theta\gamma}^2}{i_{\theta\theta} i_{\gamma\gamma}}$$

Reference: Royall [44] gives the details.

If, $\rho_{\theta\gamma} \neq 0$, the probability of misleading evidence can be large. In fact the maximum value is

$$\Phi\left(-\sqrt{1 - \rho_{\theta\gamma}^2} \sqrt{2\ln(k)}\right)$$

which approaches $\Phi(0) = \frac{1}{2}$ as $|\rho_{\theta\gamma}| \to 1$. Thus, with estimated likelihood there is no guaranteed bound on the probability of misleading evidence, even in large samples.

Example. In the $N(\mu, \sigma^2)$ problem the likelihood function is

$$L(\mu, \sigma^2) \propto \frac{1}{2\sigma^2}^{\frac{n}{2}} \exp\left\{-\frac{1}{2\sigma^2} \sum_{i=1}^{n}(x_i - \mu)^2\right\}$$

The estimated likelihood is obtained by substituting the maximum likelihood estimate of σ^2, i.e.,

$$\hat{\sigma}^2 = \frac{1}{n} \sum_{i=1}^{n}(x_i - \bar{x})^2$$

so that

$$L_e(\mu) = L(\mu, \hat{\sigma}^2) \propto \exp\left\{-\frac{n \sum_{i=1}^{n}(x_i - \mu)^2}{2 \sum_{i=1}^{n}(x_i - \bar{x})^2}\right\}$$

The estimated likelihood is given by

$$L_e \propto \exp\left\{-\frac{t^2}{n-1}\right\}$$

where t is the Student's t statistic with $n - 1$ degrees of freedom.

Note that the estimated likelihood is not invariant under reparametrization.

18.8   Profile Likelihood

18.8.1   Introduction

We consider the situation where θ is the parameter of interest and γ is the nuisance parameter (γ may be vector valued). Thus the complete likelihood is given by

$$\text{Lik}\,(\theta; \gamma, x)$$

The **profile likelihood** for θ is defined by

$$\text{Lik}_p(\theta; x) = \max_{\gamma} \text{Lik}(\theta, \gamma, x) = \text{Lik}(\theta, \widehat{\gamma}(\theta))$$

where $\widehat{\gamma}(\theta)$ denotes the value of γ which maximizes the likelihood $\text{Lik}(\theta, \gamma, x)$ for fixed θ. The profile likelihood is not a true or genuine likelihood and hence it does not obey the universal bound for the probability of misleading evidence. If the likelihood is orthogonal then use of the profile likelihood will uncover the orthogonal likelihood.

Example. Let $X_1, X_2, \ldots, X_n$ be iid each $N\,(\theta, 1)$ and let Y be independent of the X_i's with pdf which is $N\,(\lambda, \exp\{-n\theta^2\}$. The parameter of interest is θ and λ is the nuisance parameter. The joint density of $X_1, X_2, \ldots, X_n$, and Y is given by

$$f(\boldsymbol{x}, y; \theta, \lambda) = \left[(2\pi)^{-n/2} \exp\left\{ -\frac{1}{2} \sum_{i=1}^{n}(x_i - \theta)^2 \right\} \right] \left[(2\pi \exp\{-n\theta^2\})^{-1/2} \exp\left\{ -\frac{(y - \lambda)^2}{2e^{-n\theta^2}} \right\} \right]$$

$$= (2\pi)^{-(n+1)/2} \exp\left\{ -\frac{1}{2} \sum_{i=1}^{n} x_i^2 + n\overline{x}\theta - \frac{(y - \lambda)^2}{2e^{-n\theta^2}} \right\}$$

where $\overline{x}$ is the sample mean of the x_i's.

The log of the joint density is given by

$$-\frac{(n+1)}{2}\ln(2\pi) - \frac{1}{2}\sum_{i=1}^{n} x_i^2 = n\overline{x}\theta - \frac{(y - \lambda)^2}{2e^{-n\theta^2}}$$

and for fixed θ the maximum likelihood estimate of λ is given by the solution to

$$\frac{2(y - \lambda)}{2e^{-n\theta^2}} = 0$$

so that $\widehat{\lambda}(\theta) = y$.

It follows that the profile likelihood for θ is given by

$$f(\boldsymbol{x}, y; \theta, \lambda)\Big|_{\lambda=\widehat{\lambda}(\theta)} = (2\pi)^{-(n+1)/2} \exp\left\{-\frac{1}{2}\sum_{i=1}^{n} x_i^2 + n\overline{x}\theta\right\}$$

If we used the profile likelihood to measure the evidence for θ_2 vs θ_1 we would find

$$\frac{\mathrm{Lik}_p(\theta_2)}{\mathrm{Lik}_p(\theta_1)} = \frac{e^{n\overline{x}\theta_2}}{e^{n\overline{x}\theta_1}} = e^{n\overline{x}(\theta_2-\theta_1)}$$

Consider now the probability of misleading evidence when $\theta_1 = 0$ and $\theta_2 = \theta > 0$

$$P_{\theta_1}\left(\frac{\mathrm{Lik}_p(\theta_2)}{\mathrm{Lik}_p(\theta_1)} \geq k\right) = P_0\left(e^{n\overline{X}\theta} \geq k\right)$$

$$= P_0(n\overline{X}\theta \geq \ln(k))$$

$$= P_0\left(\sqrt{n}(\overline{X}) \geq \frac{\ln(k)}{\sqrt{n}}\right)$$

$$= 1 - \Phi\left(\frac{\ln(k)}{\sqrt{n}}\right)$$

which tends to $1/2$ as n increases. Thus the universal bound does not hold in general for profile likelihoods.

Note that in this example it would be foolish to use the profile likelihood for the elimination of the nuisance parameter λ. The marginal distribution of $\overline{X}$ is normal with mean θ and variance $1/n$ which does not depend on λ. Hence we may base a marginal likelihood on

$$f_{\overline{X}}(\overline{x}; \theta) = (\sqrt{2\pi/n})^{-n/2} \exp\left\{-\frac{n(\overline{x}-\theta)^2}{2}\right\}$$

This is maximized when $\theta = \overline{x}$, so a marginal likelihood for θ is given by

$$\mathrm{Lik}_p(\theta, \boldsymbol{x}, y) = \exp\left\{\frac{-n(\theta-\overline{x})^2}{2}\right\}$$

which is the normal likelihood with $\sigma^2 = 1/n$ and since $\overline{X}$ is $\mathrm{N}\,(\theta, 1/n)$ the probabilities of misleading evidence (and weak evidence) have the same properties of those derived previously for the normal distribution with known variance.

18.8.2 Misleading Evidence Using Profile Likelihoods

Despite the fact that profile likelihoods do not obey the universal bound we can consider their use as if it were a true likelihood and investigate the consequences.

Royall [44] proves that when γ has a fixed dimensional and we have

$$X_1, X_2, \ldots, X_n \text{ i.i.d. with pdf } f(x; \theta, \gamma)$$

where f is smooth, then for n large the probability of observations giving a profile likelihood ratio of k or larger is approximated by the bump function with σ^2 replaced by the first element $i^{\theta\theta}(\gamma)$ in the inverse of the information matrix for one observation.

More precisely Royall proves that

$$P_{\theta_1} \left(\frac{\text{Lik}_p(\theta_2; \boldsymbol{x}_n)}{\text{Lik}_p(\theta_1; \boldsymbol{x}_n)} \geq k \right) \longrightarrow \Phi \left(-\frac{c}{2} - \frac{\ln(k)}{c} \right)$$

where

$$|\theta_1 - \theta_2| = c \left(\frac{i^{\theta\theta}}{n} \right)^{1/2}$$

In particular this result implies that the probability of misleading evidence is approximately $\phi(-2(\ln(k))^{1/2})$ when

$$\theta_2 = \theta_1 \pm (2 \ln(k))^{1/2} \left(\frac{i^{\theta\theta}}{n} \right)^{1/2}$$

Example. Let $Y_1, Y_2, \ldots, Y_n$ be iid $N(\mu, \sigma^2)$. Then the likelihood of μ and σ^2 is given by

$$(2\pi\sigma^2)^{-\frac{n}{2}} \exp \left\{ -\frac{1}{2\sigma^2} \sum_{i=1}^n (y_i - \mu)^2 \right\}$$

for which the MLEs of μ and σ^2 are known to be

$$\hat{\mu} = \bar{y} \text{ and } \hat{\sigma}^2 = \frac{1}{n} \sum_{i=1}^n (y_i - \bar{y})^2$$

The likelihood evaluated at the MLE of μ and σ^2 is thus

$$(2\pi)^{-\frac{n}{2}} \left[\frac{\sum_{i=1}^n (y_i - \bar{y})^2}{n} \right]^{-\frac{n}{2}} \exp \left\{ -\frac{n}{2} \right\}$$

Note that Fisher's information matrix for one observation is given by

$$i(\mu, \sigma^2) = \begin{bmatrix} \frac{1}{\sigma^2} & 0 \\ 0 & \frac{1}{2\sigma^4} \end{bmatrix}$$

so that

$$i^{\mu\mu} = \sigma^2$$

The MLE of σ^2 for fixed μ is given by

$$\hat{\sigma}^2(\mu) = \frac{1}{n} \sum_{i=1}^{n} (y_i - \mu)^2$$

The likelihood evaluated at this value of σ^2 is thus

$$(2\pi)^{-\frac{n}{2}} \left[\frac{\sum_{i=1}^{n} (y_i - \mu)^2}{n} \right]^{-\frac{n}{2}} \exp\left\{ -\frac{n}{2} \right\}$$

It follows that the profile likelihood for μ is given by

$$\mathrm{Lik}_p(\mu; \boldsymbol{y}) = \left[\frac{\sum_{i=1}^{n} (y_i - \bar{y})^2}{\sum_{i=1}^{n} (y_i - \mu)^2} \right]^{\frac{n}{2}}$$

since

$$\sum_{i=1}^{n} (y_i - \mu)^2 = \sum_{i=1}^{n} (y_i - \bar{y})^2 + n(\mu - \bar{y})^2$$

the profile likelihood for μ may be written as

$$\mathrm{Lik}_p(\mu; \boldsymbol{y}) = \left[\frac{1}{1 + \frac{n(\mu - \bar{y})^2}{(n-1)s^2}} \right]^{\frac{n}{2}} = \left[\frac{1}{1 + \frac{t^2(\mu)}{n-1}} \right]^{\frac{n}{2}}$$

where $(n-1)s^2 = \sum_{i=1}^{n} (y_i - \bar{y})^2$ and

$$t^2(\mu) = \frac{n(\bar{y} - \mu)^2}{s^2}$$

is the square of Student's t statistic.

For a $\frac{1}{k}$ likelihood interval we require

$$\left[\frac{1}{1 + \frac{n(\mu-\bar{y})^2}{(n-1)s^2}}\right] \geq \left(\frac{1}{k}\right)^{\frac{2}{n}}$$

or

$$|\mu - \bar{y}| \leq \sqrt{\frac{s^2}{n}(n-1)\left[k^{\frac{2}{n}} - 1\right]}$$

which is similar to the interval obtained for the known variance case.

Example. The MLE for μ with σ^2 fixed is $\hat{\mu} = \bar{y}$. The likelihood evaluated at this value of μ is thus

$$(2\pi)^{-\frac{n}{2}}(\sigma^2)^{-\frac{n}{2}}\exp\left\{-\frac{1}{2\sigma^2}\sum_{i=1}^{n}(y_i - \bar{y})^2\right\}$$

so that the profile likelihood for σ^2 is given by

$$L_{pl}(\sigma^2; \boldsymbol{y}) = \frac{(2\pi)^{-\frac{n}{2}}(\sigma^2)^{-\frac{n}{2}}\exp\left\{-\frac{1}{2\sigma^2}\sum_{i=1}^{n}(y_i - \bar{y})^2\right\}}{(2\pi)^{-\frac{n}{2}}\left[\frac{\sum_{i=1}^{n}(y_i - \mu)^2}{n}\right]^{-\frac{n}{2}}\exp\left\{-\frac{n}{2}\right\}}$$

which reduces to

$$\left[\frac{\sum_{i=1}^{n}(y_i - \bar{y})^2}{n\sigma^2}\right]^{\frac{n}{2}}\exp\left\{-\frac{n}{2}\frac{\sum_{i=1}^{n}(y_i - \bar{y})^2}{n\sigma^2} - \frac{n}{2}\right\}$$

If we define

$$u = \frac{\sum_{i=1}^{n}(y_i - \bar{y})^2}{n\sigma^2}$$

then the $\frac{1}{k}$ likelihood interval may be written as

$$ue^u \geq ek^{-\frac{2}{n}}$$

Note that in this case the profile likelihood is very similar to the marginal likelihood for σ^2 based on the distribution of

$$\sum_{i=1}^{n}(Y_i - \overline{Y})^2$$

Which of these to use? In general use a true likelihood if it is available.

18.8.3   *General Linear Model Likelihood Functions*

Consider the general linear model

$$Y \sim \text{MVN}\left(X\beta, I\sigma^2\right)$$

where, for simplicity, we treat σ^2 as known. In this model, X is $n \times p$ of rank $p < n$ and β is a $p \times 1$ vector of unknown parameters. The following result can be established.

Theorem 18.8.1. *If $L^\top \beta$ is a set of linear functions of β, then the profile likelihood function for $L^\top \beta$ is*

$$\exp\left\{-\frac{1}{2\sigma^2}(L^\top\beta - L^\top b)^\top [L^\top(X^\top X)^{-1}L]^{-1}(L^\top\beta - \underline{L}^\top b)\right\}$$

where b is the least squares estimate of β.

Theorem 18.8.2. *If a general linear model is written in the form*

$$Y \sim \text{MVN}\left(X\beta + Z\gamma, I\sigma^2\right)$$

then the profile likelihood for γ is given by

$$\ell(\gamma; y) := \exp\left\{-\frac{1}{2\sigma^2}(\gamma - \widehat{\gamma})^\top Z^\top D Z(\gamma - \widehat{\gamma})\right\}$$

where $\widehat{\gamma}$ is any solution to the equations

$$Z^\top D Z\widehat{\gamma} = Z^\top Dy \ \text{ and } \ D = I - X(X^\top X)^{-1}X^\top$$

18.8.4   *Using Profile Likelihoods*

Given a profile likelihood for a parameter θ we define the k unit likelihood interval for θ as

$$\{\theta : \ \text{Lik}_p(\theta; y) \geq k\}$$

where typical choices of k are $\frac{1}{8}$ and $\frac{1}{32}$. Values of θ not in the k unit interval have a value of θ (the MLE) which has a likelihood $\frac{1}{k}$ greater.

Example 1. If $y_1, y_2, \ldots, y_n$ are a random sample from a normal distribution with parameters μ and σ^2 where σ^2 is known then the previous sections yield the likelihood for μ as

$$\exp\left\{-\frac{(\mu - \bar{y})^2}{2\sigma^2}\right\}$$

so that the k unit likelihood interval is given by

$$\left\{\mu : \bar{y} - \sqrt{2\log\left(\frac{1}{k}\right)}\sqrt{\frac{\sigma^2}{n}} \leq \mu \leq \bar{y} + \sqrt{2\log\left(\frac{1}{k}\right)}\sqrt{\frac{\sigma^2}{n}}\right\}$$

If we take $k = \frac{1}{8}$, then the $\frac{1}{8}$ likelihood interval becomes

$$\left\{\mu : \bar{y} - 2.04\sqrt{\frac{\sigma^2}{n}} \leq \mu \leq \bar{y} + 2.04\sqrt{\frac{\sigma^2}{n}}\right\}$$

which is clearly related to the conventional 95% confidence interval for μ.

Example 2. In a simple linear regression model in which $y_1, y_2, \ldots, y_n$ are independent with common variance σ^2 and

$$E(Y_i) = \beta_0 + \beta_1 x_i$$

where the x_i are known, the profile likelihood of β_1 is given by

$$\exp\left\{-\frac{(\beta_1 - b_1)^2 \sum_{i=1}^{n}(x_i - \bar{x})^2}{2\sigma^2}\right\}$$

where

$$b_1 = \frac{\sum_{i=1}^{n}(x_i - \bar{x})(y_i - \bar{y})}{\sum_{i=1}^{n}(x_i - \bar{x})^2}$$

It follows that the $\frac{1}{8}$ profile likelihood interval for β_1 is given by

$$\left\{\beta_1 : b_1 - 2.04\sqrt{\frac{\sigma^2}{\sum_{i=1}^{n}(x_i - \bar{x})^2}} \leq \beta_1 \leq b_1 + 2.04\sqrt{\frac{\sigma^2}{\sum_{i=1}^{n}(x_i - \bar{x})^2}}\right\}$$

Example 3. In a multiple linear regression model in which $y_1, y_2, \ldots, y_n$ are independent with common variance σ^2 and

$$E(Y_i) = \beta_0 + \beta_1 x_{i1} + \cdots + \beta_p x_{ip}$$

where the x_i are known the profile likelihood of β_j is given by

$$\exp\left\{-\frac{(\beta_j - b_j)^2}{2\sigma^2 c^{(j+1,j+1)}}\right\}$$

where b_j is the least squares estimate of β_j obtained by solving the least squares equations

$$X^T X b = X^T y$$

and $c^{(j+1,j+1)}$ is the $j+1, j+1$ element of the inverse of the matrix $X^T X$.

It follows that the $\frac{1}{8}$ profile likelihood interval for β_j is given by

$$\left\{ \beta_j : b_j - 2.04 \sqrt{\sigma^2 c^{(j+1,j+1)}} \le \beta_j \le b_j + 2.04 \sqrt{\sigma^2 c^{(j+1,j+1)}} \right\}$$

Note that this interval is different from that obtained if a simple linear regression model is used with the single covariate x_j in which case the interval is

$$\left\{ \beta_j : b_j - 2.04 \sqrt{\frac{\sigma^2}{\sum_{i=1}^n (x_{ij} - \bar{x}_{+j})^2}} \le \beta_j \le b_j + 2.04 \sqrt{\frac{\sigma^2}{\sum_{i=1}^n (x_{ij} - \bar{x}_{+j})^2}} \right\}$$

Example 4. Consider a one-way analysis of variance model in which we have the model

$$E(Y_{ij}) = \mu + \tau_i \text{ for } i = 1, 2, \ldots, p \quad j = 1, 2, \ldots, n_i$$

The canonical contrasts $\tau_i - \tau_{i'}$ are linearly estimable with maximum likelihood estimates given by

$$\widehat{\tau_i - \tau_{i'}} = \bar{y}_{i+} - \bar{y}_{i'+}$$

Since the variance of $\bar{y}_{i+} - \bar{y}_{i'+}$ is

$$\sigma^2 \left(\frac{1}{n_{i+}} + \frac{1}{n_{i'+}} \right)$$

the $\frac{1}{8}$ likelihood interval for $\tau_i - \tau_{i'}$ is given by

$$\bar{y}_{i+} - \bar{y}_{i'+} \pm 2.04 \sqrt{\sigma^2 \left(\frac{1}{n_{i+}} + \frac{1}{n_{i'+}} \right)}$$

18.8.5 Profile Likelihoods for Unknown Variance

Theorem 18.8.3. *If a general linear model is written in the form*

$$Y \sim MVN \left(X\beta + Z\gamma, I\sigma^2 \right)$$

where σ^2 is unknown, then the profile likelihood for γ is given by

$$\ell(\gamma; y) = \left\{ 1 + \frac{(\gamma - \hat{\gamma})^{\top} Z^{\top} D Z (\gamma - \hat{\gamma})}{SSE} \right\}^{-\frac{n}{2}}$$

where SSE is the error sum of squares in the full model, $D = I - X(X^{\top}X)^{-1}X^{\top}$.

Proof. The density of Y is given by

$$f_Y(y; \beta, \sigma^2, \gamma) = (2\pi\sigma^2)^{-\frac{n}{2}} \exp\left\{ -\frac{1}{2\sigma^2}(y - X\beta + Z\gamma)^{(2)} \right\}$$

Maximizing over β and σ^2 yields

$$\widetilde{\beta} = (X^{\top}X)^{-1}X^{\top}(y - Z\gamma)$$
$$n\widetilde{\sigma}^2 = (y - X\widetilde{\beta} - Z\gamma)^{(2)}$$

Note that

$$y - X\widetilde{\beta} - Z\gamma = y - X(X^{\top}X)^{-1}X^{\top}(y - Z\gamma) - Z\gamma$$
$$= D(y - Z\gamma)$$

where $D = I - X(X^{\top}X)^{-1}X^{\top}$
so that

$$n\widetilde{\sigma}^2 = [D(y - Z\gamma)]^{(2)}$$

Thus we have

$$f_Y(y; \widetilde{\beta}, \widetilde{\sigma}^2, \gamma) = (2\pi\widetilde{\sigma}^2)^{-\frac{n}{2}} \exp\left\{ -\frac{n}{2} \right\}$$

Maximizing $f_Y(y; \beta, \sigma^2, \gamma)$ over β, σ^2 and γ yields the equations

$$X^{\top}X\widehat{\beta} + X^{\top}Z\widehat{\gamma} = X^{\top}y$$
$$Z^{\top}X\widehat{\beta} + Z^{\top}Z\widehat{\gamma} = Z^{\top}y$$
$$n\widehat{\sigma}^2 = (y - X\widehat{\beta} - Z\widehat{\gamma})^{(2)}$$

It follows that

$$\widehat{\beta} = (X^{\top}X)^{-1}X^{\top}(y - Z\widehat{\gamma})$$
$$\widehat{\gamma} = (Z^{\top}DZ)^{-}Z^{\top}Dy$$

and hence

$$\begin{aligned}
y - X\widehat{\beta} - Z\widehat{\gamma} &= y - X(X^\top X)^{-1}X^\top(y - Z\widehat{\gamma}) - Z\widehat{\gamma} \\
&= D(y - Z\widehat{\gamma})
\end{aligned}$$

Thus

$$n\widehat{\sigma}^2 = [D(y - Z\widehat{\gamma})]^{(2)}$$

It follows that the profile likelihood for γ is given by

$$\frac{f_Y(y; \widetilde{\beta}, \widetilde{\sigma}^2, \gamma)}{f_Y(y; \widehat{\beta}, \widehat{\sigma}^2, \widehat{\gamma})} = \left\{ \frac{\widetilde{\sigma}^2}{\widehat{\sigma}^2} \right\}^{-\frac{n}{2}}$$

or

$$\frac{f_Y(y; \widetilde{\beta}, \widetilde{\sigma}^2, \gamma)}{f_Y(y; \widehat{\beta}, \widehat{\sigma}^2, \widehat{\gamma})} = \left\{ \frac{[D(y - Z\gamma)]^{(2)}}{D(y - Z\widehat{\gamma})]^{(2)}} \right\}^{-\frac{n}{2}}$$

Now note that

$$\begin{aligned}
[D(y - Z\gamma)]^{(2)} &= \{D[(y - Z\widehat{\gamma}) + (Z\widehat{\gamma} - Z\gamma)]\}^{(2)} \\
&= (y - Z\widehat{\gamma})^\top D(y - Z\widehat{\gamma}) \\
&\quad + (\widehat{\gamma} - \gamma)^\top Z^\top DZ(\widehat{\gamma} - \gamma) \\
&\quad + 2(\widehat{\gamma} - \gamma)^\top Z^\top D(y - Z\widehat{\gamma}) \\
&= \text{SSE} + (\widehat{\gamma} - \gamma)^\top Z^\top DZ(\widehat{\gamma} - \gamma)
\end{aligned}$$

Thus the profile likelihood for γ is given by

$$\mathscr{L}_p(\gamma; y) = \left\{ 1 + \frac{(\widehat{\gamma} - \gamma)^\top Z^\top DZ(\widehat{\gamma} - \gamma)}{\text{SSE}} \right\}^{-\frac{n}{2}}$$

as claimed.   □

18.9   Computation of Profile Likelihoods

There is an R package, developed by Leena Choi, called Profile Likelihood which can be used to find profile likelihoods for a variety of common models.

18.10 Summary

We have provided some examples that suggest that the use of pseudo-likelihoods can be fruitful in representing the evidence about a parameter of interest in the presence of nuisance parameters. A complete solution for all problems is too much to hope for. Indeed even the problem of evidence for composite hypotheses is not solved. See Zhang [57] and Bickel [4] for some possibilities.

Chapter 19
Other Inference Methods and Concepts

19.1 Fiducial Probability and Inference

R.A. Fisher introduced the concept of fiducial probability and used in to develop fiducial inference. Counterexamples though the years have lead to its lack of use in statistics.

Example. Consider a deck of N cards numbered $1, 2, \ldots, N$. One card is drawn at random, its number denoted by U. Then

$$\mathbb{P}(U = u) = \frac{1}{N} \quad u = 1, 2, \ldots, N \tag{19.1}$$

Suppose now that we add an unknown number θ to U. We are not told the observed value of U, u_{obs}, or the value of θ but we are told the observed value, $t_{obs} = u_{obs} + \theta$, of the total $T = U + \theta$. Note that we could see t_{obs} if and only if one of the following outcomes occurred:

$$(U = 1, \theta = t_{obs} - 1), (U = 2, \theta = t_{obs} - 2), \ldots, (U = N, \theta = t_{obs} - N)$$

1. Given the value of t_{obs} there is a one-to-one correspondence between the values of U and θ. If we knew θ then we could determine the value of u_{obs}.
2. If we do not know the value of θ then observing $T = t_{obs}$ will tell us nothing about u_{obs}.
3. Thus the state of uncertainty regarding u_{obs} will be the same after the observation of t_{obs} as it was before.

© Springer International Publishing Switzerland 2014
C.A. Rohde, *Introductory Statistical Inference with the Likelihood Function*, DOI 10.1007/978-3-319-10461-4_19

Therefore we assume that (19.1) holds, and we can write

$$\mathbb{P}(\theta = t_{obs} - u) = \mathbb{P}(U = u) = \frac{1}{N} \quad u = 1, 2, \ldots, N$$

which we call the **fiducial probability distribution** of θ.

Example. Assume that $X \overset{d}{\sim} N(\theta, 1)$ and define $U = T - \theta$. Then $U \overset{d}{\sim} N(0, 1)$. If we observe $T = t_{obs}$ then t_{obs} arises from a pair of values $(U = u, \theta = t_{obs} - u)$ so that given t_{obs} there is a one-to-one correspondence between the possible values of U and θ. Again, since θ is unknown we will learn nothing about which value of U occurred. Thus we may assume that $U \overset{d}{\sim} N(0, 1)$ even after $T = t_{obs}$ is observed. Thus we can calculate (fiducial) probabilities about θ by transforming them into probability statements about U, i.e.,

$$\theta \leq y \quad \Longleftrightarrow \quad U \geq t_{obs} - y$$

so that

$$\mathbb{P}_{\mathscr{F}}(\theta \leq y) = \mathbb{P}(U \geq t_{obs} - y) = \Phi(y - t_{obs})$$

where $\Phi(w) = \int_{-\infty}^{w} e^{-z^2/2}/\sqrt{2\pi}dz$. Note that such probability statements are the same as if we treated θ as a random variable with a normal distribution with mean t and variance 1. Thus the fiducial distribution of θ is $N(t_{obs}, 1)$. The fiducial density is the derivative with respect to θ, i.e.,

$$p_{\mathscr{F}}(\theta; t_{obs}) = \frac{1}{\sqrt{2\pi}} \exp\left\{ -\frac{(\theta - t_{obs})^2}{2} \right\}$$

Kalbfleisch lists sufficient conditions for the fiducial argument to apply:

1. A single real-valued parameter.
2. A minimal sufficient statistic T exists for θ.
3. There is a pivot $U(T, \theta)$ such that

   (i) For each θ, $U(t, \theta)$ is a one-to-one function of t
   (ii) For each t, $U(t, \theta)$ is a one-to-one function of θ

These assumptions which are compounded when we move to more than one parameter mean that the scope of fiducial inference is severely limited. In fact it is largely ignored in most modern treatments of statistics.

Suppose that $X_1, X_2, \ldots, X_n$ are iid each $N(\mu, \sigma^2)$ where σ^2 is known. Then, whatever the value of μ, we know that for every value of $\alpha \in [0, 1]$ we can find an upper $100(1 - \alpha)\%$ confidence interval for μ, namely

$$\overline{X} + z_{1-\alpha} \frac{\sigma}{\sqrt{n}}$$

which we know has the property that

$$\mathbb{P}\left\{\mu \le \overline{X} + z_{1-\alpha}\frac{\sigma}{\sqrt{n}}\right\} = 1 - \alpha$$

considered as a function of the random variable $\overline{X}$. Fisher noted that the left hand-side has all of the properties of a distribution function defined over the parameter space and thus proceeded to define the fiducial distribution of μ for fixed $\overline{X} = \overline{x}_{obs}$ and its derivative as the fiducial density of μ given $\overline{x}_{obs}$. Thus we can speak of the fiducial probability, $\mathbb{P}_{\mathscr{F}}(A)$ that $\mu \in A$ calculated as

$$\mathbb{P}_{\mathscr{F}}(\mu \in A) = \int_A \frac{1}{\sqrt{2\pi}} \exp\left\{-\frac{\sqrt{n}(\mu - \overline{x}_{obs})^2}{2\sigma^2}\right\} d\mu$$

As another example let $X_1, X_2, \ldots, X_n$ be iid each uniform on $(0, \theta)$. Then $Y = \max\{X_1, X_2, \ldots, X_n\}$ is the minimal sufficient statistic which has distribution function

$$F_Y(y; \theta) = \mathbb{P}_\theta(Y \le y) = [\mathbb{P}_\theta(X \le y)]^n = \left[\frac{y}{\theta}\right]^n$$

It follows that

$$\mathbb{P}\left(\frac{Y}{\theta} \le y\right) = \mathbb{P}(Y \le y\theta) = y^n$$

19.1.1   *Good's Example*

Suppose that X is a random variable with density function

$$f_X)(x; \theta) = \frac{\theta^2(x + a)e^{-x\theta}}{a\theta + 1} \quad \text{where } a > 0, \theta > 0, x \ge 0$$

which has distribution function

$$
\begin{aligned}
F(x; \theta) &= \int_0^x f(t; \theta) dt \\
&= \int_0^x \frac{\theta^2(t + a)e^{-t\theta}}{a\theta + 1} dt \\
&= \frac{\theta^2}{a\theta + 1} \int_0^x (t + a)e^{-t\theta} dt
\end{aligned}
$$

Now note that

$$\int_0^x (t+a)e^{-t\theta}\,dt = \int_0^x te^{-t\theta}\,dt + a\int_0^x e^{-t\theta}\,dt$$

$$= -\left.\frac{te^{-t\theta}}{\theta}\right|_0^x + \frac{1}{\theta}\int_0^x e^{-t\theta}\,dt + a\int_0^x e^{-t\theta}\,dt$$

$$= -\frac{xe^{-x\theta}}{\theta} + \frac{1+a\theta}{\theta}\int_0^x e^{-t\theta}\,dt$$

$$= -\frac{xe^{-x\theta}}{\theta} + \frac{1+a\theta}{\theta^2}\left[1 - e^{-x\theta}\right]$$

It follows that

$$F_X(x;\theta) = 1 - e^{-x\theta}\left[1 + \frac{x\theta}{a\theta + 1}\right]$$

The fiducial density of θ is the derivative of $F_X(x;\theta)$ with respect to θ or

$$\mathscr{F}_x(\theta) = \frac{x\theta e^{-x\theta}}{(a\theta + 1)^2}[a + (a + x)(1 + a\theta)]$$

Suppose we now observe, independently of X, another random variable Y with density

$$f_Y(y;\theta) = \frac{\theta^2(y+b)e^{-x\theta}}{b\theta + 1} \quad \text{where } b > 0, \theta > 0, x \ge 0 \text{ and } b \ne a$$

If we use the fiducial density based on X as a "prior" for θ and combine it with the density for Y the resulting posterior would be

$$\mathscr{P}_{XY}(\theta; x, y) = \mathscr{F}_x(\theta)f_Y(y;\theta)$$

which is equal to

$$\frac{x\theta e^{-x\theta}}{(a\theta + 1)^2}[a + (a + x)(1 + a\theta)]\frac{\theta^2(y+b)e^{-y\theta}}{b\theta + 1}$$

If fiducial probabilities behaved like true probabilities it should make no difference whether we observed X or Y first. If we used the fiducial density for θ based on Y and combined it with density of X the resulting posterior would be

$$\mathscr{P}_{YX}(\theta; y, x) = \mathscr{F}_y(\theta)f_X(x;\theta)$$

which is equal to

$$\frac{y\theta e^{-y\theta}}{(b\theta + 1)^2} [b + (b + x)(1 + b\theta)] \frac{\theta^2 (x + a)e^{-x\theta}}{a\theta + 1}$$

The laws of probability would say that these two expressions should be equal. They are clearly not. So fiducial probabilities are not compatible with Bayes theorem and hence are not warranted.

19.1.2 Edward's Example

Consider two hypotheses $\theta = +1$ or $\theta = -1$ and suppose that there are two possible outcomes of a random variable X, $X = +1$ or $X = -1$. The probability model for X is

$$\mathbb{P}_{\theta=+1}(X = x) = \begin{cases} p & x = +1 \\ q & x = -1 \end{cases} \quad ; \quad \mathbb{P}_{\theta=-1}(X = x) = \begin{cases} q & x = +1 \\ p & x = -1 \end{cases}$$

Since when $\theta = +1$, $X = +1$ with probability p, and when $\theta = -1$, $X = -1$ with probability p, we have that

$$\mathbb{P}(X\theta = +1) \quad \text{with probability } p.$$

This statement is true in general and when $X = +1$ is equivalent to the statement

$$\mathbb{P}(\theta = +1 | X = +1) = p$$

which is the fiducial probability statement about θ following from observing that $X = +1$.

Thus starting with no prior information and performing an experiment which is uninformative we arrive at a statement of probability for θ.

Suppose now that $p = q = \frac{1}{2}$. Then

(i) There is no information about θ a priori
(ii) The observation of X is totally uninformative about θ
(iii) The likelihood ratio for comparing $\theta = +1$ to $\theta = -1$ is 1 indicating that, based on the observation, we have no preference for $\theta = +1$ vs $\theta = -1$

However we find, using the fiducial argument, that

$$\mathbb{P}_{\mathscr{F}}(\theta = +1) = \frac{1}{2} \quad \text{whatever the value of } X$$

Thus we have another example which casts doubt on the veracity of the fiducial argument.

19.2   Confidence Distributions

Recently there has been a great deal of research on confidence distributions which reduce, in many cases, to fiducial distributions, but which are solidly in the frequentist camp.

Definition 19.2.1. A function $C_n(\theta; \boldsymbol{x}_n\ :\ \mathcal{X} \times \Theta \mapsto [0,1]$ is called a **confidence distribution** if

(i) $C_n(\theta; \boldsymbol{x}_n)$ is a distribution function over Θ for each fixed $\boldsymbol{x}_n \in \mathcal{X}$
(ii) At the true parameter point $C_n(\theta_0, \boldsymbol{x}_n)$ as a function of $\boldsymbol{x}_n \in \mathcal{X}$ has a uniform distribution over $[0,1]$

$C_n(\theta; \boldsymbol{x}_n\ :\ \mathcal{X} \times \Theta \mapsto [0,1]$ is an asymptotic confidence distribution if (ii) is satisfied only asymptotically.

The paper by Xie and Singh [55] provides a useful review of the ideas. The following graph shows the unification of frequentist ideas using the confidence density:

Confidence Density Example

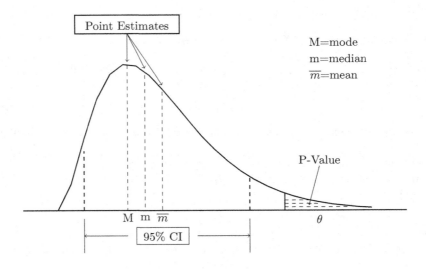

19.2.1   Bootstrap Connections

If $\widehat{\theta}$ is an estimator of θ let the bootstrap estimator be $\widehat{\theta}^*$. When the asymptotic distribution of $\widehat{\theta}$ is symmetric then the sampling distribution of $\widehat{\theta} - \theta$ is estimated by the bootstrap distribution of $\widehat{\theta}-\widehat{\theta}^*$. In this case an asymptotic confidence distribution is given by

$$C_n(\theta) = 1 - \mathbb{P}(\widehat{\theta} - \widehat{\theta}^* \leq \widehat{\theta} - \theta | \boldsymbol{x}) = \mathbb{P}(\widehat{\theta}^* \leq \theta | \boldsymbol{x})$$

the bootstrap distribution of $\widehat{\theta}$.

19.2.2 Likelihood Connections

If we normalize a likelihood function $\mathscr{L}(\theta; \boldsymbol{x})$ so that the area under the normalized likelihood function is 1, i.e., we form

$$\mathscr{L}^*(\theta; \boldsymbol{x}) = \frac{\mathscr{L}(\theta; \boldsymbol{x})}{\int_{\Theta} \mathscr{L}(\theta; \boldsymbol{x}) d\theta}$$

then, under certain conditions, we obtain an asymptotic normal confidence distribution.

Similarly, under the usual regularity conditions for maximum likelihood, we can use the normalized profile likelihood as an asymptotic confidence distribution for a parameter of interest.

It is also possible to construct approximate likelihoods using confidence distributions. Efron considered a confidence density $c(\theta; \boldsymbol{x})$ for the parameter of interest. He then considered doubling the data set by introducing another data set, considered independent of the first but having exactly the same data $\boldsymbol{x}$. Then construct the confidence density $c(\theta, \boldsymbol{x}, \boldsymbol{x})$ based on the doubled data set using the same confidence intervals to define the density. Then the implied likelihood function is

$$\mathscr{L}_{imp}(\theta; \boldsymbol{x}) = \frac{c(\theta; \boldsymbol{x}, \boldsymbol{x})}{c(\theta; \boldsymbol{x})}$$

19.2.3 Confidence Curves

Birnbaum introduced the idea of a confidence curve to summarize confidence intervals and levels of tests in one curve. In terms of confidence distributions the confidence curve is given by

$$CC(\theta) = 2 \min\{C_n(\theta; \boldsymbol{x}), 1 - C_n(\theta; \boldsymbol{x})\}$$

Thus a confidence distribution is simply a combinant such that for each $\boldsymbol{x}_n \in \mathcal{X}$ it is a distribution function as θ varies over Θ and for fixed $\theta = \theta_0$ it has a uniform distribution as $\boldsymbol{x}_n$ varies over $\mathcal{X}$.

Example. Let

$$X_i \overset{d}{\sim} N(\mu, \sigma^2) \quad i = 1, 2, \ldots, n$$

be independent with σ^2 known. Then

$$C_n(\mu; \overline{x}_{obs}) = \Phi\left(\frac{\mu - \overline{x}_{obs}}{\sigma/\sqrt{n}}\right) \quad \text{where} \quad \Phi(y) = \int_{-\infty}^{y} \frac{e^{-z^2/2}}{\sqrt{2\pi}} dz$$

is a confidence distribution for μ.

19.3   P-Values Again

Given the widespread importance of genomics P-values are now used more than ever. It is important to remember that P-values are observed values of a random variable and hence have intrinsic variability.

19.3.1   Sampling Distribution of P-Values

The P-value is defined, for a test statistic T, with distribution function $F_{H_0}(t)$ assuming the null hypothesis is true as

$$\mathbb{P}_{H_0}(T \geq t_{obs}) \quad \text{where } t_{obs} \text{ is the observed value of } T$$

Note that the P-value is given by $1 - F_{H_0}(t_{obs})$ and can be considered as an observed value of the random variable $Y = 1 - F_{H_0}(T)$. The distribution function of Y assuming the null hypothesis is true is

$$
\begin{aligned}
F_Y(y) &= \mathbb{P}_{H_0}(Y \leq y) \\
&= \mathbb{P}_{H_0}\{1 - F_{H_0}(T) \leq y\} \\
&= \mathbb{P}_{H_0}\{F_{H_0}(T) \geq 1 - y\} \\
&= 1 - \mathbb{P}_{H_0}\{F_{H_0}(T) \leq 1 - y\} \\
&= 1 - \mathbb{P}_{H_0}\{T \leq F_{H_0}^{-1}(1 - y)\} \\
&= 1 - F_{H_0}\{F_{H_0}^{-1}(1 - y)\} \\
&= 1 - (1 - y) \\
&= y
\end{aligned}
$$

for $0 < y < 1$. That is, the P-value under the null hypothesis has a uniform distribution. This fact has been known for decades, but P-values are not reported with a standard error as other statistics are.

If the alternative hypothesis is true assume that T has a distribution function $G_H(t)$. Then

$$
\begin{aligned}
F_Y(y) &= \mathbb{P}_H(Y \leq y) \\
&= \mathbb{P}_H \left\{ 1 - F_{H_0}(T) \leq y \right\} \\
&= \mathbb{P}_H \left\{ F_{H_0}(T) \geq 1 - y \right\} \\
&= 1 - \mathbb{P}_H \left\{ F_{H_0}(T) \leq 1 - y \right\} \\
&= 1 - \mathbb{P}_H \left\{ T \leq F_{H_0}^{-1}(1 - y) \right\} \\
&= 1 - G_H \left\{ F_{H_0}^{-1}(1 - y) \right\}
\end{aligned}
$$

Under suitable regularity conditions the density of Y under the alternative hypothesis is

$$
\begin{aligned}
f_Y(y) &= \frac{dF_Y(y)}{dy} \\
&= \frac{d \left[1 - G_H \left\{ F_{H_0}^{-1}(1 - y) \right\} \right]}{dy} \\
&= -g_H \left\{ F_{H_0}^{-1}(1 - y) \right\} \frac{1}{-f_{H_0} \left\{ F_{H_0}^{-1}(1 - y) \right\}} \\
&= \frac{g_H \left\{ F_{H_0}^{-1}(1 - y) \right\}}{f_{H_0} \left\{ F_{H_0}^{-1}(1 - y) \right\}}
\end{aligned}
$$

Note that for the observed value of T, t_{obs}, we have $y = 1 - F_{H_0}(t_{obs})$ and hence the density evaluated at the observed value of T, t_{obs}, is given by

$$
\frac{g_H \left\{ F_{H_0}^{-1}(1 - y) \right\}}{f_{H_0} \left\{ F_{H_0}^{-1}(1 - y) \right\}} = \frac{g_H \left\{ F_{H_0}^{-1}[F_{H_0}(t_{obs})] \right\}}{f_{H_0} \left\{ F_{H_0}^{-1}[F_{H_0}(t_{obs})] \right\}} = \frac{g_H(t_{obs})}{f_{H_0}(t_{obs})}
$$

the likelihood ratio!

P-values have been under heavy fire in the last few years for overstating the importance of effects observed in clinical and other investigations [48]. The results above due to Donahue [12] and others have been used by Boos and Stefanski [5] to explain why P-values overstate the conclusions of studies. The results of Goodman [21] are also relevant. The bottom line appears to be that use of P-values is not the way to present the evidence from studies that rely on statistical analysis to report their conclusions.

19.4   Severe Testing

Severe testing is a concept claimed to be useful for post-data inference. The ideas are best illustrated through an example and I follow the example in Mayo and Spannos [33]. Suppose that $X_1, X_2, \ldots, X_n$ are iid each $N(\mu, \sigma^2)$ where $\sigma = 2$, that $n = 100$, and we choose $\alpha = 0.025$ for a one-sided test of

$$H_0 \; : \; \mu \leq 12 \;\; \text{vs} \;\; \mu > 12$$

Since, under H_0, $\overline{X}_n \overset{d}{\sim} N(12, 2/10)$, we reject using the Neyman-Pearson theory if

$$d(\boldsymbol{x}_{obs}) = \frac{\sqrt{n}(\overline{x}_{obs} - 12)}{2} \geq 1.96 \;\; \Longleftrightarrow \;\; \overline{x}_{obs} \geq 12.4$$

Suppose now that we observe $\overline{x}_{obs} = 11.8$. Then we would not reject $H_0 \;$: $\mu = 12$. If a value of μ equal to 12.2 was deemed to be of scientific or substantive importance we can ask the question do we have evidence that $\mu < 12.2$? Mayo suggests calculating the severity with which $\mu < 12.2$ passes the test. The severity with which $\mu = 12.2$ passes the test in cases where H_0 is accepted is defined in this situation as

$$
\begin{aligned}
\mathbb{P}_\mu(\overline{X} > \overline{x}_{obs}) &= \mathbb{P}_{\mu=12.2}\left\{\overline{X} > 11.8\right\} \\
&= \mathbb{P}_{\mu=12.2}\left\{\frac{\sqrt{100}(\overline{X} - 12.2)}{2} > \frac{\sqrt{100}(11.8 - 12.2)}{2}\right\} \\
&= \mathbb{P}\left\{Z > -2\right\} \\
&= 0.977
\end{aligned}
$$

Note that the power of the test at 12.2 is

$$
\begin{aligned}
\mathbb{P}_{\mu=12.2}\left\{\overline{X} > 12.4\right\} &= \mathbb{P}_{\mu=12.2}\left\{\frac{\sqrt{100}(\overline{X} - 12.2)}{2} > \frac{\sqrt{100}(12.4 - 12.2)}{2}\right\} \\
&= \mathbb{P}\left\{Z > 1\right\} \\
&= 0.159
\end{aligned}
$$

Mayo and Spannos define the **attained power** in this situation as

$$\mathbb{P}_\mu\left\{\overline{X} > \overline{x}_{obs}\right\}$$

so that the severity with which μ passes the test is simply the attained power at μ when the observed outcome leads to acceptance of the null hypothesis.

Suppose now that the null hypothesis is rejected. In the example suppose that $\overline{x}_{obs} = 12.6$. The null hypothesis that $\mu = 12$ is rejected. Again, assuming that $\mu = 12.2$ is of scientific or substantive interest, do we have evidence of a value of μ of scientific interest? Mayo and Spannos suggest calculating the severity of $\mu > 12.2$ defined by

$$
\begin{aligned}
\mathbb{P}_\mu \left\{ \overline{X} \leq \overline{x}_{obs} \right\} &= \mathbb{P}_{\mu=12.2} \left\{ \overline{X} \leq \overline{x}_{obs} \right\} \\
&= \mathbb{P}_{\mu=12.2} \left\{ \overline{X} \leq 12.6 \right\} \\
&= \mathbb{P}_{\mu=12.2} \left\{ \frac{\sqrt{100}(\overline{X} - 12.2)}{2} \leq \frac{\sqrt{100}(12.6 - 12.2)}{2} \right\} \\
&= \mathbb{P} \left\{ Z \leq 2 \right\} \\
&= 0.977
\end{aligned}
$$

Note that in the case of a hypothesis which is rejected the severity is simply 1 minus the attained power.

Severe testing does a nice job of clarifying the issues which occur when a hypothesis is accepted (not rejected) by finding those values of the parameter (here mu) which are plausible (have high severity) given acceptance. Similarly severe testing addresses the issue of a hypothesis which is rejected by finding those values of the parameter μ which are plausible (have high severity) given rejection. Note that severity is a function of the test, T, the hypothesis, H, and the observed data, x_{obs}. Thus it is inherently a random variable and the standard results on p-values and their distributions apply to severity as well. Also note that conventions need to be established for when severity is judged to be high.

Finally note that most of the existing examples implicitly seem to require a monotone likelihood ratio so that members of the exponential family are included, but whether or not other distributions are covered under the existing theory is unknown.

19.5 Cornfield on Testing and Confidence Intervals

The following quotes by Jerry Cornfield (1966) indicate that the problems with frequentist statistics have been known for a long time.

Cornfield defines the α-postulate as "All hypotheses rejected the same critical level have equal amounts of evidence against them."

The following example will be recognized by statisticians with consulting experience as a simplified version of a very common situation. An experimenter, having made n observations in the expectation that they would permit the rejection of a particular hypothesis, at some predetermined significance level, say 0.05, finds that he has not quite attained this critical level. He still believes that the hypothesis is false and asks how many more observations would be required to have reasonable certainty of rejecting the hypothesis if the means observed after n observations are taken as the true values. He also makes it clear that had the original n observations permitted rejection he would simply have published his findings. Under these circumstances it is evident that there is no amount of additional observations, no matter how large, which would permit rejection at the 0.05 level. If the hypothesis being tested is true, there is a 0.05 chance of it having been rejected after the first round of observations. To this chance must be added the probability of rejecting after the second round, given failure to reject after the first, and this increases the total chance of erroneous rejection to above 0.05. In fact as the total number of observations in the second round is indefinitely increased the significance approaches 0.0975 ($=0.05 +0.95 \times 0.05$) if the 0.05 criteria is retained. Thus no amount of additional evidence can be collected which would provide evidence against the hypothesis equivalent to rejection at the $P = 0.05$ level and adherents of the α-postulate would presumably advise him to turn his attention to other scientific fields. The reasonableness of this advice is perhaps questionable (as is the possibility that it would be accepted). In any event it does not seem possible to argue seriously in the face of this example that all hypotheses rejected at the .05 level have equal amounts of evidence against them.

The confidence set yielded by a given body of data is the set of all hypotheses not rejected by the data, so that the relation between hypothesis test and confidence limits is close. In fact the confidence limit equivalent of the α-postulate is "All statements made with same the confidence coefficient have equal amounts of evidence in their favor." That this may be seen no more reasonable the α-postulate is suggested by the very common of inference about the ratio of two normal means. The most selective unbiased confidence set for the unknown ratio has the following curious characteristic: for every sample point there exists an $\alpha > 0$ such that all confidence limits with coefficients $\geq 1 - \alpha$ are plus to minus infinity. But to assert that the unknown ratio lies between plus and minus infinity with confidence coefficient of only $1 - \alpha$ is surely being overcautious. Even worse, the postulate asserts that there is less evidence for such an infinite interval than there is for a finite interval about a normal mean, but made with coefficient $1 - \alpha'$ where $\alpha' < \alpha$. The α-postulate cannot therefore be considered anymore reasonable than it is for hypothesis testing.

It has been proposed by proponents of confidence limits that this clearly undesirable characteristic of the limits on a ratio be avoided by redefining the sample space so as to exclude all sample points that lead to infinite limits for given α. This is equivalent to saying that if the application of a principle to given evidence leads to an absurdity then the evidence must be discarded. It is reminiscent of the heavy smoker, who, worried about the literature relating smoking to lung cancer, decided to give up reading.

Chapter 20
Finite Population Sampling

20.1 Introduction

It is fair to say that most of the information we know about contemporary society is obtained as the result of sample surveys. Real populations are finite and the branch of statistics which treats sampling of such populations is called **survey sampling**. For many years survey sampling remained the province of "survey samplers" with very little input from statisticians involved in the more traditional aspects of the subject. The decades of the 1970s, 1980s, and 1990s saw somewhat successful mergers of the two areas using new approaches to finite population sampling theory based on prediction theory and population based models.

20.2 Populations and Samples

Definition 20.2.1. A **population** is a set of N units, labeled $1, 2, \ldots, N$. With each unit is an associated characteristic Y_i.

Of interest is either the population total T or the population average $\bar{Y}$ defined by

$$T = \sum_{i=1}^{N} Y_i \quad \text{and} \quad \bar{Y} = \frac{T}{N}$$

Definition 20.2.2. A **sample** of size n from a population is an ordered subset s of the N units which define the population.

We will only consider sampling without replacement so that each element in the population can appear at most once in the sample.

© Springer International Publishing Switzerland 2014
C.A. Rohde, *Introductory Statistical Inference with the Likelihood Function*, DOI 10.1007/978-3-319-10461-4_20

20.3   Principal Types of Sampling Methods

There are a myriad of different sampling methods. Here are the most important:

Simple Random Sampling: In simple random sampling each set of n elements of the population has the same chance of being selected, i.e., each sample has the same selection probability.

Systematic Sampling: In systematic sampling we assume that the population can be labeled with the integers $1, 2, \ldots, N$ where N is the number of elements in the population:

- The sampling consists of selecting a random start and then selecting every kth element until the sample size of n is reached.
- If the population is randomly ordered then systematic sampling is equivalent to simple random sampling.

Stratified Sampling: In stratified sampling supplementary information is used to divide the population into K mutually exclusive groups called strata. A simple random sample is then selected from each stratum:

- The advantage of stratified sampling is that if the strata are internally homogeneous then the estimate of the population total or mean will have a smaller standard error than under simple random sampling.

Cluster Sampling: In cluster sampling the population is divided into K mutually exclusive groups, as in stratified sampling, called clusters:

- Unlike stratified sampling, in cluster sampling, a random sample of k clusters is selected, and a simple random sample selected from each of the selected clusters.
- The advantages of cluster sampling lie in the fact that it often gives economies of selection.
- Cluster sampling is particularly suited to situations in which the sampling frame (list of population elements) consists of clusters rather than the individual units, e.g., interest is on a sample of individuals, but we have available only a list of households.
- Cluster sampling is also called multistage sampling and it can be extended to multiple levels, i.e., a sample of clusters, then a sample of subclusters within clusters, etc.

Probability Proportional to Size: If the sample selected from each stratum or cluster is proportional to the size of the stratum or cluster the sampling is called **probability proportional to size** (PPS) sampling.

Two-Stage Sampling: In this method of sampling a large first-stage sample is selected and information obtained which is used to design the final stage sample which gathers complete information on the final selected sample.

Replicated Sampling: In this type of sampling the final sample consists of a set of samples, each selected in an identical fashion:

- The purpose of replicated sampling is to investigate non-sampling errors such as non-response and to calculate valid standard errors when the sampling process is complex.

Panel Sampling: Samples are taken at two points in time with sample overlap designed to measure possible time trends.

20.4   Simple Random Sampling

We now discuss the simplest setting which has been generalized ad nauseam to form the basis of the conventional approach to survey sampling.

Consider a population of size N

$$\mathcal{P} = \{y_1, y_2, \ldots, y_N\}$$

Of interest is the population total

$$T = \sum_{i=1}^{N} y_i$$

If we have a random sample, s, taken without replacement the natural estimator is

$$\widehat{T} = \frac{N}{n} \sum_{i \in s}^{n} y_i$$

The standard approach to this problem is to define

$$Z_i = \begin{cases} 1 & i \in s \\ 0 & \text{otherwise} \end{cases}$$

Then

$$\widehat{T} = \frac{N}{n} \sum_{i=1}^{N} y_i Z_i$$

Under simple random sampling without replacement we have that

$$\mathbb{P}(Z_i = 1) = \frac{\binom{N-1}{n-1}}{\binom{N}{n}} = \frac{\frac{(N-1)!}{(N-n)!(n-1)!}}{\frac{N!}{n!(N-n)!}} = \frac{n}{N} = \mathbb{E}(Z_i)$$

It follows that

$$\mathbb{E}(Z_i^2) = \mathbb{P}(Z_i = 1) = \frac{n}{N}$$

and hence

$$\text{var}(Z_i) = \frac{n}{N} - \frac{n^2}{N^2} = \frac{n}{N^2}(N - n)$$

Now note that for $i \neq j$

$$\mathbb{E}(Z_i Z_j) = \mathbb{P}(Z_i = 1, Z_j = 1) = \mathbb{P}(Z_i = 1)\mathbb{P}(Z_j = 1 | Z_i = 1) = \frac{n}{N}\frac{n-1}{N-1}$$

It follows that

$$\text{cov}(Z_i, Z_j) = \frac{n}{N}\frac{n-1}{N-1} - \left(\frac{n}{N}\right)^2 = \frac{n}{N}\left(\frac{n-1}{N-1} - \frac{n}{N}\right) = -\frac{n}{N^2(N-1)}(N-n)$$

Thus

$$\text{Var}(\widehat{T}) = \frac{N^2}{n^2}\text{Var}(\sum_{i=1}^{n} y_i Z_i)$$

$$= \frac{N^2}{n^2}\sum_{i=1}^{n}\sum_{j=1}^{n} y_i y_j \text{cov}(Y_i, Y_j)$$

$$= (N - n)\frac{S^2}{n}$$

where

$$S^2 = \frac{1}{N-1}\sum_{i=1}^{N}(y_i - \overline{y})^2$$

We now have an estimate of the total and, by replacing S^2 by its natural estimate the sample value s^2 an estimate of the variance. There are central limit theorems for finite populations, Lehmann [28], so that the usual methods allow the formation of a confidence interval for the population total.

20.5 Horvitz–Thompson Estimator

A general approach to the problem of finite population sampling is provided by the Horvitz–Thompson estimator [22] and its generalizations which also appear in a variety of other problems.

Consider a population of N objects, each with an associated characteristic y_i. Using a sample $s = \{i_1, i_2, \ldots, i_n\}$ it is desired to estimate the population total T defined by

$$T = \sum_{i=1}^{N} y_i$$

The **selection probabilities** are denoted by

$$(\pi_1, \pi_2, \ldots, \pi_N)$$

and are assumed known. That is,

$$\pi_i = \mathbb{P}(\text{object } i \text{ selected})$$

Similarly the probabilities of selecting i and j of the objects are assumed known and given by

$$\pi_{ij} \quad i \neq j$$

The Horvitz–Thompson estimator is defined by

$$\widehat{T} = \sum_{i \in s} \frac{y_i}{\pi_i}$$

If we define Bernoulli random variables by

$$Z_i = \begin{cases} 1 \text{ if object } i \text{ is in the sample } s \\ 0 \text{ otherwise} \end{cases}$$

then we have that

$$\mathbb{E}(Z_i) = \pi_i \ \text{ and } \ \mathbb{V}(Z_i) = \pi_i(1 - \pi_i)$$

and

$$\mathbb{C}(Z_i, Z_j) = \mathbb{E}(Z_i Z_j) - \mathbb{E}(Z_i)\mathbb{E}(Z_j) = \mathbb{P}(Z_i = 1, Z_j = 1) - \pi_i \pi_j = \pi_{ij} - \pi_i \pi_j$$

for $i \neq j$.

The Horvitz–Thompson estimator can be written in terms of the Z_i's as

$$\widehat{T} = \sum_{i=1}^{N} \frac{y_i}{\pi_i} Z_i$$

Note that the only randomness is given by the Z_i's.

It is clear that $\widehat{T}$ is unbiased since

$$\mathbb{E}(\widehat{T}) = \mathbb{E}\left(\sum_{i=1}^{N} \frac{y_i}{\pi_i} Z_i\right) = \sum_{i=1}^{N} \frac{y_i}{\pi_i} \mathbb{E}(Z_i) = \sum_{i=1}^{N} y_i = T$$

Similarly

$$\mathbb{V}(\widehat{T}) = \mathbb{V}\left(\sum_{i=1}^{N} \frac{y_i}{\pi_i} Z_i\right)$$

$$= \sum_{i=1}^{N} \left(\frac{y_i}{\pi_i}\right)^2 \mathbb{V}(Z_i) + \sum_{(i,j);j\neq i}^{N} \left(\frac{y_i y_j}{\pi_i \pi_j}\right) \mathbb{C}(Z_i, Z_j)$$

$$= \sum_{i=1}^{N} \left(\frac{y_i^2}{\pi_i}\right)(1 - \pi_i) + \sum_{(i,j);j\neq i}^{N} y_i y_j \left(\frac{\pi_{ij} - \pi_i \pi_j}{\pi_i \pi_j}\right)$$

If sampling is at random without replacement, then we have that

$$\pi_i = \frac{\binom{N-1}{n-1}}{\binom{N}{n}} = \frac{n}{N}$$

and

$$\pi_{ij} = \mathbb{P}(Z_i = 1, Z_j = 1)$$
$$= \mathbb{P}(Z_j = 1 \mid Z_i = 1)\mathbb{P}(Z_i = 1)$$
$$= \frac{(n-1)}{(N-1)} \frac{n}{N}$$

Thus we have that

$$\mathbb{V}(\widehat{T}) = \sum_{i=1}^{N} \left(\frac{y_i^2}{\pi_i}\right)(1 - \pi_i) + \sum_{(i,j);j\neq i}^{N} y_i y_j \left(\frac{\pi_{ij} - \pi_i \pi_j}{\pi_i \pi_j}\right)$$

$$= \sum_{i=1}^{N} \left(\frac{y_i^2}{n/N}\right)(1 - n/N) + \sum_{(i,j);j\neq i}^{N} y_i y_j \left(\frac{\left[\frac{n-1}{N-1}\right]\left[\frac{n}{N}\right] - \left[\frac{n}{N}\right]\left[\frac{n}{N}\right]}{\left[\frac{n}{N}\right]\left[\frac{n}{N}\right]}\right)$$

$$= \frac{N-n}{n} \sum_{i=1}^{N} y_i^2 - \frac{N-n}{n(N-1)} \sum_{(i,j);j\neq i}^{N} y_i y_j$$

$$= \frac{N-n}{n} \left[\sum_{i=1}^{N} y_i^2 - \frac{1}{N-1} \sum_{i=1}^{N} y_i \left(\sum_{j=1}^{N} y_j - y_i \right) \right]$$

$$= \frac{N-n}{n(N-1)} \left[N \sum_{i=1}^{N} y_i^2 - \left(\sum_{i=1}^{N} y_i \right)^2 \right]$$

$$= \frac{N(N-n)}{n(N-1)} \left(\sum_{i=1}^{N} y_i^2 - N\overline{y}^2 \right)$$

$$= \frac{N(N-n)}{n} S^2$$

where

$$S^2 = \frac{1}{N-1} \left[\sum_{i=1}^{N} (y_i^2 - N\overline{y}^2) \right] = \frac{1}{N-1} \sum_{i=1}^{N} (y_i - \overline{y})^2$$

$$\overline{y} = \frac{1}{N} \sum_{i=1}^{N} y_i$$

Thus we recover the results of the first section.

The Horvitz–Thompson estimator provides a unifying approach to finite population sampling theory from a frequentist or sampling theory perspective Overton and Stehman [36].

20.5.1 Basu's Elephant

However, the Horvitz–Thompson estimator cannot be used uncritically as Basu's elephant example shows.

The circus owner is planning to ship his 50 adult elephants and so he needs a rough estimate of the total weight of his elephants. As weighing an elephant is a cumbersome process, the owner wants to estimate the total weight by weighing just one elephant. Which elephant should he weigh? So the owner looks back on his records and discovers a list of the elephant's weights taken 3 years ago. He finds that 3 years age Sambo the middle sized elephant was the average (in weight) elephant in his herd. He checks with the elephant trainer who reassures him (the owner) that Sambo may still be considered the average elephant in the herd. Therefore, the owner plans to weigh Sambo and take 50 y (where y is the present weight of Sambo) as an estimate of the total weight

$$Y = Y_1 + Y_2 + \ldots Y_{50}$$

of the 50 elephants. But the circus statistician is horrified when he learns of the owner's purposive sampling plan. "How can you get an unbiased estimate of Y this way?" protests the statistician. So, together they work out a compromise sampling plan. With the help of a table of random numbers they devise a plan that allots a selection probability of $\frac{99}{100}$ to Sambo and equal selection probabilities of $\frac{1}{4900}$ to each of the other elephants. Naturally Sambo is selected and the owner is happy. "How are you going to estimate Y?, asks the statistician. "Why? The estimate ought to be $50y$ of course", says the owner. "Oh! no! That cannot possibly be right," says the statistician, "I recently read an article in the Annals of Mathematical Statistics where it is proved that the Horvitz–Thompson estimator is the unique hyper-admissable estimator in the class of all generalized polynomial unbiased estimators." What is the Horvitz–Thompson estimator in this case?" asks the owner, duly impressed. "Since the selection probability for Sambo in our plan was $\frac{99}{100}$," says the statistician, the proper estimate of Y is $\frac{100y}{99}$ and not $50y$." "And how would you have estimated Y," inquires the incredulous owner, "if our sampling plan made us select, say, the big elephant Jumbo?". "According to what I understand of the Horvitz–Thompson estimation method," says the unhappy statistician, " the proper estimate of Y would then have been $4900y$, where y is Jumbo's weight." That is how the circus statistician lost his circus job and perhaps became a teacher of statistics!

[1]

Basu's elephant example has been criticized by many as being "too extreme" to be useful in practice. However the following passage from Einbeck et al. [13] shows that this may be hasty.

The goal of this paper was to show that there exists an striking analogy between the theories of sampling and smoothing, leading to a similar discrepancy between theoretically optimal and practically useful weighting schemes. We believe that this tells us an important lesson about statistical methods in general: weighting is performed in virtually all statistical disciplines, and a usual way of motivating such weights is to look at theoretical, bias-minimizing criteria. These criteria will often suggest to choose weights inversely proportional to some kind of selection probability (density). This however makes the estimator extremely sensitive to extreme observations (which correspond to Jumbo in Sect. 1 and the outlying predictors in Sect. 2). Hence, we advise to be careful with bias-minimizing estimators if there are any observations which might be labeled by the terms "extreme," "undesired," "outlying," "weak," "needy," and the like, and it is likely that this holds far beyond the scope of sampling and smoothing.

20.5.2 An Unmentioned Assumption

Suppose now that the population is

$$\mathcal{C} = \{y_1, y_2, \ldots, y_N\}$$

where one of the y_i's is of the order $10^{10^{10}}$ and all the other y's are equal to $1 + \delta_i$ where $|\delta_i| < \epsilon$ and ϵ is very small, say .01. Then the probability that a random sample of size n does **not** contain the large y is

$$\frac{(N-1)}{N}\frac{(N-2)}{(N-1)}\frac{(N-3)}{(N-2)}\cdots\frac{(N-n)}{(N-n+1)} = 1 - \frac{n}{N}$$

Thus if $N = 1000$ and $n = 100$ the probability the a random sample will not contain the large y is 0.9. Thus even though random sampling ensures that on average we get an unbiased estimator of the population total 90 % of the random samples are truly bad, i.e., they greatly underestimate the population total.

The point is that having a random sample is no guarantee that it is a good sample. Why then is random sampling so popular and advocated by almost everyone? There seems to be a tacit assumption that the population being sampled consists of "similar objects." Then situations such as just discussed do not arise. The model-based approach to sampling legitimizes this by placing a model on the y's not the randomization process and bases sampling theory and practice on predicting the unobserved y's. Advocates of the randomization procedure (and there are many) protest the validity of the model assumptions. Fortunately the differences in practical settings are small, but it again points out the frailness of statistical theory: something must be assumed.

20.6 Prediction Approach

Suppose we have a sample from a population (often called the target population), how do we estimate the total T?

One way to understand the problem is to decompose the population total as follows:

$$T = \sum_{i=1}^{N} Y_i = \sum_{s} Y_i + \sum_{s^c} Y_i = T_s + T_{s^c}$$

where s^c is the complement of s with respect to the sample s, i.e., s^c consists of those units in the population which are not in the sample, T_s is the total of the observed sample, and T_{s^c} is the total of the unobserved values of Y.

Thus the problem of estimating T is reduced to one of **predicting** the total of the unobserved values, T_{s^c}, using the observed total T_s. It is natural to do this by estimating the average value of Y using the sample data by computing $\bar{y}$ and then using $(N - n)\bar{y}$ as the estimate of the total of the unobserved Y's. The estimate of the total is then taken to be

$$\hat{T} = T_s + (N - n)\bar{y} = T_s + \frac{(N - n)}{n}T_s = \frac{N}{n}T_s$$

As appealing as the approach seems it is useful to have a formal statement of its validity so that in more complex situations we may develop analogous procedures under more general models.

Let us assume that $Y_1, Y_2, \ldots, Y_N$ are generated by a random process such that

$$E(Y_i) = \mu \; ; \text{var}\,(Y_i) = \sigma^2; \quad \text{and the Y's are independent}$$

This simple model reflects the fact that the unobserved Y values have "something in common" with the observed values which will allow us to make inferences about them using the observed data.

It can be shown that under these assumptions, $\hat{T} = \frac{N}{n}T_s$, is that estimator of T which minimizes $E(\hat{T} - T)^2$ among all linear functions of the observed data which are unbiased, i.e., satisfy $E(\hat{T} - T) = 0$. This result generalizes to more complicated linear models relating the observed and unobserved values and provides a convenient framework for discussing finite population sampling.

The estimator $\hat{T} = \frac{N}{n}T_s$ is often called the "expansion" estimator of T.

Under the model assumptions the estimator $\hat{T}$ satisfies $E(\hat{T} - T) = 0$ and is thus an unbiased estimator of the population total. The expected squared error is thus the variance which of $\hat{T} - T$ under the model is given by

$$
\begin{aligned}
E(\hat{T} - T)^2 &= \operatorname{var}(\hat{T} - T) \\
&= \operatorname{var}\left(\frac{(N-n)}{n}T_s - T_{s^c}\right) \\
&= \frac{(N-n)^2}{n^2}n\sigma^2 + (N-n)\sigma^2 \\
&= (N-n)\left(\frac{N-n}{n}+1\right)\sigma^2 \\
&= N^2\left(1 - \frac{n}{N}\right)\frac{\sigma^2}{n}
\end{aligned}
$$

The expected squared error thus provides a natural measure of variability for the estimator. The term $(1 - \frac{n}{N})$ is called the **finite population correction factor**. Note that if the sample size equals the population size ($n = N$) then the variance of the estimator is zero since we know the population total in this case. An approximate 95 % confidence interval for the population total is given by

$$
\hat{T} \pm 2N\sqrt{1 - \frac{n}{N}}\,\frac{\sigma}{\sqrt{n}}
$$

20.6.1   *Proof of the Prediction Result*

Assume that $Y_1, Y_2, \ldots, Y_N$ are random variables generated by a random process $\mathcal{R}$. The problem is to use the sampled items, $\bar{y}_s$ to predict $\theta = \sum_{i=1}^{N}\ell_i Y_i$, i.e., a linear function of the Y's. The simplest, most natural predictor, L, satisfies

(i)   Linearity, i.e., $L = \sum_{i \in s} h_i Y_i$
(ii) Unbiasedness, i.e, $\mathbb{E}(L - \theta)^2 = 0$
(iii) Minimum mean square error, i.e., choose h_i to minimize $\mathbb{E}(L - \theta)^2$

The simplest assumption on the random process is that the Y's are uncorrelated with mean μ and variance σ^2. In this case unbiasedness requires that

$$\mathbb{E}[\sum_{i \in s} h_i Y_i - \sum_{i=1}^{N} \ell_i Y_i] = \sum_{i \in s} h_i \mu - \sum_{i=1}^{N} \ell_i \mu$$

$$= \left[\sum_{i \in s} h_i - \sum_{i=1}^{N} \ell_i \right] \mu$$

$$= 0$$

i.e., $\sum_{i \in s} h_i = \sum_{i=1}^{N} \ell_i$. The mean square error of the predictor is the same as its variance because of the unbiasedness condition and we have

$$\mathbb{E}[L - \theta]^2 = \mathbb{V}\left[\sum_{i \in s} h_i Y_i - \sum_{i=1}^{N} \ell_i Y_i \right]$$

$$= \mathbb{V}\left[\sum_{i \in s} (h_i - \ell_i) Y_i - \sum_{i \notin s} \ell_i Y_i \right]$$

$$= \sum_{i \in s} (h_i - \ell_i)^2 \sigma^2 + \sum_{i \notin s} \ell_i^2 \sigma^2$$

Thus we need to minimize (using Lagrange multipliers)

$$g(\mathbf{h}, \lambda) = \sum_{i \in s} (h_i - \ell_i)^2 \sigma^2 + \sum_{i \notin s} \ell_i^2 \sigma^2 + \lambda(\sum_{i \in s} h_i = \sum_{i=1}^{N} \ell_i)$$

It follows that

$$\frac{\partial g(\mathbf{h}, \lambda)}{\partial h_i} = 2 h_i \sigma^2 + \lambda$$

and

$$\frac{\partial g(\mathbf{h}, \lambda)}{\partial \lambda} = \sum_{i \in s} h_i - \sum_{i=1}^{N} \ell_i$$

It follows that

$$2 \sum_{i \in s} h_i \sigma^2 + n\lambda = 0$$

and hence

$$\lambda = -\frac{2\sigma^2}{n} \sum_{i=1}^{N} \ell_i$$

Thus

$$h_i = -\frac{1}{2\sigma^2}\lambda = \frac{1}{n} \sum_{i=1}^{N} \ell_i = \frac{\Delta}{n}$$

and the predictor is

$$\frac{\Delta}{n} \sum_{i \in s} y_i = \Delta \overline{y}_s$$

Note that if each $\ell_i = 1$ then the predictor is $N\overline{y}_s/n$, the expansion estimator.

20.7 Stratified Sampling

One of the most important methods of sampling finite populations is called
stratified sampling. In stratified sampling the population is divided into K mutually
exclusive subsets, called **strata**, and a simple random sample drawn from each.
In essence then stratified sampling may be viewed as taking K independent
simple random samples, one from each stratum. The reasons for using stratified
sampling are:

1. Under certain conditions the standard error of the estimates obtained using
   stratified sampling may be much smaller than using simple random sampling.
   This leads to shorter confidence intervals for parameters of interest and more
   precise inferences.
2. The estimation procedures are no more complicated since we simply combine
   simple random samples over strata, weighting inversely as the variance.
3. The costs involved in taking a stratified sample may not be substantially greater
   than those for a simple random sample and the resulting reduction in standard
   errors may be worthwhile.

20.7.1 Basic Results

We assume that there are N_i units in the ith stratum with associated characteristics
$Y_{i1}, Y_{i2}, \ldots, Y_{iN_i}$. The total for the ith stratum is $T_i = \sum_{j=1}^{N_i} Y_{ij}$. Assuming simple
random sampling, with a sample of size n_i in the ith stratum:

1. The estimate of the total in the ith stratum is given by

$$\hat{T}_i = T_{s_i} + \frac{(N_i - n_i)}{n_i} T_{s_i} = \frac{N_i}{n_i} T_{s_i}$$

where s_i denotes the sample in the ith stratum.

2. It follows that the estimate of the population total is given by

$$\hat{T} = \sum_{i=1}^{K} \frac{N_i}{n_i} \hat{T}_{s_i}$$

In order to determine the standard error of $\hat{T}$ we must make some model assumptions:

(a) The Y_{ij} are assumed independent.
(b) $E(Y_{ij}) = \mu_i$.
(c) $\text{var}(Y_{ij}) = \sigma_i^2$.

Under these assumptions we have that

$$\hat{T} - T = \sum_{i=1}^{K} \left[T_{s_i} + \frac{(N_i - n_i)}{n_i} T_{s_i} \right] - \sum_{i=1}^{K} (T_{s_i} + T_{s_i^c})$$

$$= \sum_{i=1}^{K} \left[\frac{(N_i - n_i)}{n_i} T_{s_i} - T_{s_i^c} \right]$$

Since each term in brackets has expected value equal to zero it follows that $E(\hat{T} - T) = 0$. The expected squared error thus satisfies

$$E(\hat{T} - T)^2 = \sum_{i=1}^{K} \left[\left(\frac{(N_i - n_i)}{n_i} \right)^2 n_i \sigma_i^2 + (N_i - n_i)\sigma_i^2 \right]$$

$$= \sum_{i=1}^{K} N_i(N_i - n_i) \frac{\sigma_i^2}{n_i}$$

$$= \sum_{i=1}^{K} N_i^2 (1 - \frac{n_i}{N_i}) \frac{\sigma_i^2}{n_i}$$

20.8   Cluster Sampling

Assume that the population of N individuals is arranged into K clusters of sizes $N_1, N_2, \ldots, N_K$, respectively. The value of the response variable Y for individual j in cluster i is denoted by Y_{ij}.

Cluster sampling proceeds by first selecting a random sample of k clusters and then selecting a random sample from each of the selected clusters. In order to develop expressions for the estimate and its variance we need a model describing the process which generates the response variable:

1. One simple model which appears to capture the principal features of clustering is as follows:

$$E(Y_{ij} = \mu$$

$$\text{cov}\,(Y_{ij}, Y_{lm}) = \begin{cases} \sigma_i^2 & i = l,\; j = m \\ \rho_i \sigma_i^2, & i = l,\; j \neq m \\ 0 & i \neq l \end{cases}$$

2. This simple model appears to capture the fact that objects within clusters (e.g., households) may not be independent.
3. Let s denote the sample of k clusters and s_i denote the sample of size n_i drawn from the ith selected cluster.

The population total can then be written as the sum of three components:

$$T = \sum_{i \in s} \sum_{j \in s_i} Y_{ij} + \sum_{i \in s} \sum_{j \in s_i^c} y_{ij} + \sum_{i \in s^c} \sum_{j=1}^{N_i} Y_{ij}$$

1. The first term represents the observed total of the units in the selected sample of clusters.
2. The second term represents the total of the unobserved units in the selected sample of clusters
3. The third term represents the total of the units in the unobserved clusters.

The estimator $\hat{T}_{opt}$ is unbiased and has minimum mean square prediction error under the model given by

$$\hat{T}_{opt} = \sum_{i \in s} \sum_{j \in s_i} Y_{ij} + \sum_{i \in s} (N_i - n_i) \left[\omega_i \bar{Y}_{s_i} + (1 - \omega_i)\hat{\mu} \right] + \sum_{i \in s^c} N_i \hat{\mu}$$

where

$$\omega_i = \frac{\rho_i n_i}{(1 - \rho_i + n_i \rho_i)}$$

$$\hat{\mu} = \sum_{i \in s} u_i \bar{y}_{s_i}$$

$$u_i = \frac{\frac{\omega_i}{\rho_i \sigma_i^2}}{\sum_{j \in s} \frac{\omega_j}{\rho_j \sigma_j^2}}$$

See Lohr [30] for an introductory treatment of finite population sampling from both the randomization and modeling point of view.

20.9 Practical Considerations

20.9.1 Sampling Frame Problems

The basic requirement of a sampling frame is that each element in the population should appear once and only once to ensure that correct probability calculations can be made. Consider the problems connected with a telephone survey:

- Missing elements, an individual does not have a telephone or it is an unlisted number.
- The elements are clustered since there is usually one number per family.
- Individuals can be listed more than once, e.g., at home and with a car phone.
- Some numbers are inapplicable, e.g., the numbers for time, weather, etc.

Of the problems with the sampling frame the most important is the problem of non-coverage.

20.9.2 Nonresponse

In any real sampling situation the problem of non-response is extremely important:

- **Total nonresponse** means that some individuals fail to respond to any of the survey.
- **Item nonresponse** means that some individuals fail to respond to part of the survey.
- The effect of nonresponse is to invalidate standard errors of estimates and thus to cast doubt on the conclusions reached from the survey.
- For item response there are a variety of imputation or "missing data" procedures which can be used, under model assumptions to obtain estimates in the presence of nonresponse. This is currently a very active research area in statistics.

20.9.3 Sampling Errors

Sampling errors, described by the standard errors of estimates, are part of every survey and can be reduced by careful use of supplementary information to increase the precision of the sample.

20.9.4   Non-sampling Errors

Non-sampling errors are much more damaging than sampling errors since they cannot be quantified and consist mainly of non-coverage errors and nonresponse errors. Any sample survey should try to minimize the total survey error defined as the sum of the sampling errors and the non-sampling errors.

20.10   Role of Finite Population Sampling in Modern Statistics

As statisticians and big data scientists accumulate more and more data from the web the principles of finite population sampling will become more important; in particular the notion of population sampled will become paramount to inference.

Chapter 21
Appendix: Probability and Mathematical Concepts

21.1 Probability Models

21.1.1 Definitions

Definition 21.1.1. A **statistical experiment** is a "random" phenomenon which yields a unique outcome called a **sample point** or an **elementary event**.

Definition 21.1.2. A **sample space** Ω is the collection of all sample points relative to a statistical experiment. We denote sample points by ω.

Definition 21.1.3. An **event** is a collection of sample points.

Definition 21.1.4. An **event space** is a nonempty collection of events

In probability theory we assume that every event space is a σ-algebra. That is,

Definition 21.1.5. Let Ω be set. A class of subsets of Ω, $\mathcal{W}$, is said to be a σ-**algebra** if the following conditions are satisfied:

  (i) $\mathcal{W}$ is nonempty.
  (ii) $E \in \mathcal{W}$ implies $E^C \in \mathcal{W}$.
 (iii) If $E_1, E_2, \ldots$ is a denumerable collection of sets in $\mathcal{W}$ then $\cup_{i=1}^{\infty} E_i \in \mathcal{W}$.

If the sample space is the set of real numbers, $\mathbb{R}$, or $\mathbb{R}^n$ the event space is taken to the collection of all **Borel sets** which includes sets of the form $(a, b]$, open sets, closed sets, etc. It is very hard to find a non-Borel set.

Definition 21.1.6. Let Ω be a sample space and let $\mathcal{W}$ be a σ-algebra over Ω. A **probability measure** $\mathbb{P}$ on $\mathcal{W}$ is a function $\mathbb{P} : \mathcal{W} \mapsto [0, 1]$ such that

  (i) $\mathbb{P}(\Omega) = 1$
  (ii) $\mathbb{P}(E) \geq 0$ for all $E \in \mathcal{W}$

© Springer International Publishing Switzerland 2014
C.A. Rohde, *Introductory Statistical Inference with the Likelihood Function*, DOI 10.1007/978-3-319-10461-4_21

(iii) If $E_1, E_2, \ldots$ is a finite or denumerable collection of mutually exclusive events $(E_i \cap E_j = \emptyset; \; i \neq j)$ in $\mathcal{W}$ then

$$\mathbb{P}(\cup_{i=1}^{\infty} E_i) = \sum_{i=1}^{\infty} \mathbb{P}(E_i)$$

Definition 21.1.7. A **probability space** or **probability model** is the triple $(\Omega, \mathcal{W}, \mathbb{P})$ where Ω is a sample space, $\mathcal{W}$ is a σ-algebra, and $\mathbb{P}$ is a probability measure on $\mathcal{W}$.

21.1.2 Properties of Probability

1. If $E \in \mathcal{W}$ then $\mathbb{P}(E^C) = 1 - \mathbb{P}(E)$
2. $\mathbb{P}(\emptyset) = 0$
3. If $E_1, E_2 \in \mathcal{W}$ and $E_1 \subseteq E_2$ then $\mathbb{P}(E_1) \leq \mathbb{P}(E_2)$
4. $\mathbb{P}(E_1 \cup E_2) = \mathbb{P}(E_1) + \mathbb{P}(E_2) - \mathbb{P}(E_1 \cap E_2)$
5. (Boole's Inequality) If $E_1, E_2, \ldots$ is a denumerable collection of events in $\mathcal{W}$ then

$$\mathbb{P}(\cup_{i=1}^{\infty} E_i) \leq \sum_{i=1}^{\infty} \mathbb{P}(E_i)$$

21.1.3 Continuity Properties of Probability Measures

Definition 21.1.8. A sequence of sets $E_1, E_2, \ldots$, is said to be increasing (non-decreasing) if $E_n \subseteq E_{n+1}$ for $n = 1, 2, \ldots$ and decreasing (non-increasing) if $E_n \supseteq E_{n+1}$ for $n = 1, 2, \ldots$.

Theorem 21.1.1. *If $\{E_n\}$ is a increasing or decreasing sequence of sets we have*

$$\mathbb{P}(\lim_{n \to \infty} E_n) = \lim_{n \to \infty} \mathbb{P}(E_n)$$

21.1.4 Conditional Probability

Definition 21.1.9. The **conditional probability** of B given A, $\mathbb{P}(B \mid A)$, is defined as

$$\mathbb{P}(B \mid A) = \frac{\mathbb{P}(B \cap A)}{\mathbb{P}(A)}$$

provided $\mathbb{P}(A) > 0$.

21.1.5 Properties of Conditional Probability

1. Let $(\Omega, \mathcal{W}, \mathbb{P})$ be a probability space, let $\mathbb{P}(A) > 0$, and define $\mathbb{P}(\bullet \mid A)$ to be the conditional probability given A for any event in $\mathcal{W}$. Then $(\Omega, \mathcal{W}, \mathbb{P}(\bullet \mid A))$ is a probability space.
2. (**Multiplication Rule**) If $\mathbb{P}(\cap_{i=1}^{k} E_i) > 0$ then

$$\mathbb{P}(\cap_{i=1}^{k} E_i) = \mathbb{P}(E_1)\mathbb{P}(E_2 \mid E_1) \times \cdots \times \mathbb{P}(E_k \mid \cap_{i=1}^{k-1} E_i)$$

3. A **partition**, $\mathcal{P}$, of a sample space, Ω, is a non-empty denumerable collection of mutually exclusive events in $\mathcal{W}$ such that $\Omega = \cup_{i=1}^{\infty} E_i$.
4. (**Law of Total Probability**) If $E_1, E_2, \ldots$ is a partition of Ω such that $\mathbb{P}(E_i) > 0$ for all i then for any event E in $\mathcal{W}$

$$\mathbb{P}(E) = \sum_{i=1}^{\infty} \mathbb{P}(E \mid E_i)\mathbb{P}(E_i)$$

5. (**Bayes Theorem**) If $\mathbb{P}(E) > 0$ and $\mathcal{P}$ is a partition of Ω such that $\mathbb{P}(E_i) > 0$ for all i then

$$\mathbb{P}(E_i \mid E) = \frac{P(\mathbb{P} \mid E_i)\mathbb{P}(E_i)}{\sum_{j=1}^{\infty} \mathbb{P}(E \mid E_j)\mathbb{P}(E_j)}$$

6. (**Simpson's Paradox**) It is possible to have

$$\mathbb{P}(A \mid B \cap C) \geq \mathbb{P}(A \mid B^C \cap C) \text{ and } \mathbb{P}(A \mid B \cap C^C) \geq \mathbb{P}(A \mid B^C \cap C^C)$$

and yet

$$\mathbb{P}(A \mid B) < \mathbb{P}(A \mid B^C)$$

21.1.6 Finite and Denumerable Sample Spaces

If Ω is finite or denumerable we can assign probabilities to all events $E \in \mathcal{W}$ by defining

$$\mathbb{P}(E) = \sum_{\omega \in E} p(\omega)$$

where $p(\omega)$ is called a **probability density function** and has the properties

(i) $p(\omega) \geq 0$ for all $\omega \in \Omega$

(ii) $\sum_{\omega \in \Omega} p(\omega) = 1$

Such probability models are called **discrete** probability models.

21.1.6.1   Random Sampling from a Population

A population of size N is a set of N objects.

Definition 21.1.10. A **sample** of size n from a population is an n-tuple of the form

$$(a_1, a_2, \ldots, a_n)$$

where a_i is an object in the population for each i.

Definition 21.1.11. A sample is said to be

1. **With replacement** if each element in the population can appear **more than once** in the sample
2. **Without replacement** if each element in the population can appear **at most once** in the sample

Definition 21.1.12. A sample is said to be a **random sample** if the probability of its selection is equal to the reciprocal of the number of possible samples.

21.1.6.2   Combinatorics

1. Given two sets A and B having m and n, elements respectively, there are $m \times n$ ordered pairs of the form (a_i, b_j) where $a_i \in A$ and $b_j \in B$.
2. Given r sets $A_1, A_2, \ldots, A_r$ containing $m_1, m_2, \ldots, m_r$ elements, respectively, there are $m_1 \times m_2 \times \cdots \times m_r$ r-tuples of the form

$$(a_1, a_2, \ldots, a_r); \quad a_i \in A_i \ \text{for} \ i = 1, 2, \ldots, r$$

3. A **permutation** of a set containing n elements is an arrangement of the elements of the set to form an n-tuple. There are n! permutations of a set containing n elements where $n!$ is defined as $n(n-1) \cdots 3 \cdot 2 \cdot 1$. By convention $0! = 1$. This convention is related to the Gamma function.
4. Given a set containing n elements the number of subsets of size x is given by

$$\binom{n}{x} = \frac{n!}{x!(n-x)!} = \frac{(n)_x}{x!}$$

where $(n)_x = n(n-1)\cdots(n-x+1) = \prod_{i=0}^{x-1}(n-i)$. This expression is read as n choose x and is called the number of **combinations** of n items taken x at a time.

Result 21.1.1. Given a population of size N there are

(i) N^n samples of size n with replacement
(ii) $N(N-1) \times \cdots \times (N-n+1) = (N)_n$ samples of size n without replacement

21.1.6.3   Two Important Discrete Probability Models

Result 21.1.2. Given a population of size N containing D objects of type A and $N - D$ objects of type $\overline{A}$ the probability that a random sample of size n contains x objects of type A is

(i)

$$p(x) = \binom{n}{x} p^x (1-p)^{n-x} \ \ \text{for} \ \ x = 0, 1, \ldots, n$$

if sampling is **with replacement** where $p = D/N$. This probability model is called the **binomial** probability distribution with parameters n and p.

(ii)

$$p(x) = \binom{n}{x} \frac{(D)_x (N-D)_{(n-x)}}{(N)_n} \ \ \text{for} \ \ x = 0, 1, \ldots, \min{(n, D)}$$

if sampling is **without replacement**. This probability model is called the **hypergeometric** probability distribution with parameters N, D, and n.

21.1.7   Independence

Definition 21.1.13. Events A and B are **independent** if

$$\mathbb{P}(A \cap B) = \mathbb{P}(A)\mathbb{P}(B)$$

Theorem 21.1.2. *Events A and B are independent if and only if*

$$\mathbb{P}(B \mid A) = \mathbb{P}(B)$$

Definition 21.1.14. Events $E_1, E_2, \ldots, E_n$ are independent if

$$\mathbb{P}(\cap_{i \in S} E_i) = \prod_{i \in S} \mathbb{P}(E_i) \text{ where } S \text{ is any subset of } \{1, 2, \ldots, n\}$$

21.1.7.1   Independent Trial Models

Let $\mathcal{W}_1, \mathcal{W}_2, \ldots, \mathcal{W}_n$ be σ-algebras over $\Omega_1, \Omega_2, \ldots, \Omega_n$, respectively. Define

$$\Omega = \Omega_1 \times \Omega_2 \times \cdots \times \Omega_n$$

On Ω define events E by

$$E = \{\omega : \omega = (\omega_1, \omega_2, \ldots, \omega_n) \text{ where } \omega_1 \in E_1, \omega_2 \in E_2, \ldots, \omega_n \in E_n\}$$

and $E_1 \in \mathcal{W}_1, E_2 \in \mathcal{W}_2, \ldots, E_n \in \mathcal{W}_n$. Finally let $\mathcal{W}$ be the σ-algebra generated by events of the form E.

Definition 21.1.15. The experimental setup just defined is called an experiment with n trials.

Definition 21.1.16. If $\mathbb{P}$ is a probability on $\mathcal{W}$ then the experiment with n trials is said to be an experiment with n independent trials if

$$\mathbb{P}(E) = \prod_{i=1}^{n} \mathbb{P}_i(E_i)$$

where $E_i \in \mathcal{W}_i$ for i=1,2,...,n, $E \in \mathcal{W}$, and $\mathbb{P}_i$ is a probability measure on $\mathcal{W}_i$ for i=1,2,...,n.

21.1.7.2   Bernoulli Trial Models

Definition 21.1.17. An experiment is said to be Bernoulli trial experiment if

(i) Each Ω_i consists of two sample points, ω_1, ω_2, the same for each i
(ii) The trials are independent
(iii) The probabilities are homogeneous from trial to trial, i.e.,

$$\mathbb{P}_i(\{\omega_1\}) = \mathbb{P}(\{\omega_1\}) \text{ for } i = 1, 2, \ldots, n$$

We call the two events in a Bernoulli trial model success and failure.

21.1.7.3 Results on Bernoulli Trial Models

1. The number of successes, x, in n Bernoulli trials has probability distribution given by

$$p(x) = \binom{n}{x} p^x (1-p)^{n-x} \ \text{ for } \ x = 0, 1, \ldots, n$$

   i.e., the binomial distribution with parameters n and p where p is the probability of a success on any trial.
2. The probability distribution of the trial number, x, on which the first success occurs (waiting time until the first success) is

$$p(x) = (1-p)^{x-1} p \ \text{ for } \ x = 1, 2, \ldots$$

   This probability distribution is called the **geometric** distribution with parameter p.
3. The probability distribution of the trial number, x, on which the rth success occurs (waiting time until the rth success) is

$$p(x) = \binom{x+r-1}{r-1} (1-p)^{x-r} p^r \ \text{ for } \ x = r, r+1, \ldots$$

   This probability distribution is called the **negative binomial** distribution with parameters r and p.
4. Given k successes in n Bernoulli trials the probability that a particular trial resulted in a success is k/n.

21.1.7.4 Multinomial Trial Models

Definition 21.1.18. An experiment is said to be multinomial trial experiment if

 (i) Each Ω_i consists of $k \geq 2$ sample points, $\omega_1, \omega_2, \ldots, \omega_k$, the same for each i
 (ii) The trials are independent
(iii) The probabilities are homogeneous from trial to trial, i.e.,

$$\mathbb{P}_i(\{\omega_j\}) = \mathbb{P}(\{\omega_j\}) \ \text{ for } i = 1, 2, \ldots, n \text{ and } j = 1, 2, \ldots, k$$

21.2   Random Variables and Probability Distributions

21.2.1   Measurable Functions

Definition 21.2.1. Let Ω be a set and let $\mathcal{W}$ be a σ-algebra over Ω. A function f: $\Omega \mapsto R$ is said to be $\mathcal{W}$- measurable if the inverse image of every Borel set is in $\mathcal{W}$, i.e.,

$$X^{-1}(B) = \{\omega :\; f(\omega) \in B\} \in \mathcal{W}\}$$

for every Borel set B.

21.2.2   Random Variables:Definitions

Definition 21.2.2. Let $(\Omega, \mathcal{W}, P)$ be a probability space. A random variable X is a real-valued measurable function on Ω:

1. X is a random variable if and only if $\{\omega : X(\omega) \leq x\}$ is in $\mathcal{W}$.
2. If X and Y are random variables so are cX, X^2, $X + Y$, XY and $\mid X \mid$.

21.2.3   Distribution Functions

Definition 21.2.3. If X is a random variable on $(\Omega, \mathcal{W}, \mathbb{P})$ then $(R, \mathcal{B}, \mathbb{Q})$ is a probability space where

$$\mathbb{Q}(B) = P(X^{-1}(B)) = \mathbb{P}(\{\omega : X(\omega) \in B\}) \text{ for } B \in \mathcal{B}$$

$\mathbb{Q}$ is called the probability measure induced (on R) by X and is called the **probability distribution of X** or the **distribution of X**.

Definition 21.2.4. The **distribution function**, F, of X is defined as

$$F(x) = \mathbb{P}(\{\omega : X(\omega) \leq x\}) \text{ for all } x \in R$$

21.2.3.1   Properties of Distribution Functions

1. $F(-\infty) = 0$, $F(+\infty) = 1$.
2. F is non-decreasing.
3. F is right continuous, i.e., $\lim_{\Delta \to 0} F(x + \Delta) = F(x)$ where $\Delta > 0$.
4. The set of discontinuity points of F is at most denumerable.
5. We write $F(x) = \mathbb{P}(X \leq x)$ even though it is misleading.

Definition 21.2.5. Any real-valued function F defined on R which is non-decreasing, right continuous, and for which $F(-\infty) = 0$; $F(+\infty) = 1$ is called a distribution function.

Result 21.2.1. Given a distribution function F, there exists a unique probability measure $\mathbb{P}$ on $\mathcal{B}$ such that $(R, \mathcal{B}, \mathbb{P})$ is a probability space. Thus a distribution function determines the underlying probability measure and conversely. The probability measure $\mathbb{P}$ on $\mathcal{B}$ is defined by

$$\mathbb{P}(\, (-\infty, x] \,) = F(x) \ \text{ for } x \in R$$

21.2.4   Discrete Random Variables

Definition 21.2.6. A random variable X on $(\Omega, \mathcal{W}, \mathbb{P})$ is said to be discrete if there exists a countable set $\mathcal{C} = \{x_1, x_2, \ldots\} \subset R$ such that

$$\mathbb{P}(X \in \mathcal{C}) = \mathbb{P}(\{\omega : X(\omega) \in \mathcal{C}\}) = 1$$

The points of $\mathcal{C}$ are called **discrete points** or **mass points**. For a discrete random variable the function f: $R \mapsto [0, 1]$, where

$$f(x) = \mathbb{P}(X = x) = P(\{\omega : X(\omega) = x\})$$

is called the probability density function (pdf) of X.

21.2.4.1   Results and Examples—Discrete Random Variables

1. The distribution function for a discrete random variable is a step function with step height equal to $f(x) = \mathbb{P}(X = x) = F(x) - F(x-)$ where $F(x-) = \lim_{\Delta \to 0} F(x - \Delta)$; $\Delta > 0$
2. X has a **Bernoulli** pdf if

$$f(x) = p^x(1-p)^{1-x} \ \ x = 0, 1$$

3. X has a **binomial** pdf with parameters n and p if

$$f(x) = \binom{n}{x} p^x(1-p)^{n-x} \ \text{ for } x = 0, 1, \ldots, n$$

4. X has a **geometric** pdf with parameter p if

$$f(x) = (1 - p)^{x-1}p \ \text{ for } \ x = 1, 2, \ldots$$

5. X has a **negative binomial** distribution with parameters r and p if

$$f(x) = \binom{x-1}{r-1}p^{x-r}p^r \ \text{ for } \ x = r, r + 1, \ldots$$

6. X has a **Poisson** pdf with parameter λ if

$$f(x) = \frac{\lambda^x e^{-\lambda}}{x!} \ \text{ for } \ x = 0, 1, \ldots$$

21.2.5 *Continuous Random Variables*

Definition 21.2.7. The random variable X defined on $(\Omega, \mathcal{W}, P)$ is said to be an (absolutely) continuous random variable if its distribution function can be written as

$$F(x) = \int_{-\infty}^{x} f(u)du \ .$$

where

$$f(x) \geq 0 \ \text{ and } \ \int_{-\infty}^{+\infty} f(x)dx = 1$$

f(x) is called the pdf (probability density function) of X.

21.2.5.1 **Properties and Examples of Continuous Random Variables**

1. The distribution function of a continuous random variable is differentiable almost everywhere and

$$\frac{dF(x)}{dx} = f(x)$$

2. X has a **uniform** distribution if

$$f(x) = 1 \ \text{ for } \ 0 \leq x \leq 1 \ \text{ and } \ 0 \ \text{ elsewhere}$$

3. X has a **rectangular** distribution with parameter $\theta > 0$ if

$$f(x) = \frac{1}{\theta} \quad \text{for} \ \ 0 \leq x \leq \theta \ \ \text{and} \ \ 0 \ \ \text{elsewhere}$$

4. X has a bf exponential distribution with parameter $\theta > 0$ if

$$f(x) = \frac{1}{\theta} e^{-\theta x} \quad \text{for} \ \ x \geq 0 \ \ \text{and} \ \ 0 \ \ \text{elsewhere}$$

5. Z has a **standard normal** or Gaussian(0,1) distribution if

$$f(z) = \frac{1}{\sqrt{2\pi}} e^{-z^2/2} \quad \text{for} \ \ -\infty < z < +\infty$$

6. X has a **Gamma** distribution with parameters $\alpha > 0$ and $\beta > 0$ if

$$f(x) = \frac{x^{\alpha-1} e^{-x/\beta}}{\Gamma(\alpha)\beta^\alpha} \quad \text{for} \ \ x \geq 0 \ \ \text{and} \ \ 0 \ \ \text{elsewhere}$$

where

$$\Gamma(\alpha) = \int_0^\infty x^{\alpha-1} e^{-x} dx$$

7. X has a **Beta** distribution with parameters $\alpha > 0$ and $\beta > 0$ if

$$f(x) = \frac{x^{\alpha-1}(1-x)^{\beta-1}}{B(\alpha,\beta)} \quad \text{for} \ \ 0 \leq x \leq 1 \ \ \text{and} \ \ 0 \ \ \text{otherwise}$$

where

$$B(\alpha,\beta) = \int_0^1 x^{\alpha-1}(1-x)^{\beta-1} dx = \frac{\Gamma(\alpha)\Gamma(\beta)}{\Gamma(\alpha+\beta)}$$

8. The **survival function** associated with a distribution function is defined as

$$S(x) = \mathbb{P}(X > x) = 1 - F(x)$$

Definition 21.2.8. X has a distribution which belongs to the **exponential family** if

$$f(x) = \exp\left\{\sum_{j=1}^k a_j(\theta) t_j(x) - c(\theta) + h(x)\right\}$$

where θ is a k-dimensional vector of real-valued parameters and the set of values of x for which $f(x) > 0$ (called the support of f) does not depend on θ.

21.2.6   *Functions of Random Variables*

Result 21.2.2. If X is a random variable on $(\Omega, \mathcal{W}, \mathbb{P})$ and $g : \quad R \mapsto R$ is a measurable function on $(R, \mathcal{B})$ then $Y = g(X) = (g \circ X)(\omega)$ is a random variable on $(\Omega, \mathcal{W}, \mathbb{P})$.

• The distribution of Y is given by

$$\mathbb{P}(B) = \mathbb{P}(X \in g^{-1}(B)) = \mathbb{P}(\{\omega : \omega \in X^{-1}(g^{-1}(B))\}) \text{ for } B \in \mathcal{B}$$

• The distribution function of Y is given by

$$F_Y(y) = \mathbb{P}(\{x : \ g(x) \le y\}) = \mathbb{P}(\{\omega : \ g(x(\omega)) \le y\})$$

The pdf of $Y = g(X)$ if it exists is obtained as follows:

(i) If X is discrete then $Y = g(X)$ is discrete and

$$f_Y(y) = \sum_S f(x) \text{ where } S = \{x : \ y = g(x)\}$$

(ii) If X is continuous and $Y = g(X)$ is discrete then

$$f_Y(y) = \int_S f(x)dx \text{ where } S = \{x : \ y = g(x)\}$$

(iii) If X is continuous and $Y = g(X)$ is continuous then

$$F_Y(y) = \int_S f(x)dx \text{ where } S = \{x : \ g(x) \le y\} \text{ and } f_Y(y) = \frac{dF_Y(y)}{dy}$$

(iv) If X is continuous and g is differentiable and one to one then

$$f_Y(y) = f_X[g^{-1}(y)]J(x,y)$$

where

$$J(x,y) = \left| \frac{dx}{dy} \right|_{x=g^{-1}(y)}$$

$J(x, y)$ is called the Jacobian of the transformation.

Example 21.2.1. 1. If Z has a standard normal distribution and $X = \mu + \sigma Z$ then X has a $N(\mu, \sigma^2)$ distribution and

$$f(x) = \frac{1}{\sigma\sqrt{2\pi}} \exp -\frac{(x-\mu)^2}{2\sigma^2}$$

2. If Z has a standard normal distribution and $X = Z^2$ then X has a chi-square distribution with one degree of freedom. The chi-square distribution with r degrees of freedom is defined as the Gamma distribution with parameters $\alpha = r/2$ and $\beta = 2$.

21.3 Random Vectors

21.3.1 Definitions

Definition 21.3.1. Let $(\Omega, \mathcal{W}, \mathbb{P})$ be a probability space. A random vector **X** is a function $\mathbf{X} : \Omega \mapsto R^k$ such that the inverse image of every Borel set in $\mathcal{B}^k$ is in $\mathcal{W}$ We write $\mathbf{X} = (X_1, X_2, \ldots, X_k)$ and call X_i the ith **coordinate** or the ith **projection** of **X**.

21.3.1.1 Properties of Random Vectors

1. If **X** is a random vector then each coordinate is a random variable.
2. If $X_1, X_2, \ldots, X_k$ are random variables on the same probability space then $\mathbf{X} = (X_1, X_2, \ldots, X_k)$ is a random vector.
3. The joint probability distribution of **X** is defined by

$$\mathbb{Q}(B) = \mathbb{P}(\mathbf{X}^{-1}(B)) = \mathbb{P}(\{\omega : \mathbf{X}(\omega) \in B\}) \ \ for \ B \in \mathcal{B}^k$$

4. The joint distribution function of **X** is defined as

$$F(\mathbf{x}) = \mathbb{P}(\mathbf{X} \leq \mathbf{x})$$
$$= \mathbb{P}(X_1 \leq x_1, X_2 \leq x_2, \ldots, X_k \leq x_k)$$
$$= \mathbb{P}(\{\omega : X_1(\omega) \leq x_1, X_2(\omega) \leq x_2, \ldots, X_k(\omega) \leq x_k\})$$

5. Properties of joint distribution functions: in two dimensions we have

(i) $F(x_1, x_2) = \mathbb{P}(X_1 \leq x_1, X_2 \leq x_2)$
(ii) $0 \leq F(x_1, x_2) \leq 1)$

(iii) $F(x_+h_1, x_2 + h_2) - F(x_1 + h_1, x_2) - F(x_1, x_2 + h_2) + F(x_1, x_2) \geq 0$
      for $h_1 \geq 0, h_2 \geq 0$
(iv) $F(-\infty, x_2) = F(x_1, -\infty) = 0$
(v) $F(+\infty, +\infty) = 1$

21.3.2   Discrete and Continuous Random Vectors

Definition 21.3.2. A random vector $\mathbf{X}$ is discrete if there exists a countable set $\mathcal{C} = \{\mathbf{x}_1, \mathbf{x}_2, \ldots\} \subset R$ such that $\mathbb{P}(\mathbf{X} \in \mathcal{C}) = 1$.

The function $f(\mathbf{x}) = \mathbb{P}(\mathbf{X} = \mathbf{x})$ is called the joint pdf of $\mathbf{X}$ and satisfies

$$0 \leq f(\mathbf{x} \leq 1 \text{ and } \sum_{x_1} \sum_{x_2} \cdots \sum_{x_k} f(x_1, x_2, \ldots, x_k) = 1$$

Definition 21.3.3. A random vector $\mathbf{X}$ is continuous if there exists a function f such that the distribution function of $\mathbf{X}$ is given by

$$F(x_1, x_2, \ldots, x_k) = \int_{-\infty}^{x_k} \cdots \int_{-\infty}^{x_1} f(u_1, \ldots, u_k) du_1 \cdots du_k$$

f is called the joint pdf of $\mathbf{X}$ and satisfies

$$f(\mathbf{x}) > 0 \text{ and } \int_{-\infty}^{+\infty} \cdots \int_{-\infty}^{+\infty} f(x_1, \ldots, x_k) dx_1 \cdots dx_k = 1$$

21.3.3   Marginal Distributions

Let S_1 and S_2 be nonempty subsets of the integers 1,2,...,k containing p and q elements, respectively, where $p + q = k$, such that

$$S_1 \cup S_2 = \{1, 2, \ldots, k\} \text{ and } S_1 \cap S_2 = \emptyset$$

If $\mathbf{X}$ is a k-dimensional random vector, write

$$\mathbf{X} = (\mathbf{X}_1, \mathbf{X}_2)$$

where

$$\mathbf{X}_1 = (X_{i_1}, X_{i_2}, \ldots, X_{i_p}) \text{ and } \mathbf{X}_2 = (X_{j_1}, X_{j_2}, \ldots, X_{j_q})$$

and

$$S_1 = \{i_1, i_2, \ldots, i_p\} \; ; \; S_2 = \{j_1, j_2, \ldots, j_q\}$$

Definition 21.3.4. The marginal distribution function of $\mathbf{X}_1$ is given by $F(\mathbf{x}_1, \infty)$ where $F(\mathbf{x}_1, \mathbf{x}_2)$ is the distribution function of $(\mathbf{X}_1, \mathbf{X}_2)$. In particular, the marginal distribution function of X_i is obtained when $S_1 = \{i\}$

If $\mathbf{X}$ is a discrete random vector then the pdf of $\mathbf{X}_1$ is given by

$$f_{\mathbf{X}_1}(\mathbf{x}_1) = \sum_{\text{all } \mathbf{x}_2} f(\mathbf{x}_1, \mathbf{x}_2)$$

where $f(\mathbf{x}_1, \mathbf{x}_2)$ is the joint pdf of $\mathbf{X}$. Similarly if $\mathbf{X}$ is a continuous random vector then the pdf of $\mathbf{X}_1$ is given by

$$f_{\mathbf{X}_1}(\mathbf{x}_1) = \int_{\text{all } \mathbf{x}_2} f(\mathbf{x}_1, \mathbf{x}_2)$$

where $f(\mathbf{x}_1, \mathbf{x}_2)$ is the joint pdf of $\mathbf{X}$.

If $\mathbf{X} = (X, Y)$ these two formulas reduce to

$$f_X(x) = \sum_{\text{all } y} f(x, y) \;\text{ and }\; f_X(x) = \int_{-\infty}^{+\infty} f(x, y) dy$$

21.3.4 The Multinomial Distribution

Definition 21.3.5. The random vector $\mathbf{X}$ is said to have a multinomial distribution with parameters $n, p_1, p_2, \ldots . p_k$ if its pdf is given by

$$f_{\mathbf{X}}(\mathbf{x}) = n! \prod_{i=1}^{k} \frac{p_i^{x_i}}{x_i!} \;\text{ for } \mathbf{x} \in S$$

where

$$S = \{\mathbf{x} : \; x_i = 0, 1, \ldots, n \;\; x_1 + x_2 + \cdots + x_k = n\}$$

and

$$0 \le p_i \le 1 \; ; \; p_1 + p_2 + \cdots + p_k = 1$$

21.3.4.1 Multinomial Results

1. The multinomial distribution gives the probability of the number of times outcomes $\omega_1, \omega_2, \ldots, \omega_k$ occur in n multinomial trials.
2. The marginal distribution of any subset of the multinomial is also multinomial. In particular the marginal distribution of X_i is binomial (n, p_i).

21.3.5 Independence of Random Variables

Definition 21.3.6. The random variables $X_1, X_2, \ldots, X_n$ are independent if

$$\mathbb{P}(X_1 \in B_1, X_2 \in B_2, \ldots, X_n \in B_n) = \prod_{i=1}^{n} \mathbb{P}(X_i \in B_i)$$

for all Borel sets B_i

21.3.5.1 Properties of Independent Random Variables

1. If $X_1, X_2, \ldots, X_n$ are independent, $A \subset \{X_1, X_2, \ldots, X_n\}$, and g and h are measurable functions then $g(A)$ and $h(A^C)$ are independent.
2. If $\mathbf{X}$ is a random vector its components $X_1, X_2, \ldots, X_n$ are independent if and only if the joint distribution function of $\mathbf{X}$ satisfies

$$F_{\mathbf{X}}(\mathbf{x}) = \prod_{i=1}^{n} F_{X_i}(x_i)$$

where F_{X_i} is the marginal distribution function of X_i for i=1,2,...,n.
3. If $\mathbf{X}$ has a pdf then its components are independent if and only if the joint pdf satisfies

$$f_{\mathbf{X}}(\mathbf{x}) = \prod_{i=1}^{n} f_{X_i}(x_i)$$

where f_{X_i} is the marginal pdf of X_i for i=1,2,...,n.
4. If $\mathbf{X} = (\mathbf{X_1}, \mathbf{X_2})$ then $\mathbf{X_1}$ and $\mathbf{X_2}$ are independent if and only if

$$F_{\mathbf{X_1},\mathbf{X_2}}(\mathbf{x_1}, \mathbf{x_2}) = F_{\mathbf{X_1}}(\mathbf{x_1})F_{\mathbf{X_2}}(\mathbf{x_2})$$

21.3.6 Conditional Distributions

Definition 21.3.7. Let $\mathbf{X}$ be a k-dimensional random vector with pdf $f(\mathbf{x})$. Let $A \subset R^k$ be an event such that $\mathbb{P}(\mathbf{X} \in A) > 0$. Then the conditional pdf of $\mathbf{X}$ given $\mathbf{X} \in A$ is defined as

$$f(\mathbf{x} \mid \mathbf{X} \in A) = \frac{f(\mathbf{x})\mathbf{1}_A(\mathbf{x})}{\mathbb{P}(\mathbf{X} \in A)}$$

where $\mathbf{1}_A$ is the indicator function of the set A.

Definition 21.3.8. Let $\mathbf{X}$ and $\mathbf{Y}$ have joint distribution specified by the joint pdf $f_{\mathbf{X},\mathbf{Y}}$ and let the marginal pdf of $\mathbf{X}$ be $f_{\mathbf{X}}$. Then the conditional pdf of $\mathbf{Y}$ given $\mathbf{X} = \mathbf{x}$ is defined as

$$f(\mathbf{y} \mid \mathbf{x}) = \frac{f_{\mathbf{X},\mathbf{Y}}(\mathbf{x},\mathbf{y})}{f_{\mathbf{X}}(\mathbf{x})}$$

21.3.6.1 Properties and Examples of Conditional Distributions

1. For fixed $\mathbf{x}$, $f(\mathbf{y} \mid \mathbf{x})$ is a pdf.
2. (Generalization of the Law of Total Probability) The marginal pdf of $\mathbf{Y}$ is given by

$$f_{\mathbf{Y}}(\mathbf{y}) = \int_{\text{all } \mathbf{x}} f(\mathbf{y} \mid \mathbf{x}) f_{\mathbf{X}}(\mathbf{x}) d\mathbf{x}$$

3. If $\mathbf{X}$ is multinomial then the conditional distribution of any subset of $\mathbf{X}$ given another subset of $\mathbf{X}$ is also multinomial.

21.3.7 Functions of a Random Vector

Definition 21.3.9. If $\mathbf{X}$ is a k-dimensional random vector and $g : R^k \mapsto R^p$ where $p \leq k$ is a measurable function then $\mathbf{Y} = g(\mathbf{X})$ is a random vector with probability distribution given by

$$\mathbb{P}_{\mathbf{Y}}(B) = \mathbb{P}(\{\mathbf{x} : g(\mathbf{x}) \in B\})$$

and distribution function given by

$$F_{\mathbf{Y}}(\mathbf{y}) = \mathbb{P}(\{\mathbf{x} : g(\mathbf{x}) \leq \mathbf{y}\})$$

Result 21.3.1. If $\mathbf{X}$ has pdf $f_{\mathbf{X}}$ then $\mathbf{Y}$ has pdf $f_{\mathbf{Y}}$ given by :

(i) $f_{\mathbf{Y}}(\mathbf{y}) = \sum_{B_{\mathbf{y}}} f_{\mathbf{X}}(\mathbf{x})$ if $\mathbf{X}$ is discrete where $B_{\mathbf{y}} = \{\mathbf{x} : g(\mathbf{x}) = \mathbf{y}\}$.

(ii) $f_{\mathbf{Y}}(\mathbf{y}) = \int_{B_{\mathbf{y}}} f_{\mathbf{X}}(\mathbf{x})d\mathbf{x}$ if $\mathbf{X}$ is continuous and $\mathbf{Y}$ is discrete where

$$B_{\mathbf{y}} = \{\mathbf{x} : g(\mathbf{x}) = \mathbf{y}\}$$

(iii) $f_{\mathbf{Y}}(\mathbf{y}) = \frac{\partial F_{\mathbf{Y}}(\mathbf{y})}{\partial \mathbf{y}}$ where

$$F_{\mathbf{Y}}(\mathbf{y}) = \int_{B_{\mathbf{y}}} f_{\mathbf{X}}(\mathbf{x})d\mathbf{x}$$

if $\mathbf{X}$ is continuous, $\mathbf{Y}$ is continuous, and $B_{\mathbf{y}} = \{\mathbf{x} : g(\mathbf{x}) \leq \mathbf{y}\}$.

(iv) If $\mathbf{X}$ has joint pdf $f_X(\mathbf{x})$ and $\mathbf{Y} = \mathbf{g}(\mathbf{x})$, assume that $\mathbf{x}$ and $\mathbf{y}$ are n-dimensional and that $\mathbf{g}$ is one-one. The density of $\mathbf{Y}$ at $\mathbf{y}$ is given by

$$f_Y(\mathbf{y}) = f_X[\mathbf{g}^{-1}(\mathbf{y})] \left| \det[\mathbf{J}(\mathbf{x},\mathbf{y})]_{\mathbf{x}=\mathbf{g}^{-1}(\mathbf{y})} \right|$$

where

$$\mathbf{J}(\mathbf{x},\mathbf{y}) = \begin{bmatrix} \frac{\partial x_1}{\partial y_1} & \frac{\partial x_1}{\partial y_2} & \cdots & \frac{\partial x_1}{\partial y_n} \\ \frac{\partial x_2}{\partial y_1} & \frac{\partial x_2}{\partial y_2} & \cdots & \frac{\partial x_2}{\partial y_n} \\ \vdots & \vdots & \ddots & \vdots \\ \frac{\partial x_n}{\partial y_1} & \frac{\partial x_n}{\partial y_2} & \cdots & \frac{\partial x_n}{\partial y_n} \end{bmatrix}$$

is the Jacobian (matrix) of the transformation.
Note that $\mathbf{J}(\mathbf{x},\mathbf{y})$ is often easier to calculate using the relationship

$$\mathbf{J}(\mathbf{x},\mathbf{y}) = [\mathbf{J}(\mathbf{y},\mathbf{x})]^{-1}$$

where

$$\mathbf{J}(\mathbf{y},\mathbf{x}) = \begin{bmatrix} \frac{\partial y_1}{\partial x_1} & \frac{\partial y_1}{\partial x_2} & \cdots & \frac{\partial y_1}{\partial x_n} \\ \frac{\partial y_2}{\partial x_1} & \frac{\partial y_2}{\partial x_2} & \cdots & \frac{\partial y_2}{\partial x_n} \\ \vdots & \vdots & \ddots & \vdots \\ \frac{\partial y_n}{\partial x_1} & \frac{\partial y_n}{\partial x_2} & \cdots & \frac{\partial y_n}{\partial x_n} \end{bmatrix}$$

Example 21.3.1. 1. If X and Y are independent binomial random variables with parameters n_1, n_2, p, respectively then $X + Y$ has a binomial distribution with parameters $n_1 + n_2, p$.

2. If X and Y are independent Poisson random variables with parameters λ_1, λ_2, respectively then $X + Y$ has a Poisson distribution with parameters $\lambda_1 + \lambda_2$.

3. If X is $N(\mu_1, \sigma_1^2)$, Y is $N(\mu_2, \sigma_2^2)$ and X and Y are independent then $X + Y$ is $N(\mu_1 + \mu_2, \sigma_1^2 + \sigma_2^2)$.
4. If X is Gamma(α_1, β) and Y is Gamma(α_2, β) and X and Y are independent, then $X + Y$ is Gamma$(\alpha_1 + \alpha_2, \beta)$.
5. If X is $N(0, 1)$ and Y is $N(0, 1)$ and X and Y are independent then X/Y has a Cauchy distribution with parameters 0 and 1.
6. If X is Cauchy(μ_1, σ_1) and Y is Cauchy(μ_2, σ_2) and they are independent then $X + Y$ has a Cauchy distribution with $\mu = \mu_1 + \mu_2$ and $\sigma + \sigma_1 + \sigma_2$.

21.3.8 The Multivariate Normal Distribution

Definition 21.3.10. If $\mathbf{X}$ is a k-dimensional random vector its matrix representation is the k by 1 vector given by

$$\mathbf{X} = \begin{bmatrix} X_1 \\ X_2 \\ \vdots \\ X_k \end{bmatrix}$$

Definition 21.3.11. If $Z_1, Z_2, \ldots, Z_k$ are independent each normal with parameters 0 and 1 the k-dimensional random vector $\mathbf{Z}$ defined by $\mathbf{Z} = (Z_1, Z_2, \ldots, Z_k)$ is said to have a standard multivariate normal distribution with parameters $\mathbf{0}$ and $\mathbf{I}$. Here $\mathbf{0}$ is a k by 1 vector of 0's and $\mathbf{I}$ is the k by k identity matrix.

Definition 21.3.12. If $\mathbf{Z}$ is **standard multivariate normal** then its pdf is given by

$$f_{\mathbf{Z}}(\mathbf{z}) = \frac{1}{(2\pi)^{k/2}} exp\{-\frac{1}{2}\mathbf{z}^\top\mathbf{z}\} \text{ for } -\infty < z < +\infty$$

Definition 21.3.13. $\mathbf{X}$ has a multivariate normal distribution in k dimensions with parameters $\boldsymbol{\mu}$ and $\boldsymbol{\Sigma}$ if

$$\mathbf{X} = \boldsymbol{\mu} + \mathbf{BZ}$$

where $\mathbf{Z}$ is standard multivariate normal in k dimensions and $\boldsymbol{\Sigma} = \mathbf{BB}^\top$.

Result 21.3.2. The pdf of the k-dimensional multivariate normal with parameters $\boldsymbol{\mu}$ and $\boldsymbol{\Sigma}$ written as MVN $(\boldsymbol{\mu}, \boldsymbol{\Sigma})$ is given by

$$f_{\mathbf{X}}(\mathbf{x}) = \frac{1}{(2\pi)^{k/2}(\det \boldsymbol{\Sigma})^{1/2}} \exp\left\{-\frac{1}{2}(\mathbf{x} - \boldsymbol{\mu})^\top \boldsymbol{\Sigma}^{-1}(\mathbf{x} - \boldsymbol{\mu})\right\}$$

21.3.8.1   Properties of the Multivariate Normal Distribution

1. If $\mathbf{X}$ is MVN $(\boldsymbol{\mu}, \boldsymbol{\Sigma})$ then

$$\mathbf{Y} = \mathbf{a} + \mathbf{C}\mathbf{X}$$

   is MVN$(\mathbf{a} + \mathbf{C}\boldsymbol{\mu}, \mathbf{C}\boldsymbol{\Sigma}\mathbf{C}^{\top})$ where $\mathbf{Y}$ is p dimensional, $p \leq k$, $\mathbf{a}$ is a p by 1 vector, and $\mathbf{C}$ is a p by p matrix of rank p.
2. If $(\mathbf{X}, \mathbf{Y})$ is MVN $(\boldsymbol{\mu}, \boldsymbol{\Sigma})$ where

$$\boldsymbol{\mu} = \begin{bmatrix} \boldsymbol{\mu}_x \\ \boldsymbol{\mu}_y \end{bmatrix} \quad \text{and} \quad \boldsymbol{\Sigma} = \begin{bmatrix} \boldsymbol{\Sigma}_{\mathbf{xx}} & \boldsymbol{\Sigma}_{\mathbf{xy}} \\ \boldsymbol{\Sigma}_{\mathbf{yx}} & \boldsymbol{\Sigma}_{\mathbf{yy}} \end{bmatrix}$$

   then the marginal distribution of $\mathbf{X}$ is MVN $(\boldsymbol{\mu}_x, \boldsymbol{\Sigma}_{xx})$.
3. The conditional distribution of $\mathbf{Y}$ given $\mathbf{X} = \mathbf{x}$ is

$$\text{MVN} \left(\boldsymbol{\mu}_y + \boldsymbol{\Sigma}_{yx}\boldsymbol{\Sigma}_{xx}^{-1}(\mathbf{x} - \boldsymbol{\mu}_x), \boldsymbol{\Sigma}_{yy} - \boldsymbol{\Sigma}_{yx}\boldsymbol{\Sigma}_{xx}^{-1}\boldsymbol{\Sigma}_{xy} \right)$$

21.4   Expected Values

21.4.1   Expected Value of a Random Variable

Definition 21.4.1. If X is a random variable with pdf f then the expected value of X, $\mathbb{E}(X)$, is defined as follows:

(i) If X is discrete then

$$\mathbb{E}(X) = \sum_{x \in S} x f(x) \quad \text{where} \quad S \text{ is the set of discrete(mass) points of X}$$

(ii) If X is a continuous random variable then

$$\mathbb{E}(X) = \int_{-\infty}^{+\infty} x f(x) dx$$

provided both the sum and the integral converge absolutely.

Definition 21.4.2. The expected value of a random variable exists (is finite) if and only if both $\mathbb{E}(X^+)$ and $\mathbb{E}(X^-)$ are finite where

$$X^+ = X \cdot \mathbf{1}_{X \geq 0} \quad \text{and} \quad X^- = X \cdot \mathbf{1}_{X < 0}$$

and $\mathbf{1}$ is the indicator function. In this case

$$\mathbb{E}(X) = \mathbb{E}(X^+) + \mathbb{E}(X^-)$$

21.4.1.1 Notation

We sometimes write

$$\mathbb{E}(X) = \int x dF(x) \quad \text{or} \quad \mathbb{E}(X) = \int x f(x) d\mu(x)$$

to denote the expected value of X, which covers both the discrete and the continuous case using a single notation. In this notation μ denotes counting measure if X is discrete and Lebesgue measure if X is continuous.

Result 21.4.1. If X is a random variable with expected value equal to μ then

1. If X is discrete with mass points $0, 1, 2, \ldots$

$$\mu = \sum_{x=0}^{\infty} [1 - F(x)] = \sum_{x=0}^{\infty} P(X > x)$$

2. If X is a continuous random variable with distribution function F

$$\mu = \int_{0}^{+\infty} [1 - F(x)] dx - \int_{-\infty}^{0} F(x) dx$$

3. If $Y = g(X)$ where $g : R \mapsto R$ is measurable then the expected value of Y is given by

$$\mathbb{E}(Y) = \int y f_Y(y) d\mu(y) = \int g(x) f_X(x) d\mu(x)$$

which has been called the **Law of the Unconscious Statistician**.

21.4.1.2 Properties of Expected Values

1. If c is a constant then $\mathbb{E}(c) = c$
2. If c is a constant then $\mathbb{E}[cg(X)] = c\mathbb{E}[g(X)]$
3. If c_1, c_2 are constants then

$$\mathbb{E}[c_1 g_1(X) + c_2 g(X)] = c_1 \mathbb{E}[g_1(X)] + c_2 \mathbb{E}[g_2(X)]$$

and more generally

$$\mathbb{E}\left[\sum_{i=1}^{n} c_i g_i(X) \right] = \sum_{i=1}^{n} c_i \mathbb{E}[g_i(X)]$$

4. If $g_1(X) \leq g_2(X)$ for all values of X then $\mathbb{E}[g_1(X)] \leq \mathbb{E}[g_2(X)]$
5. If $X \geq 0$ then $\mathbb{E}(X) \geq 0$

21.4.2   Distributions and Expected Values

Theorem 21.4.1. *Two distribution functions F and G are equal if and only if*

$$\mathbb{E}_F[u(X)] = \mathbb{E}_G[u(X)] \quad \text{for all bounded continuous functions } u$$

21.4.3   Moments

Definition 21.4.3. The rth moment of the random variable X, μ_r' is defined as $\mathbb{E}(X^r)$ provided $\mathbb{E}(\mid X \mid^r)$ is finite.

Definition 21.4.4. The rth central moment of the random variable X, μ_r, is defined as
$\mathbb{E}(X - \mu)^r$ provided $\mathbb{E}[(\mid (X - \mu) \mid^r)]$ is finite where μ is the expected value of X.

21.4.4   Properties and Results on Expected Values and Moments

1. The mean of X is defined as $\mu = \mathbb{E}(X)$.
2. The variance, $\mathbb{V}(X)$, of X is defined as $\mathbb{E}[(X - \mu)^2]$.
3. $\mathbb{V}(X) = \mathbb{E}(X^2) - [\mathbb{E}(X)]^2$.
4. The mean, μ, of X minimizes $\mathbb{E}(X - c)^2$.
5. If X is random variable with $\mathbb{E}(X) = \mu$ and $\mathbb{V}(X) = \sigma^2$ then the **standardized version** of X is defined as

$$Z = \frac{X - \mu}{\sigma}$$

   and $\mathbb{E}(Z) = 0$ and $\mathbb{V}(Z) = 1$.
6. **Markov's Inequality**: For any positive random variable Y we have

$$\mathbb{P}(Y \geq k) \leq \frac{\mathbb{E}(Y)}{k} \quad \text{for any positive k}$$

7. **Chebyshev Inequality**. Let X be random variable and assume that $\mu = \mathbb{E}(X)$ and $\mathbb{V}(X) = \sigma^2$ exist. Then

$$\mathbb{P}(\mid X - \mu \mid) \geq \gamma\sigma) \leq \frac{1}{\gamma^2}$$

8. **Jensen's Inequality**. If $g : R \mapsto R$ is a convex function then

$$\mathbb{E}[g(X)] \geq g(\mathbb{E}(X))$$

21.4.5 Other Functionals of a Distribution

Definition 21.4.5. The **pth quantile** of the distribution F, or the random variable X, is defined as any number η_p satisfying

$$F(\eta_p-) \leq p \leq F(\eta_p) \quad \text{or} \quad \mathbb{P}(X < \eta_p) \leq p \leq \mathbb{P}(X \leq \eta_p)$$

Result 21.4.2. 1. The **median** of X is the 0.5 quantile, i.e., the median, η, satisfies

$$\mathbb{P}(X < \eta) \leq 1/2 \leq \mathbb{P}(X \leq \eta)$$

2. The median, η, minimizes $\mathbb{E}(|X - c|)$.
3. The **quartiles** of X are the 0.25 and 0.75 quantiles.
4. The **deciles** of X are the $0.1, 0.2, \ldots, 0.9$ quantiles.

21.4.6 Probability Generating Functions

Definition 21.4.6. If X is a discrete random variable with sample space $\{0,1,2,\ldots\}$ the **probability generating function** of X is

$$P(s) = \sum_{k=0}^{\infty} s^k p_k$$

where $p_k = P(X = k)$. P(s) converges for $|s| \leq 1$

21.4.6.1 Properties of Probability Generating Functions

1. The pgf uniquely determines the pdf.
2. The moments of a random variable with pgf P(s), if they exist, can be found by differentiating the pgf, more precisely,

$$\mathbb{E}[X(X-1)\cdots(X-r+1)] = \frac{d^r P(s)}{d^r s}\bigg|_{s=1}$$

3. $\mathbb{E}[X(X-1)\cdots(X-r+1)]$ is called the rth **factorial moment** of X.

21.4.7 Moment-Generating Functions

Definition 21.4.7. The **moment-generating function** of a random variable X is defined as

$$M(t) = \mathbb{E}(e^{tX})$$

provided the expectation is finite for some $t \in T$ where T is an interval of real numbers containing 0.

21.4.7.1 Properties of Moment-Generating Functions

1. If the mgf exists it uniquely determines the pdf.
2. If the mgf exists then $M(t) = P(e^t)$ where P(s) is the pgf.
3. If the mgf of X exists then the moments of X can be found by differentiating the mgf, more precisely,

$$\left. \frac{d^r M(t)}{d^r t} \right|_{t=0} = \mathbb{E}(X^r)$$

4. If the moment-Generating function of X exists then

$$M(t) = \sum_{r=0}^{\infty} \frac{\mu'_r t^r}{r!}$$

5. If the moment-Generating function of X exists, then

$$e^{-\mu t} M(t) = \sum_{r=0}^{\infty} \frac{\mu_r t^r}{r!}$$

21.4.8 Cumulant Generating Functions and Cumulants

Definition 21.4.8. If the mgf function of X exists then the **cumulant generating function**, cgf, of X, $K(t)$, is defined as $K(t) = \ln M(t)$.

Definition 21.4.9. The rth cumulant of X is defined as coefficient of $t^r/r!$ in the expansion of $K(t)$ around t=0 and is denoted by κ_r.

21.4.8.1 Properties of Cumulants

(i) The first four cumulants in terms of the first four central moments are

(1) $\kappa_1 = \mu_1$
(2) $\kappa_2 = \mu_2$
(3) $\kappa_3 = \mu_3$
(4) $\kappa_4 = \mu_4 - 3\mu_2^2$

(ii) The first four central moments in terms of the first four cumulants are

(1) $\mu_1 = \kappa_1$
(2) $\mu_2 = \kappa_2$
(3) $\mu_3 = \kappa_3$
(4) $\mu_4 = \kappa_4 + 3\kappa_2^2$

(iii) For symmetric distributions all odd cumulants are zero.

Definition 21.4.10. The **skewness** of X is defined as

$$\kappa_3/\sigma^3 = \mu_3/\sigma^3$$

Definition 21.4.11. The **kurtosis** of X is defined as

$$\kappa_4/\sigma^4 = \frac{\mu_4 - 3\mu_2^2}{\sigma^4}$$

21.4.9 Expected Values of Functions of Random Vectors

Definition 21.4.12. If **X** is a random vector and $g : R^k \mapsto R$ is a Borel measurable function then the expected value of $Y = g(\mathbf{X})$ is given by

$$\mathbb{E}(Y) = \int_{\text{all } y} y f_Y(y) d\mu(y) = \int_{\text{all } \mathbf{x}} g(x) f_{\mathbf{X}}(\mathbf{x}) d\mu(\mathbf{x})$$

where $f_Y(y)$ is the pdf of Y and $f_{\mathbf{X}}$ is the pdf of **X**.

21.4.9.1 Properties and Definitions

1. The expected value of $\sum_{i=1}^{n} a_i X_i$ is given by

$$\mathbb{E}(\sum_{i=1}^{n} a_i X_i) = \sum_{i=1}^{n} a_i \mathbb{E}(X_i)$$

where $a_1, a_2, \ldots, a_n$ are constants.

2. The **covariance** of X and Y is defined as

$$\mathbb{C}\left(X,Y\right) = \mathbb{E}[(X - \mu_X)(Y - \mu_Y)] = \mathbb{E}(XY) - \mu_X\mu_Y$$

where $\mu_X = \mathbb{E}(X)$ and $\mu_Y = \mathbb{E}(Y)$.

3. $\mathbb{C}\left(X,Y\right) = \mathbb{C}\left(Y,X\right)$.

4. $\mathbb{C}\left(X,X\right) = \mathbb{V}\left(X\right)$.

5. $\mathbb{C}\left(X,c\right) = 0$ where c is a constant.

6. (Cauchy-Schwarz Inequality) $[\mathbb{C}(X,Y)]^2 \leq \mathbb{V}(X)\mathbb{V}(Y)$ with equality holding if and only if $Y = a + bX$ for some constants a and b.

7. The **correlation** of X and Y is defined as

$$\operatorname{corr}\left(X,Y\right) = \rho_{XY} = \frac{\mathbb{C}\left(X,Y\right)}{\sqrt{\mathbb{V}\left(X\right)\mathbb{V}\left(Y\right)}}$$

where $\mathbb{V}\left(X\right)$ is the variance of X and $\mathbb{V}\left(Y\right)$ is the variance of Y.

8. $|\operatorname{corr}\left(X,Y\right)| \leq 1$ with equality holding if and only if $Y = a + bX$ for some constants a and b.

9. Variance of a linear combination

$$\mathbb{V}\left(\sum_{i=1}^{n} a_i X_i\right) = \sum_{i=1}^{n}\sum_{j=1}^{n} a_i a_j \mathbb{C}\left(X_i, X_j\right)$$

10. Covariance of two linear combinations

$$\mathbb{C}\left(\sum_{i=1}^{n} a_i X_i, \sum_{j=1}^{m} b_j Y_j\right) = \sum_{i=1}^{n}\sum_{j=1}^{m} a_i b_j \mathbb{C}\left(X_i, Y_j\right)$$

11. $\mathbb{C}\left(aX + bY, cX + dY\right) = (ac)\mathbb{V}\left(X\right) + (bd)\mathbb{V}\left(Y\right) + (ad + bc)\mathbb{C}\left(X,Y\right)$.

12. $\mathbb{V}\left(X + Y\right) = \mathbb{V}\left(X\right) + \mathbb{V}\left(Y\right) + 2\mathbb{C}\left(X,Y\right)$.

13. $\mathbb{V}\left(X - Y\right) = \mathbb{V}\left(X\right) + \mathbb{V}\left(Y\right) - 2\mathbb{C}\left(X,Y\right)$.

14. X and Y are **uncorrelated** if $\mathbb{C}\left(X,Y\right) = 0$.

15. If X and Y are independent then they are uncorrelated but not conversely.

16. If $X_1, X_2, \ldots, X_n$ are pairwise uncorrelated ($\mathbb{C}\left(X_i, X_j\right) = 0$ for $i \neq j$) and $\mathbb{E}(X_i) = \mu$; $\mathbb{V}\left(X\right) = \sigma^2$ then

$$\mathbb{E}(\overline{X}) = \mu \ \text{ and } \ \mathbb{V}\left(\overline{X}\right) = \frac{\sigma^2}{n}$$

where

$$\bar{X} = \frac{\sum_{i=1}^{n} X_i}{n}$$

17. If X and Y are independent then $\mathbb{E}(XY) = \mathbb{E}(X)\mathbb{E}(Y)$

18. If $X_1, X_2, \ldots, X_n$ are independent with X_i having mgf $M_i(t)$ then the mgf of the sum $S_n = \sum_{i=1}^{n} X_i$ is given by

$$M_{S_n}(t) = \prod_{i=1}^{n} M_i(t)$$

21.4.10 Conditional Expectations and Variances

1. The **conditional expectation** of Y given $\mathbf{X} = \mathbf{x}$ is defined as

$$\mathbb{E}(Y \mid \mathbf{X} = \mathbf{x}) = \int_{-\infty}^{+\infty} y f(y \mid \mathbf{x}) d\mu(y)$$

2. The function $\mathbb{E}(Y \mid \mathbf{X})$ whose value at $\mathbf{x}$ is $\mathbb{E}(Y \mid \mathbf{X} = \mathbf{x})$ is a random variable.
3. $\mathbb{E}[\mathbb{E}(Y \mid \mathbf{X})] = \mathbb{E}(Y)$.
4. The **conditional variance** of Y given $\mathbf{X} = \mathbf{x}$ is defined as

$$\mathbb{V}(Y \mid \mathbf{X} = \mathbf{x}) = \int_{-\infty}^{+\infty} (y - \mu_{Y|\mathbf{x}})^2 f(y \mid \mathbf{x}) d\mu(y)$$

   where $\mu_{Y|\mathbf{x}}$ is the conditional expectation of Y given $\mathbf{X} = \mathbf{x}$.
5. The function $\mathbb{V}(Y \mid \mathbf{X})$ whose value at $\mathbf{x}$ is $\mathbb{V}(Y \mid \mathbf{X} = \mathbf{x})$ is a random variable.
6. **Conditional variance formula**

$$\mathbb{V}(Y) = \mathbb{E}[\mathbb{V}(Y \mid \mathbf{X})] + \mathbb{V}[\mathbb{E}(Y \mid \mathbf{X})]$$

7. The **conditional covariance** of Y and Z given $\mathbf{X} = \mathbf{x}$ is defined as

$$\mathbb{C}((Y, Z) \mid \mathbf{X}) = \int_{-\infty}^{+\infty} \int_{-\infty}^{+\infty} (y - \mu_{Y|\mathbf{x}})(z - \mu_{Z|\mathbf{x}}) f(y, z \mid \mathbf{x}) d\mu(y, z)$$

8. The function $\mathbb{C}((Y, Z) \mid \mathbf{X})$ whose value at $\mathbf{x}$ is $\mathbb{C}((Y, Z) \mid \mathbf{X} = \mathbf{x})$ is a random variable.
9. **Conditional covariance formula**

$$\mathbb{C}(Y, Z) = \mathbb{E}[\mathbb{C}((Y, Z) \mid \mathbf{X})] + \mathbb{C}[\mathbb{E}(Y \mid \mathbf{X}), \mathbb{E}(Z \mid \mathbf{X})]$$

21.5   What Is Probability?

Bruno de Finetti, one of the foremost probabilists of the twentieth century, wrote:

> Probability does not exist.

De Finetti's statement has something to do with the many different ways we use probability, i.e., the different kinds of A for which we make statements such as

$$\text{the probability of } A \text{ is } \mathbb{P}(A)$$

Examples of A include

- A is the event that a coin will come up heads in 20 tosses.
- A is the statement that a defendant is guilty.
- A is the statement that a treatment cures a disease.
- A is the statement that it will rain tomorrow.
- A is the event that the mean of n iid normal(0,1) random variables will exceed $1/\sqrt{n}$.

Consider a situation in which we have a coin which consists of a euro and a quarter, the heads being the euro and the tail the quarter. Does this new coin have an intrinsic probability, θ, of falling heads if tossed? If so what does it mean? If not what do we mean by inference about θ?

Probabilists view de Finetti's statement as almost irrelevant as do many statisticians who adopt the view that probability is a measure with norm 1 on a σ-field of events, subsets of a sample space, i.e., a probability space consists of $(\Omega, \mathcal{W}, \mathbb{P})$ where Ω is a sample space, $\mathcal{W}$ is a σ-field of subsets of Ω, and $\mathbb{P}$ has the properties:

(i) $P(\Omega) = 1$
(ii) $0 \le P(E) \le 1$ for all $E \in \mathcal{W}$
(iii) If $E_1, E_2, \ldots$ is a denumerable collection of mutually exclusive sets in $\mathcal{W}$ then

$$P\left(\cup_{i=1}^{\infty} E_i\right) = \sum_{i=1}^{\infty} P(E_i)$$

the so-called axiom of countable additivity.

As is well known these axioms imply the entire array of probability results useful in statistics.

However

- They do not tell us how to interpret probabilities.
- Nor how we can convey the results of statistical analyses to scientists and the public, e.g., how do we convey the meaning of a confidence interval or a Bayesian interval when the "event" is a statement about a parameter?

The "three" standard interpretations of probability are:

1. **Frequency interpretation**
2. **Belief interpretation**
3. **Logical interpretation**

The first interpretation leads to "classical" or "frequentist" statistics while the second and third lead to "Bayesian" statistics both "subjective" and "objective."

21.5.1   Frequency Interpretation

> ... the probability of an event is the long-run frequency with which the event occurs in a certain experimental setup or in a certain population

Shafer [47]

For example if an experiment is performed n times and an event A occurs k times then the relative frequency of A is $\frac{k}{n}$. If this fraction converges to say, p, as n increases, then p is the probability of A in the frequency interpretation.

- Note that the frequency interpretation only applies when the experiment can be repeated and we have convergence of the relative frequency.
- The scope is narrow.
- What about conditional probability and independence?
- What about the convergence of $\frac{k}{n}$?
- Which trials?
- How long a run?
- Real or hypothetical trials?

Any event occurs exactly once (in all its detail) so only non-trivial frequencies can be defined unless the event is considered as one of a "more general" type of event. How to choose this type is called "typing" Granularity is also an issue, i.e., in n trials relative frequencies can only be of the form c/n and yet some physical events can have irrational probabilities. We can always transform into "single case," e.g., 1,000 trials of a coin toss can be considered as one trial of 1,000 tosses.

If we allow infinite number of trials we need to consider the "order" of the trials to obtain relative frequency, e.g., an even number among the non-negative integers has frequency $1/2$ if the order is

$$(1, 2, 3, 4, 5, \ldots)$$

and frequency $1/4$ if the order is

$$(1, 3, 5, 2, 7, 9, 11, 4, 13, 15, 17, 6, 19, 21, 23, 8, \ldots)$$

This is called the *reference sequence problem*:

- No evidence in favor of any event implies equal probability for each of the events.
- Circular and implies symmetry.
- Different kinds of symmetry imply different probabilities for the same phenomenon.

> Thus the probability is considered to be a value independent of the observer. It gives the approximate value of the relative frequency of an event in a long sequence of experiments.
> . . .
> As the probability of a random event is an objective value which does not depend on the observer, one can approximately calculate the long run behaviour of such events, and the calculations can be empirically verified.
> In everyday life we often make subjective judgements concerning the probability of a random event. The mathematical theory of probability, however, does not deal with these subjective judgements but with objective probabilities.

Renyi [40]

21.5.2   *Belief Interpretations*

Consider collections of propositions or sentences and new sentences made by combining sentences according to certain rules. A sentence or proposition is either true or false and the rules for building new sentences are such that the truth of a new sentence is determined by the truth of the combining sentences and the type of rule.

The logical structure of the combinations are **"and," "or,"** and **"not."** These are represented as follows:

$$
\begin{array}{ll}
\text{and} & \text{\& or } \wedge \\
\text{or} & \vee \\
\text{not} & \sim \text{ or } \neg
\end{array}
$$

Consider two sentences A and B. The truth value of the combinations is as follows:

Sentence		Truth-value		
A	B	A & B	A $\vee$ B	$\neg$ A
T	T	T	T	F
T	F	F	T	F
F	T	F	T	T
F	F	F	F	T

Consider now a collection of sentences (or events or hypotheses) $E_1, E_2, \ldots$.

- A **betting strategy** between you, Y, and nature, N, is a setup in which you pay $p(E_i)$ units to nature to play and receive 1 unit from nature if E_i occurs.
- The strategy is defined as **fair** if you are not certain to have a positive gain or a positive loss.

Howson and Urbach [23] prove the following:

Theorem 21.5.1 (Ramsey, deFinetti).   *In order for a betting strategy to be fair, the $p(E_i)$ (called betting prices) must have the following properties:*

1. $0 \leq p(E_i)$ for all i.
2. If E is always true $p(E) = 1$.
3. If E_1 and E_2 are mutually exclusive then $p(E_1 \vee E_2) = p(E_1) + p(E_2)$.

To prove (1) we have the following payoff matrix:

Event E_i	Payoff to Y
T	$1 - p(E_i)$
F	$-p(E_i)$

If $p(E_i) < 0$ then you are certain to gain either $|p(E_i)|$ or $1 + |p(E_i)|$ so $p(E_i)$ must be nonnegative.

To prove (2) we note that if E is certain to occur your payoff is $1 - p(E)$ which is a certain loss if $p(E) > 1$ and a certain gain if $p(E) < 1$. Hence $p(E) = 1$

To prove (3) let E_1 and E_2 be mutually exclusive with betting prices p_1 and p_2. If you bet on both E_1 and E_2 then the payoff matrix is

Event status		
E_1	E_2	Payoff to Y
T	F	$1 - p(E_1) - p(E_2)$
F	T	$1 - p(E_1) - p(E_2)$
F	F	$-[p(E_1) + p(E_2)]$

(E_1 and E_2 are mutually exclusive so E_1 and E_2 cannot both be true).

This is equivalent to the following bet on $E_1 \vee E_2$:

Event $E_1 \vee E_2$ status	Payoff to Y
T	$1 - p(E_1) - p(E_2)$
F	$-p(E_1) - p(E_2)$

For another bet on $E_1 \vee E_2$ with stake r the payoff matrix would be

Event $E_1 \vee E_2$ status	Payoff to Y
T	$1 - r$
F	$-r$

Combining these two bets into one strategy shows that the difference in payoffs would be

Event $E_1 \vee E_2$ status	Payoff difference to Y
T	$r - p(E_1) - p(E_2)$
F	$r - p(E_1) - p(E_2)$

which is certain to result in a gain or loss unless $r = p(E_1) + p(E_2)$.

Hence betting prices must obey the laws of probability.

How one decides their specific personal or subjective probability of a particular event can be done using the following scheme:

Suppose that you are interested in determining the probability of an event E. Consider two wagers defined as follows:

Wager 1 :   You receive $100 if the event E occurs and nothing if it does not occur.
Wager 2 :   There is a jar containing x white balls and $N - x$ red balls. You receive $100 if a white ball is drawn and nothing otherwise.

You are required to make one of the two wagers. Your probability of E is taken to be the ratio x/N at which you are indifferent between the two wagers.

- The belief interpretation is a gambling interpretation, e.g., if your probability of event A is p then your odds on a gamble for which you receive 1 unit if A occurs is $p/(1-p)$ to 1. Conversely if you are willing to bet on A with odds a to 1 then your probability is $a/(1+a)$. Similarly bets against A are defined and required to be consistent with those for bets on A.
- Probabilities so defined obey Kolmogorov's axioms **provided** you act in such a way to avoid certain loss (Dutch book argument).
- Conditional probabilities for B given A are simply probabilities so assigned under the additional condition that A has occurred.
- Linearity of money, i.e., betting amount may depend on the units involved which may mean the result does not hold.
- In the definition of conditional probability, rewritten as

$$\mathbb{P}(A \cap B) = \mathbb{P}(A)\mathbb{P}(B|A)$$

and called the **Rule of Compound Probability** there is the assumption that B follows A and that its probability under these circumstances is well defined.

Is the interpretation **normative** or **descriptive**, i.e.,

1. Do the probabilities describe how we should behave (normative)?
2. Do they describe how we actually behave (descriptive)? Lots of work shows that people don't behave according to the axioms.
3. While not important to statistical analysis it is important to consumers of statistical results.

21.5.3   Rational Belief Interpretation

- The probability of A is the degree to which we should believe that A will occur based on our evidence.
- This interpretation can be made precise. Derivation assumes "reasonable" properties of belief.

Cox [10] develops the properties of probability for propositions. A **proposition** is a statement denoted by **a**. A proposition may be true or false. There are three methods of working with propositions to form new propositions:

1. **Contradictory** denoted by $\sim$ and defined by

$$\sim a = \text{not } a$$

2. **Conjunction** of a and b denoted by $a \wedge b$ and defined by

$$a \wedge b = \text{a and b}$$

3. **Disjunction** of a and b denoted by $a \vee b$ and defined by

$$a \vee b = \text{a or b}$$

These methods have properties which Cox uses to develop the basic properties of probability using just two axioms:

Axiom 21.5.1. The probability of an event on given evidence determines the probability of its contradictory on the same evidence.

Axiom 21.5.2. The probability on given evidence that both of two events are true is determined by their separate probabilities, one on the given evidence, the other on this evidence with the additional assumption that the first event is true.

Thus we have the properties of probability derived from two axioms.
Some problems with this interpretation are:

- Why should belief for A or B depend only on beliefs for A and B?
- Conditional belief in B given A may depend on how we learned about A, i.e., there is a uniqueness question for $\mathbb{P}(B|A)$.

21.5.4 Countable Additivity Assumption

The axiom of countable additivity cannot be justified in the frequency definition of probability. Under an additional assumption it can be justified in the subjective approach.

Let $\{E_1, E_2, \ldots\}$ be a collection of mutually exclusive events whose union is the sample space Ω. Let $p_i = P(E_i)$ and let $\Delta_i \Theta_i$ be the corresponding stakes where

$$\Delta_i = \pm 1 \quad \text{and} \quad \Theta_i \geq 0 \quad \text{for } i = 1, 2, \ldots,$$

The loss that would occur if E_k is true would be given by

$$L_k = \sum_{i=1}^{\infty} p_i \Delta_i \Theta_i - \Delta_k \Theta_k$$

Thus, a loss is certain if $L_k > 0$ for all $k = 1, 2, \ldots$.

Theorem 21.5.2. *If only a finite amount of money changes hands* then the *probabilities are coherent (certain loss is not possible) if and only if $\sum_{i=1}^{\infty} p_i = 1$.*

21.5.5 Lindley's Wheel

Imagine a perfectly balanced roulette wheel of diameter $1/2\pi$ so that the circumference is 1. If the pointer on this wheel is spun where it stops produces a point which is equally likely to lie anywhere on the circumference. Call this a random point. If we cut the circle we have a line of unit length and a point which is equally likely, to be anywhere on the line. (By equally likely we mean that a bet as to whether the point will lie in a subinterval A depends only on the length of the interval and not its position).

If we now consider the spin of another identical wheel, similarly cut, we have a unit square with the property that any region of area A is as equally likely as any other region of area A. This leads to defining the probability of the event that the point is in A as the area of A. The total area is 1.

It is easily seen that probability so defined has the properties we assume, i.e.,

1. $P(\Omega) = 1$
2. $0 \leq P(A) \leq 1$ for any A
3. $P(A \cup B) = P(A) + P(B)$ if $A \cap B = \emptyset$

21.5.6 Probability via Expectations

This approach is due to Peter Whittle [53]. Whittle uses expectation as the basic concept. Let Ω be a sample space (set) of points ω and let $\mathcal{W}$ be a σ-algebra over Ω. Define a **random variable** to be a real-valued function from the sample space such that the inverse image of every Borel set is in the σ-algebra $\mathcal{W}$.

Define the **expectation operator**, $\mathbb{E}$, to be a function from the set of all random variables to the real line which satisfies the following axioms:

Axiom 1: If $X \geq 0$ then $\mathbb{E}(X) \geq 0$
Axiom 2: If c is a constant then $\mathbb{E}(cX) = c\mathbb{E}(X)$
Axiom 3: $\mathbb{E}(X_1 + X_2) = \mathbb{E}(X_1) + \mathbb{E}(X_2)$
Axiom 4: $\mathbb{E}(1) = 1$

Axiom 5:   If a sequence of random variables $\{X_n : n = 1, 2, \ldots\}$ increases monotonically to a limit X then $\mathbb{E}(X_n) = \mathbb{E}(X)$

The probability of an event A, $\mathbb{P}(A)$, is then defined as

$$\mathbb{P}(A) = \mathbb{E}(\mathbf{1}_A) \text{ for any } A \in \mathcal{W}$$

The motivation for the use of expectations is based on a concept of average. Suppose that we have a collection (set) of N individuals. Assume that to each individual ω_i there is an associated value of a real-valued quantity X which we call a random variable. Suppose further that there are n_k individuals with value x_k. Then the population average of X is given by

$$\mathbb{A}v(X) = \frac{1}{N} \sum_k n_k x_k = \sum_k p_k x_k$$

where p_k is the proportion of the individuals having value x_k. Averages such as these are a facet of everyday life and understood by all.

It is easy to see that $\mathbb{A}v$, as just defined, satisfies the first four of the axioms. The fifth axiom is added as a continuity condition and allows probability to satisfy the axiom of countable additivity.

Consider a large population (size N) from which we have selected a "random" sample of size $n \ll N$. We find that x individuals in the sample have incomes satisfying condition C. Of interest is the proportion D/N in the population which have condition C.

Belief, logical, and frequentists agree (well mostly agree) that a reasonable probability model for the observed data is the binomial, i.e.,

$$\mathbb{P}(x) = \binom{n}{x} \theta^x (1 - \theta)^{n-x}$$

for $x = 0, 1, 2, \ldots, n$ (provided we assume $n < D$).

While agreeing on the basic model advocates of the different interpretations of probability differ on the manner in which x provides information on θ:

1. The frequentist or classical statistician assumes that θ is fixed and uses properties of those values of x not observed to make inferences. These are the usual P-value and confidence interval statements.
2. The belief and the logical approaches to interpretation of probabilities are willing to assume knowledge of θ in the form of a probability distribution **prior** and then calculate the **posterior** distribution of θ and base inferences on this.

Why is it such a "big deal" that inferences are interpreted differently? Because each approach can show the other is inadequate, i.e., the frequentists stridently demand to know how a prior can be justified while the Bayesian can demonstrate incoherence of some frequentist statements not to mention that the frequentist is silent with respect to single case situations. That being said, the frequentist some-times use, Bayesian ideas to develop procedures and evaluates using frequentist methods and the Bayesian checks procedures to see their frequentist properties.

21.6   Final Comments

- The philosophy of probability is concerned with how the definition can be related to real events (i.e., interpretation of probabilities) and how the properties indicated in the definition can be justified (derivation of probability axioms). These are necessarily related.
- The philosophy of statistics is concerned with how one should use a probability model for a given observed data to make inferences about the model (usually the model is specified by a few unknown parameters and inference is intended to answer questions about these parameters).

In most statistical settings we need to know only the first two interpretations of probability. Of these the frequency interpretation is the best known but least capable of justifying while the subjective interpretation is easily justified but hard to apply in many scientific contexts.

Two quotes illustrating differing points of view toward applications of probability:

Probability only works if we do not attempt to define what probability means in the real world.

Williams [54]

The probability of an event is the relative frequency with which I expect the event to occur.

Anonymous

21.7   Introduction to Stochastic Processes

21.7.1   Introduction

Definition 21.7.1. A **stochastic process** is an indexed collection of random vari-ables or vectors usually written as

$$\{X_t;\ t \in T\}$$

Clearly a random variable is a stochastic process as is a random vector or a sequence of random variables. In short the study of random variables is a special case of the study of stochastic processes.

What makes stochastic processes useful is

- Modeling of dependent random variables
- Richness of potential applications
- Richness of the theory
- Potential for inference research
- Applications to Bayesian inference

21.7.2 Types of Stochastic Processes

Usually we think of the index set T as **time** so that we are interested in modelling random phenomena that evolve over time. This leads to the first major classification of the types of stochastic processes: that based on the nature of the the index set and the nature of the sample space called the **state space**.

This later notion reflects the type of thinking about phenomena occurring over time: the state of the process at time t.

Index set (Time)	State space	
	Discrete	Continuous
Discrete		
Continuous		

- n Bernoulli trials or an infinite sequence of Bernoulli trials is a discrete time, discrete state stochastic process.
- A sequence of continuous random variables is a discrete time, continuous state stochastic process.
- The Poisson process is a continuous time, discrete state stochastic process.
- The Weiner process is a continuous time, continuous state stochastic process.

By definition a stochastic process is an indexed collection of random variables. Since a random variable is a function defined on a probability space a stochastic process may be viewed as a function of two variables, the state space and the time index. If time is fixed at t the value of the stochastic process is X_t a random variable. If the value of the state space is fixed at $\omega \in \Omega$ then the value of the stochastic process is

$$\{x_t(\omega) \ : \ \omega \in \Omega\}$$

which is called the **sample path** or **realization** of the stochastic process. (Recall the distinction between a random variable and its observed value).

A second way of classifying stochastic processes is by their evolution over time, i.e., how properties of the joint distribution of a subset of the random variables change over time.

If we consider a sequence of independent identically distributed random variables with 0 expected value, i.e.,

$$X_1, X_2, \ldots, X_n, \ldots \text{ or } \{X_t : t = 1, 2, \ldots\}$$

where

$$E(X_t) = 0, \ t \in T$$

then we know that

- The distribution of X_{n+1} is independent of the preceding random variables $X_1, X_2, \ldots, X_n$
- The distribution of X_n does not depend on n
- If $S_{n+1} = X_1 + X_2 + \cdots + X_{n+1}$ then

$$E(S_{n+1}|X_1, X_2, \ldots, X_n) = S_n$$

These three properties lead to definitions of three major classes of stochastic processes.

- **Markov processes** (the distribution at time $t + \Delta$ depends only on the present, X_t, not on the history of the process)
- **Stationary processes** (certain properties of the distribution of the process remain constant over time)
- **Martingales** (the expected value of the process at time t depends only on the state of the process at the immediately preceding time point).

Each of these classes of processes has a well-developed theory and a broad range of "applications."

21.7.3   Markov Processes

To set some notation define the **history**, $\mathcal{H}_{t-}$, of the stochastic process as

$$\mathcal{H}_{t-} = \{X_1, X_2, \ldots, X_{t-}\}$$

Thus for example

$$E[X_t|\mathcal{H}_{t-}]$$

is the expected value of X_t given the history of the process up to the present time and

$$f_{X_t, X_{t+s}}(x_t, x_{t+s} | \mathcal{H}_{t-})$$

is the joint density of X_t and X_{t+s} ($s > 0$) given the history of the process up to t.

Roughly speaking a **Markov process** is a stochastic process in which the present state determines the future evolution of the process. More formally a sequence $X_1, X_2, \ldots$ is a (discrete time) Markov process if

$$P(X_{n+1} \le x | \mathcal{H}_n) = P(X_{n+1} \le x | X_1, X_2, \ldots, X_n)$$
$$= P(X_{n+1} \le x | X_n)$$

for all x.

If, in addition, this probability does not depend on n the Markov process is said to be (time) **homogeneous**. Much of the development of the theory of Markov processes hinges on a careful use of the law of total probability and the multiplication rule.

Suppose that the random variables have densities (discrete or continuous). Then the Markov condition is

$$f_{X_{n+1} | \mathcal{H}_n}(x) = f_{X_{n+1} | X_n}(x)$$

Thus if the process is Markov and homogeneous we have that the joint density of $X_1, X_2, \ldots, X_{n+1}$ is given by

$$f_{X_1}(x_1) f_{X_2 | X_1}(x_2 | x_1) \cdots f_{X_{n+1} | X_n}(x_{n+1} | x_n)$$

using the multiplication rule.

Suppose now that $1 \le n_1 < n$ and $n_1 < n_2 < n$. Then the law of total probability says that

$$f_{X_{n+1} | X_{n_1}}(x | y)$$

is given by

$$\int_{\mathscr{X}} f_{X_{n+1} | X_{n_2}}(x | x_{n_2}, z) f_{X_{n_2} | X_{n_1}}(z | x_{n_1} = y) dm(z)$$

which is called the **Chapman–Kolmogorov** equation. It is a direct consequence of the law of total probability.

21.7.4 Markov Chains

When the state space is discrete a Markov process is said to be a Markov chain.

Definition 21.7.2. A **Markov chain** is a discrete state, discrete time stochastic process which satisfies

$$P(X_{n+1} = x | \mathcal{H}_n) = P(X_n = x | X_i = x_i; i = 0, \ldots, n)$$
$$= P(X_{n+1} = x | X_n = x_n)$$

For all $n \geq 1$, all values of $x_0, x_1, \ldots, x_n$ and x.

The evolution of a Markov chain is thus described by the collection of **transition probabilities**

$$P(X_{n+1} = x | X_n = x_n)$$

Since the sample space is countable with no loss of generality we assume that the state space is

$$\Omega = \{1, 2, \ldots\}$$

i.e., the integers. As useful terminology we say that the chain is in state i if $X_n = i$ and has visited state j if $X_t = j$ for some $t = 1, 2, \ldots, n - 1$.

In general the transition probabilities depend on n.

Definition 21.7.3. A Markov chain is (time) **homogeneous** if

$$P(X_{n+1} = j | X_n = i) = P(X_1 = j | X_0 = i) = p_{ij}$$

The matrix whose elements are the p_{ij} is called the **matrix of transition probabilities**. It is easy to see that a matrix of transition probabilities has the following properties:

$$p_{ij} \geq 0 \quad \text{and} \quad \sum_j p_{ij} = 1 \quad \text{for each } i$$

Consider the case where the chain has two states, 0 and 1. The transition matrix is thus

$$\mathbf{P} = \begin{bmatrix} 1 - p_{01} & p_{01} \\ p_{10} & 1 - p_{10} \end{bmatrix}$$

If we assume that the initial probabilities are p_0 and p_1 then the probability of state 0 at time 1 is given by

$$p_1(0) = p_0 p_{00} + p_1 p_{10} = p_0(1 - p_{01}) + p_1 p_{10}$$

Similarly the probability of being in state 1 at time 1 is

$$p_1(1) = p_0 p_{01} + p_1 p_{11} = p_0 p_{01} + p_1(1 - p_{10})$$

In general the probability of state 0 at time $n + 1$ given state 0 at time n is given by

$$p_{n+1}(0) = p_n(0) p_{00} + p_n(1) p_{10} = p_n(0)(1 - p_{01}) + p_n(1) p_{10}$$

and the probability of state 1 at time $n + 1$ given state 0 at time n

$$p_{n+1}(1) = p_n(0) p_{01} + p_n(1) p_{11} = p_n(0) p_{01} + p_n(1)(1 - p_{10})$$

again using the law of total probability.

In matrix notation we thus have

$$[p_{n+1}(0) , \; p_{n+1}(1)] = [p_n(0) , \; p_n(1)] \begin{bmatrix} 1 - p_{01} & p_{01} \\ p_{10} & 1 - p_{10} \end{bmatrix}$$

and it follows that

$$[p_{n+1}(0) , \; p_{n+1}(1)] = [p_0 , \; p_1] \begin{bmatrix} 1 - p_{01} & p_{01} \\ p_{10} & 1 - p_{10} \end{bmatrix}^n$$

Consider

$$\det \left(\begin{bmatrix} 1 - p_{01} - \lambda & p_{01} \\ p_{10} & 1 - p_{10} - \lambda \end{bmatrix} \right) = 0$$

which defines the eigenvalues of $\mathbf{P}$. The above equation is equivalent to

$$[(1 - p_{01}) - \lambda][(1 - p_{01}) - \lambda] - p_{01} p_{10} = 0$$

which reduces to

$$\lambda^2 - (2 - p_{01} - p_{10})\lambda + 1 - p_{01} - p_{10} = 0$$

so that

$$\lambda = \frac{1}{2} \left[2 - p_{01} - p_{10} \pm \sqrt{(2 - p_{01} - p_{10})^2 - 4(1 - p_{01} - p_{10}}\right]$$

$$= \frac{1}{2} \left[(2 - p_{01} - p_{10}) \pm (p_{01} + p_{10}) \right]$$

Hence the two characteristic roots are given by

$$\lambda = 1 \quad \text{and} \quad \lambda = 1 - p_{01} - p_{10}$$

The equation

$$\begin{bmatrix} 1 - p_{01} & p_{01} \\ p_{10} & 1 - p_{10} \end{bmatrix} \begin{bmatrix} x_1 \\ x_2 \end{bmatrix} = \begin{bmatrix} x_1 \\ x_2 \end{bmatrix}$$

reduces to

$$(1 - p_{01})x_1 + p_{01}x_2 = x_1 p_{10}x_1 + (1 - p_{10})x_2 = x_2$$

so that

$$p_{01}(x_2 - x_1) = 0 \quad p_{10}(x_2 - x_1) = 0, \quad \text{i.e.,} \quad x_1 = x_2$$

If $\lambda = 1 - p_{01} - p_{10}$ the equation

$$\begin{bmatrix} 1 - p_{01} & p_{01} \\ p_{10} & 1 - p_{10} \end{bmatrix} \begin{bmatrix} x_1 \\ x_2 \end{bmatrix} = \lambda \begin{bmatrix} x_1 \\ x_2 \end{bmatrix}$$

reduces to

$$p_{01}x_2 = -p_{10}x_1$$

i.e., we can let

$$x_1 = p_{01} \quad \text{and} \quad x_2 = -p_{10}$$

Then we have that

$$\begin{bmatrix} 1 - p_{01} & p_{01} \\ p_{10} & 1 - p_{10} \end{bmatrix} \begin{bmatrix} 1 & p_{01} \\ 1 & -p_{10} \end{bmatrix} = \begin{bmatrix} 1 & \lambda p_{01} \\ 1 & -\lambda p_{10} \end{bmatrix}$$

i.e.,

$$\mathbf{PQ} = \begin{bmatrix} 1 & \lambda p_{01} \\ 1 & -\lambda p_{10} \end{bmatrix}$$

where

$$\mathbf{Q} = \begin{bmatrix} 1 & p_{01} \\ 1 & -p_{10} \end{bmatrix}$$

Note that

$$\mathbf{Q}^{-1} = -\frac{1}{p_{01} + p_{10}} \begin{bmatrix} -p_{10} & -p_{01} \\ -1 & 1 \end{bmatrix}$$

and hence

$$\mathbf{Q}^{-1}\mathbf{PQ}$$

is equal to

$$-\frac{1}{p_{01} + p_{10}} \begin{bmatrix} -p_{10} & -p_{01} \\ -1 & 1 \end{bmatrix} \begin{bmatrix} 1 & \lambda p_{01} \\ 1 & -\lambda p_{10} \end{bmatrix}$$

or

$$\mathbf{Q}^{-1}\mathbf{PQ} = \mathbf{D}$$

where

$$\mathbf{D} = \begin{bmatrix} 1 & 0 \\ 0 & \lambda \end{bmatrix}$$

and $\lambda = 1 - p_{01} - p_{10}$.

It follows that

$$\mathbf{p} = \mathbf{QDQ}^{-1} \quad \text{and hence} \quad \mathbf{P}^n = \mathbf{QD}^n\mathbf{Q}^{-1}$$

Thus we have that

$$[p_{n+1}(0) , p_{n+1}(1)] = [p_0 , p_1]\mathbf{P}^n$$
$$= [p_0 , p_1]\mathbf{QD}^n\mathbf{Q}^{-1}$$

Matrix multiplication shows that

$$[p_{n+1}(0) ,\ p_{n+1}(1)] = \left[\frac{p_{01}}{p_{01} + p_{10}} ,\ \frac{p_{10}}{p_{01} + p_{10}}\right] + \frac{\lambda^n}{p_{01} + p_{10}}\ [a ,\ -a]$$

where

$$a = p_0 p_{01} - p_1 p_{10} = p_0(p_{01} + p_{10}) - p_{10}$$

If $p_{01} + p_{10} < 1$ we have that $\lambda < 1$ and hence

$$[p_{n+1}(0) ,\ p_{n+1}(1)] \longrightarrow \left[\frac{p_{01}}{p_{01} + p_{10}} ,\ \frac{p_{10}}{p_{01} + p_{10}}\right]$$

which is called the **stationary distribution** of the chain.

Definition 21.7.4. A state i is said to be **persistent** or **recurrent** if the probability that the process returns to i is 1; i.e.,

$$P(X_n = i \text{ for some } n \geq 1 \mid X_0 = i) = 1$$

Otherwise, the state is said to be **transient**:

- A state i in a Markov chain can communicate with state j written $i \rightarrow j$ if $p_{ij}(n) > 0$ for some n; i.e., it is possible to eventually get to state j having started from state i.
- Two states intercommunicate if i communicates with j and conversely. In this case we write $i \leftrightarrow j$.
- It can be shown that the state space of a Markov chain can be written as

$$S = T \cup C_1 \cup C_2 \cup \ldots$$

where T is the collection of transient states and the sets of states $C_1, C_2, \ldots$ consist of distinct sets of states which intercommunicate (such a set of states is called an irreducible set of states).
- If all states in the chain are irreducible the chain is said to be irreducible.

The structure of a Markov chain can be simple or complicated. For example, the chain with transition matrix

$$\mathbf{P} = \begin{bmatrix} p_{00} & p_{01} & p_{02} \\ p_{10} & p_{11} & p_{12} \\ p_{20} & p_{21} & p_{22} \end{bmatrix}$$

can exhibit dramatically different behavior depending on the p_{ij}'s.

If $p_{02} = 0, p_{12} = 0, p_{20} = 0, p_{21}$ with all other entries positive, i.e.,

$$\mathbf{P} = \begin{bmatrix} p_{00} & p_{01} & 0 \\ p_{10} & p_{11} & 0 \\ 0 & 0 & 1 \end{bmatrix}$$

It is clear that if the process starts in state 0 or 1 it stays in those two states while if it starts in state 2 it stays there. State 2 is called an absorbing state.

If $p_{02} = 10^{-6}, p_{12} = 10^{-6}, p_{20} = 10^{-6}, p_{21} = 10^{-6}$, i.e., positive, i.e.,

$$\mathbf{P} = \begin{bmatrix} p_{00} & p_{01} - 10^{-6} & 10^{-6} \\ p_{10} & p_{11} & 0 \\ 10^{-6} & 10^{-6} & 1 - 2 \times 10^{-6} \end{bmatrix}$$

then the process reaches every state infinitely often, but the times between visits from 2 to 0 or 1 and conversely are very long.

If

$$\mathbf{P} = \begin{bmatrix} 0 & 1 & 0 & 0 & \dots \\ 0 & 0 & 1 & 0 & \dots \\ 0 & 0 & 0 & 1 & \dots \\ \vdots & \vdots & \vdots & \ddots & \vdots \end{bmatrix}$$

then no matter where the process starts it never returns to that state.

A major result in Markov chain theory is that if a chain is irreducible with all states persistent with finite mean recurrence times then there is a unique stationary distribution π given by the solution to

$$\pi^\top \mathbf{P} = \pi^\top$$

Moreover the mean recurrence time of state i is π_i^{-1}.

21.8 Convergence of Sequences of Random Variables

21.8.1 Introduction

In this section we consider two types of convergence of a sequence of random variables: convergence in probability and convergence in distribution (often called convergence in law or weak convergence). These two types of convergence suffice for most statistical applications.

Definition 21.8.1. Let $X_1, X_2, \ldots, X_n$ and X be random variables

(i) X_n **converges to X in probability** written $X_n \overset{p}{\longrightarrow} X$ if

$$\mathbb{P}(|X_n - X| > \epsilon) \to 0 \text{ as } n \to \infty \text{ for every } \epsilon > 0$$

(ii) X_n **converges to X in distribution** written $X_n \overset{d}{\longrightarrow} X$ if

$$\mathbb{P}(X_n \leq x) \to \mathbb{P}(X \leq x) \text{ as } n \to \infty \text{ for all continuity points } x \text{ of } F$$

i.e.,

$$\lim_{n\to\infty} F_n(x) = F(x) \text{ if } F \text{ is continuous at } x$$

where F_n is the distribution function of X_n and F is the distribution function of X.

21.8.2   Basic Techniques

There are two basic limit theorems used to show convergence in probability and convergence in distribution. Both relate to the behavior of the sample average

$$\overline{X}_n = \frac{S_n}{n} \text{ where } S_n = X_1 + X_2 + \cdots + X_n$$

Theorem 21.8.1 (Weak law of large numbers). *If $X_1, X_2, \ldots, X_n$ are uncorrelated with mean μ and finite variance σ^2 then*

$$\overline{X}_n = \frac{S_n}{n} \overset{p}{\longrightarrow} \mu$$

Theorem 21.8.2 (Central limit theorem). *If $X_1, X_2, \ldots, X_n$ are independent and identically distributed with mean μ and variance σ^2 then*

$$\frac{S_n - E(S_n)}{\sqrt{var(S_n)}} = \frac{\sqrt{n}\,(\overline{X}_n - \mu)}{\sigma} \overset{d}{\longrightarrow} N(0,1)$$

21.8.3   Convergence in Probability

Definition 21.8.2. X_n **converges in probability** to a constant c, written $X_n \overset{p}{\longrightarrow} c$ if for every $\epsilon > 0$

$$\lim_{n\to\infty} \mathbb{P}(|X_n - c| < \epsilon) = \lim_{n\to\infty} \mathbb{P}(\{\omega : |X_n(\omega) - c| < \epsilon\}) = 1$$

More precisely, X_n converges to c in probability if for every $\epsilon > 0$ and $\delta > 0$ there exists a positive integer $N(\epsilon, \delta)$ such that $n > N(\epsilon, \delta)$ implies

$$\mathbb{P}(\{\omega : \mid X_n(\omega) - c \mid < \epsilon\}) \geq 1 - \delta$$

Definition 21.8.3. X_n **converges to** X **in probability**, written $X_n \xrightarrow{p} X$, if

$$\mid X_n - X \mid \xrightarrow{p} 0$$

Theorem 21.8.3. *If $X_n \xrightarrow{p} c$ and g is continuous at c then*

$$g(X_n) \xrightarrow{p} g(c)$$

Theorem 21.8.4. *If g is a continuous function and $X_n \xrightarrow{p} X$ then*

$$g(X_n) \xrightarrow{p} g(X)$$

21.8.3.1 o_p, O_p Definitions and Results

For convergence in probability of sequences of random variables there are useful analogues to o and O for sequences of numbers.

Definition 21.8.4. $X_n = o_p(b_n)$ if for all $\delta > 0, \epsilon > 0$ there exists an integer $N(\delta, \epsilon)$ such that $n > N(\delta, \epsilon)$ implies

$$\mathbb{P}(\mid X_n \mid < \epsilon \mid b_n \mid) \geq 1 - \delta$$

Definition 21.8.5. $X_n = O_p(b_n)$ if for all $\delta > 0$, there exists an integer $N(\delta)$ and a constant $K(\delta)$ such that $n > N(\delta)$ implies

$$\mathbb{P}(\mid X_n \mid < K(\delta) \mid b_n \mid) \geq 1 - \delta$$

21.8.3.2   Special Cases

1. $X_n = o_p(1)$ means **convergence in probability to** 0.
2. $X_n = O_p(1)$ means **bounded in probability**.

Result 21.8.1.   1. $X_n = o_p(a_n), Y_n = o_p(b_n)$ implies $X_n Y_n = o_p(a_n b_n)$.
2. $X_n = O_p(a_n), Y_n = O_p(b_n)$ implies $X_n Y_n = O_p(a_n b_n)$.
3. $X_n = o_p(a_n), Y_n = O_p(b_n)$ implies $X_n Y_n = o_p(a_n b_n)$.

Result 21.8.2. If r is a real-valued function defined on D such that $r(0) = 0$ and T_n (defined on D) converges in probability to 0, then for every $m > 0$:

1. If $r(h) = o(|h|^m)$ as $h \to 0$, then $r(T_n) = o_p(|h|^m)$.
2. If $r(h) = O(|h|^m)$ as $h \to 0$, then $r(T_n) = O_p(|h|^m)$.

21.8.4 Convergence in Distribution

Definition 21.8.6. $X_1, X_2, \ldots$ **converges in distribution** to X, written

$$X_n \xrightarrow{d} X$$

if for every continuity point of F, the distribution function of X,

$$\lim_{n \to \infty} F_n(x) = F(x)$$

where F_n is the distribution function of X_n.

Result 21.8.3. If $X_n \xrightarrow{d} X$ then $X_n = O_p(1)$.

Result 21.8.4. If Z denotes the standard normal distribution with expected value 0 and variance 1 and

$$\frac{X_n - \mu_n}{\sigma_n} \xrightarrow{d} Z \quad \text{for some } \mu_n, \sigma_n$$

then

$$\frac{X_n - \mu_n}{\sigma_n} = O_p(1) \quad \text{and hence} \quad X_n = \mu_n + O_p(\sigma_n)$$

21.8.5 Extension to Vectors

By defining

$$||\mathbf{a}|| = \sqrt{\sum_{i=1}^{k} a_i^2}$$

for any vector a with coordinates $a_1, a_2, \ldots, a_n$ the sequence of random vectors $\mathbf{X}_n$ converges in probability to the random vector $\mathbf{X}$ written $\mathbf{X}_n \xrightarrow{p} \mathbf{X}$ if

$$\lim_{n \to \infty} P(||\mathbf{X}_n - \mathbf{X}|| > \epsilon) = 1$$

All of the results on convergence in probability are true for the vector-valued case since this type of convergence is obviously equivalent to convergence of each of the coordinates. The definitions of o_p and O_p are the same with the understanding that $\|\mathbf{a}_n\|$ replaces $|a_n|$.

For convergence in distribution in the vector case the situation is a little more complicated because of the difficulty in dealing with distribution functions in k dimensions. The Cramer-Wold device is used to deal with this situation.

Theorem 21.8.5 (Cramer-wold device). $\mathbf{X}_n \xrightarrow{d} \mathbf{X}$ *if and only if*

$$\sum_{i=1}^{k} t_i X_n(i) \xrightarrow{d} \sum_{i=1}^{k} t_i X(i) \text{ for all } \mathbf{t} \in R^k$$

where t_i is the ith coordinate of $\mathbf{t}$, $X_n(i)$ is the ith coordinate of $\mathbf{X}_n$ and $X(i)$ is the ith coordinate of $\mathbf{X}$.

The vector central limit theorem is

Theorem 21.8.6. *Let $\mathbf{X}_1, \mathbf{X}_2, \ldots, \mathbf{X}_n$ be independent and identically distributed with mean vector $\boldsymbol{\mu}$ and variance covariance matrix $\boldsymbol{\Sigma}$ then*

$$\sqrt{n}(\overline{\mathbf{X}_n} - \boldsymbol{\mu}) \xrightarrow{d} MVN(\mathbf{0}, \boldsymbol{\Sigma})$$

21.8.6 Results on Convergence in Probability and in Distribution

Result 21.8.5. If $|X_n - Y_n| \xrightarrow{p} 0$ and $Y_n \xrightarrow{d} Y$ then $X_n \xrightarrow{d} Y$.

This result may be stated as: If $Y_n \xrightarrow{d} Y$ and $X_n - Y_n = o_p(1)$ then $X_n \xrightarrow{d} Y$.

Theorem 21.8.7. *Convergence in probability implies convergence in distribution, i.e.,*

$$\text{if } X_n \xrightarrow{p} X \text{ then } X_n \xrightarrow{d} X$$

Result 21.8.6. If $X_n \xrightarrow{d} X$ and $Y_n \xrightarrow{p} 0$ then

$$X_n Y_n \xrightarrow{p} 0$$

This result may be stated as: If $X_n \xrightarrow{d} X$ and $Y_n = o_p(1)$ then $Y_n X_n = o_p(1)$.

Theorem 21.8.8 (Slutsky's theorem).

(i) If $X_n \xrightarrow{d} X$ *and* $S_n \xrightarrow{p} c$ *then*

$$S_n + X_n \xrightarrow{d} c + X$$

(ii) If $X_n \xrightarrow{d} X$ *and* $S_n \xrightarrow{p} c$ *then*

$$S_n X_n \xrightarrow{d} cX$$

(iii) If $X_n \xrightarrow{d} X$ *and* $S_n \xrightarrow{p} c$ *then*

$$X_n / S_n \xrightarrow{d} X/c$$

21.8.7   The Delta Method

Result 21.8.7 (Univariate delta method). If

$$\sqrt{n}(Y_n - \mu) \xrightarrow{d} N(0, \sigma^2)$$

and $g : R \mapsto R$ is differentiable at $x = \mu$ with derivative $g'(\mu)$ then

$$\sqrt{n}(g(Y_n) - g(\mu)) \xrightarrow{d} N(0, [g'(\mu)]^2 \sigma^2)$$

Result 21.8.8 (Multivariate delta method). If

$$\sqrt{n}(\mathbf{Y_n} - \boldsymbol{\mu}) \xrightarrow{d} \text{MVN}(\mathbf{0}, \boldsymbol{\Sigma})$$

where $\mathbf{Y_n}$ and $\boldsymbol{\mu}$ are k dimensional and $\mathbf{g} : R^k \mapsto R^s$ has components

$$g_1(\mathbf{x}), g_2(\mathbf{x}), \ldots, g_s(\mathbf{x})$$

such that each g_i has continuous partial derivatives at $\mathbf{x} = \boldsymbol{\mu}$ then

$$\sqrt{n}(\mathbf{g}(\mathbf{Y_n}) - \mathbf{g}(\boldsymbol{\mu})) \xrightarrow{d} \text{MVN}(\mathbf{0}, \mathbf{V})$$

where

$$\mathbf{V} = (\nabla \mathbf{g}(\boldsymbol{\mu})) \boldsymbol{\Sigma} (\nabla \mathbf{g}(\boldsymbol{\mu}))^T$$

and

$$(\nabla \mathbf{g}(\boldsymbol{\mu}))$$

is the s by k matrix with i-j element equal to the partial derivative of $g_i(\mathbf{x})$ with respect to x_j evaluated at $\mathbf{x} = \boldsymbol{\mu}$.

The most important special case occurs when $s = 1$. Then

$$\nabla \mathbf{g}(\boldsymbol{\mu}) = \left[\frac{\partial g(\mathbf{x})}{\partial x_1}, \frac{\partial g(\mathbf{x})}{\partial x_2}, \ldots, \frac{\partial g(\mathbf{x})}{\partial x_k} \right]_{\mathbf{x}=\boldsymbol{\mu}}$$

21.9 Sets

21.9.1 Definitions

Definition 21.9.1. A set is a collection of points or elements:

1. The empty set $\emptyset$ is the set containing no points.
2. All sets under consideration are assumed to consist of points of a fixed nonempty set Ω (called a space).
3. Points of Ω are denoted by ω or x.
4. Capital letters such as $E_1, E_2, \ldots$ denote sets and $\{\omega\}$ denotes the set consisting of the single point ω.
5. If ω is a point in the set E, we write $\omega \in E$ while if ω is not a point in the set E we write $\omega \notin E$.
6. To describe a set E we write

$$E = \{\omega : \ S(\omega)\}$$

i.e., E is the set of all points such that the statement $S(\omega)$ is true. Alternatively we shall write $\{\ldots\ldots\}$ where all points in E are written down inside the brackets.

Definition 21.9.2. A set of sets is called a *class*. Classes are denoted by script letters, e.g., $\mathcal{W}$. The set of all subsets of Ω is called the *power set* of Ω and is denoted by 2^Ω.

Definition 21.9.3 (Set inclusion). A set E is said to be contained in a set F if $\omega \in E$ implies $\omega \in F$. This relation is written $E \subset F$.

Note that $\emptyset \subset E \subset \Omega$ for every set E and that the relation of set inclusion is reflexive and transitive, i.e.,

$$E \subset E \ ; \ E \subset F, \ F \subset G \Rightarrow E \subset G$$

Definition 21.9.4 (Set equality). Sets E and F are said to be equal if $E \subset F$ and $F \subset E$.

Note that set equality is reflexive, symmetric, and transitive, i.e.,

$$E = E, \ E \doteq F \Rightarrow F = E \ \text{ and } \ E = F, \ F = G \Rightarrow E = G$$

Definition 21.9.5 (Difference of two sets). The *difference* of two sets $E - F$ is the set defined as

$$E - F = \{\omega : \ \omega \in E \ \text{ and } \ \omega \notin F\}$$

Definition 21.9.6 (Complement). The *complement* of E is denoted by E^c and is equal to $\Omega - E$.

Definition 21.9.7 (Intersection of two sets). The *intersection* of two sets E and F is defined as

$$E \cap F = \{\omega : \ \omega \in E \ \text{ and } \ \omega \in F\}$$

Definition 21.9.8 (Mutually exclusive). If $E \cap F = \emptyset$, E and F are said to be *disjoint* or *mutually exclusive*.

Definition 21.9.9 (Union of two sets). The *union* of two sets E and F is defined as

$$E \cup F = \{\omega : \ \omega \in E \ \text{ or } \ \omega \in F\}$$

Definition 21.9.10. More generally if T is any set then

$$\cup_{t \in T} E_t = \{\omega : \omega \in E_t \ \text{ for some } \ t \in T\}$$

$$\cap_{t \in T} E_t = \{\omega : \omega \in E_t \ \text{ for all } \ t \in T\}$$

21.9.2   Properties of Set Operations

1. $(E \cup F) \cup G = E \cup (F \cup G)$ and $(E \cap F) \cap G = E \cap (F \cap G)$
2. $E \cup F = F \cup E$ and $E \cap F = F \cap E$
3. $(E \cup F) \cap G = (E \cap G) \cup (F \cap G)$ and $E \cup (F \cap G) = (E \cup F) \cap (E \cup G)$
4. $E \cup E^c = \Omega$ and $E \cap E^c = \emptyset$
5. $(E \cup F)^c = E^c \cap F^c$
6. $E - F = E \cap F^c$
7. $(E^c)^c = E$
8. $\Omega^c = \emptyset$ and $\emptyset^c = \Omega$
9. $E \subset F \Rightarrow F^c \subset E^c$

10. $(E_1 \times E_2) \cap (E_3 \times E_4) = (E_1 \cap E_3) \times (E_2 \cap E_4)$
11. $(E \times F)^c = (E^c \times F^c) \cup (E \times F^c) \cup (E^c \times F)$
12. $(\cup_{t \in T} E_t)^c = \cap_{t \in T} E_t$
13. $(\cap_{t \in T} E_t)^c = \cup_{t \in T} E_t$

21.9.3 Indicator Functions

Definition 21.9.11. If A is a set, its **indicator function** is

$$\mathbf{1}_A(\omega) = \begin{cases} 1 & \omega \in A \\ 0 & \text{otherwise} \end{cases}$$

21.9.3.1 Properties of Indicator Functions

(i) $\mathbf{1}_{A^c} = 1 - \mathbf{1}_A$
(ii) $\mathbf{1}_{A \cap B} = \mathbf{1}_A \mathbf{1}_B$
(iii) $\mathbf{1}_{A \cup B} = \mathbf{1}_A + \mathbf{1}_B - \mathbf{1}_A \mathbf{1}_B$

21.9.4 Counting and Combinatorics

Definition 21.9.12 (n-tuple). If $E_1, E_2, \ldots, E_n$ are sets, an *n-tuple* is an element of the form

$$(a_1, a_2, \ldots, a_n) \text{ where } a_1 \in E_1, a_2 \in E_2, \ldots, a_n \in E_n$$

a_i is called the ith *coordinate* of the n-tuple.

Two n-tuples are said to be equal if each coordinate of one is equal to the corresponding coordinate of the other.

Note. An ordered pair with first coordinate a and second coordinate b is an element of the form (a, b). Also note that $(a, b) = (c, d)$ if and only if $a = c$ and $b = d$. n-tuples are natural generalizations of this concept. A formal (set) definition of an ordered pair is

$$(a, b) = \{\{a\}, \{a, b\}\}.$$

Definition 21.9.13 (Cartesian product). If $E_1, E_2, \ldots, E_n$ are sets then their *Cartesian product* is defined as

$$E_1 \times E_2 \times \cdots \times E_n = \{(\omega_1, \omega_2, \ldots, \omega_n) : \omega_1 \in E_1, \omega_2 \in E_2, \ldots, \omega_n \in E_n\}$$

Definition 21.9.14. A set will be said to be:

1. *Finite* if its elements can be put into a one to one correspondence with the integers $1, 2, \ldots, n$ for some finite integer n
2. *Denumerable* if its elements can be put into a one to one correspondence with the natural numbers N where $N = \{1, 2, 3, \ldots\}$
3. *Non-denumerable* otherwise.

Result 21.9.1 (Elementary counting rules).

1. Given two sets A and B having m and n elements, respectively, there are $m \times n$ ordered pairs of the form (a_i, b_j) where $a_i \in A$ and $b_j \in B$
2. Given r sets $A_1, A_2, \ldots, A_r$ containing $m_1, m_2, \ldots, m_r$ elements, respectively, there are $m_1 \times m_2 \times \cdots \times m_r$ r-tuples of the form

$$(a_1, a_2, \ldots, a_r); \quad a_i \in A_i \text{ for } i = 1, 2, \ldots, r$$

3. A **permutation** of a set containing n elements is an arrangement of the elements of the set to form an n-tuple. There are n! permutations of a set containing n elements where $n!$ is defined as $n(n - 1) \cdots 3 \cdot 2 \cdot 1$. By convention $0! = 1$. This convention is related to the Gamma function.
4. Given a set containing n elements the number of subsets of size x is given by

$$\binom{n}{x} = \frac{n!}{x!(n - x)!} = \frac{(n)_x}{x!}$$

where

$$(n)_x = (n - x + 1) \cdots n = \prod_{i=0}^{x-1} (n - i)$$

This expression is read as n choose x and is called the number of **combinations** of n items taken x at a time.

5. Given a set, $\mathcal{P}$, containing N objects, a sample of size $n < N$ is an n tuple each element of which is an object in the set. If duplicates are allowed the sampling is said to be with replacement. If not allowed the sampling is said to be without replacement:

   (i) N^n samples of size n with replacement.
   (ii) $N \times (N - 1) \times \cdots \times (N - (n - 1)) = \prod_{i=0}^{n-1}(N - i) \equiv (N)_n \equiv N^{\underline{n}}$ samples of size n without replacement. The symbol $N^{\underline{n}}$ is called the falling factorial or Pochhammer symbol.

21.10 σ-Algebras and Borel Sets

21.10.1 σ-Algebras

Definition 21.10.1. Let Ω be set. A class of subsets of Ω, $\mathcal{W}$, is said to be a σ-**algebra** if the following conditions are satisfied:

(i) $\mathcal{W}$ is nonempty.
(ii) $E \in \mathcal{W}$ implies $E^C \in \mathcal{W}$.
(iii) If $E_1, E_2, \ldots$ is a denumerable collection of sets in $\mathcal{W}$, then $\cup_{i=1}^{\infty} E_i \in \mathcal{W}$.

21.10.1.1   Properties and Examples of σ-Algebras

1. The set of all subsets of Ω is a σ-algebra called the **power set** of Ω and denoted by 2^{Ω}.
2. The trivial σ-algebra is $\{\emptyset, \Omega\}$.
3. The intersection of any collection of σ-algebras is a σ-algebra.
4. If $\mathcal{C}$ is a collection of subsets of Ω the intersection of all σ-algebras containing $\mathcal{C}$ is called the σ-algebra generated by $\mathcal{C}$.

21.10.2   Borel σ-Algebras

Definition 21.10.2. The **Borel** σ-**algebra** is the σ-field over R, the set of real numbers, generated by the class of sets of the form

$$(a, b] \; ; \; a, b \in R \; ; \; a < b$$

1. We denote the Borel σ-algebra by $\mathcal{B}$.
2. The elements of $\mathcal{B}$ are called Borel sets.
3. The Borel σ-algebra in R^n, denoted by $\mathcal{B}^n$, is the σ-algebra generated by rectangles of the form

$$(a_1, b_1] \times (a_2, b_2] \times \cdots \times (a_n, b_n]$$

where $a_i < b_i$ for $i = 1, 2, \ldots, n$.

21.10.3   Properties and Examples of Borel Sets

1. Every open interval $(a, b), a, b \in R$ is a Borel set.
2. Every one point set $\{a\}$ is in $\mathcal{B}$.
3. $[a, b] = (a, b] \cup \{a\} \in \mathcal{B}$.
4. $(-\infty, a] \in \mathcal{B}$.

21.10.4   Measurable Functions

1. A constant function is measurable.
2. The indicator function, 1_E, of a set in $\mathcal{W}$ is measurable where

$$1_E(\omega) = \begin{cases} 1 & \omega \in E \\ 0 & \omega \notin E \end{cases}$$

3. If f and g are measurable functions and c is a constant then the functions cf, f^2, f + g, fg and $\mid f \mid$ are also measurable functions.
4. A function f is a measurable function if and only if

$$\{\omega : f(\omega) \in (-\infty, b]\,\} \in \mathcal{W} \quad \text{for} \quad b \in R$$

21.10.5   Borel Sets in n Dimensions

Definition 21.10.3. The Borel algebra, $\mathcal{B}^k$ on R^k, is the σ-algebra generated by the class of sets of the form

$$C = (a_1, b_1] \times (a_2, b_2] \times \cdots \times (a_k, b_k] \quad \text{such that} \quad a_i < b_i \;\; a_i, b_i \in R \quad \text{for} \quad i = 1, 2, \ldots, k$$

21.11   Background: Limits, o, and O Notation

The study of limit theorems and asymptotic results of interest in probability and statistics requires a reasonably careful attention to convergence of sequences of real numbers, sequences of events, and limits of functions.

21.11.1   Notation

1. $\{a_n : n \in N\}$ where $N = \{1, 2, \ldots\}$ is the set of natural numbers will denote a sequence of real numbers. For brevity we write a_n to denote such a sequence.
2. $\mid a_n \mid$ will denote the absolute value of a_n.
3. A sequence is an element of the set R^N of all functions from the set of integers to the set of real numbers.

21.11.2 Limits of Sequences

Definition 21.11.1. Let a_n for $n = 1, 2, \ldots$ denote a sequence of real numbers. The sequence is said to have a **limit** a as $n \to \infty$ if for every $\epsilon > 0$ there is an integer, $N(\epsilon)$, such that

$$n \geq N(\epsilon) \implies |a_n - a| < \epsilon$$

Definition 21.11.2. The sequence a_n is said to be **bounded** if there exists a $K > 0$ and an integer, $N(K)$, such that

$$n \geq N(K) \implies |a_n| \leq K$$

Definition 21.11.3. The sequence a_n is said to be monotone non-decreasing (nonincreasing) if $a_n \leq a_{n+1}$; $n = 1, 2, \ldots$ ($a_{n+1} \leq a_n$; $n = 1, 2, \ldots$).

A fundamental property of the set of real numbers is that a bounded monotone sequence has a limit.

21.11.3 liminf and limsup

Definition 21.11.4 (infimum). The **infimum** or **greatest lower bound** ℓ, of a set S of real numbers, is the number ℓ satisfying

(i) $\ell \leq x$ for all $x \in S$.
(ii) for all $x > \ell$ there is a $x_1 \in S$ less than x.

Definition 21.11.5 (supremum). The **supremum** υ or **least upper bound** of a set of real numbers S is the number υ satisfying

(i) $\upsilon \geq x$ for all $x \in S$ and
(ii) for all $x < \upsilon$ there is a $x_1 \in S$ greater than x.

Definition 21.11.6 (limsup). Let $\{a_n\}$ be a sequence of real numbers which is bounded above. Then

$$A = \limsup a_n = \inf_m \left\{ \sup_{n \geq m} a_n \right\} = \lim_{m \to \infty} B_m$$

since $B_m = \sup_{n \geq m} a_n$ is a monotone non-increasing sequence. If a_n is not bounded above then we define $\limsup a_n = +\infty$.

Definition 21.11.7 (liminf). Let $\{a_n\}$ be a sequence of real numbers which is bounded below. Then

$$a = \liminf a_n = \sup_m \left\{ \inf_{n \geq m} a_n \right\} = \lim_{m \to \infty} b_m$$

since $b_m = \inf_{n \geq m} a_n$ is a monotone nondecreasing sequence. If a_n is not bounded below we define $\liminf a_n = -\infty$.

21.11.3.1   Results on liminf and limsup

Result 21.11.1. 1. $\liminf a_n \leq \limsup a_n$
2. $\liminf a_n = \limsup a_n \Longleftrightarrow \lim a_n$ exists and in this case the three are equal.
3. $\liminf a_n + \liminf b_n \leq \liminf (a_n + b_n)$
4. $\limsup (a_n + b_n) \leq \limsup a_n + \limsup b_n$
5. If $x > \limsup a_n$ then $a_n < x$ for all but a finite number of values of n i.e.,

$$a_n < x \text{ eventually}$$

6. If $x < \limsup a_n$ then $a_n > x$ for infinitely many values of n, i.e.,

$$a_n > x \text{ infinitely often (i.o.)}$$

7. If $x < \liminf a_n$ then $a_n > x$ for all but a finite number of values of n, i.e.,

$$a_n > x, \text{ eventually,}$$

8. If $x > \liminf a_n$ then $a_n < x$ for infinitely many values of n, i.e.,

$$a_n > x \text{ infinitely often(i.o.)}$$

21.11.4   Sequences of Events

Definition 21.11.8. If $\{E_n\}$ is a sequence of events we define

$$\limsup E_n = \cap_{m=1}^{\infty} \cup_{n=m}^{\infty} E_n = \{\omega : \omega \in E_n \text{ for infinitely many } n\}$$

i.e, $\limsup E_n$ is the set $\{E_n, \text{ i.o.}\}$.

Definition 21.11.9. If $\{E_n\}$ is a sequence of events we define

$$\liminf E_n = \cup_{m=1}^{\infty} \cap_{n=m}^{\infty} E_n = \{\omega : \omega \in E_n \text{ for all but a finite number of } n\}$$

i.e., $\liminf E_n$ is the set $\{E_n, \text{ eventually}\}$.

Definition 21.11.10. If E_n is a sequence of events and

$$\liminf E_n = \limsup E_n$$

the common limit is called the limit of E_n written as $\lim E_n$

Result 21.11.2. Let $I_E(\omega)$ be the indicator function of E. Then for all ω

$$I_{\limsup E_n}(\omega) = \limsup[I_{E_n}(\omega)]$$

$$I_{\liminf E_n}(\omega) = \liminf[I_{E_n}(\omega)]$$

21.11.5 o, O Definitions and Results

Definition 21.11.11. $a_n = o(b_n)$ if for every $\epsilon > 0$ there exists an integer $N(\epsilon)$ such that

$$n \geq N(\epsilon) \implies |a_n| < \epsilon |b_n|$$

In particular $a_n = o(1)$ means that the limit of a_n is equal to 0.

Definition 21.11.12. $a_n = O(b_n)$ if there exists a number $K > 0$ and an integer $N(K)$ such that

$$n > N(K) \implies |a_n| < K |b_n|$$

In particular $a_n = O(1)$ means that a_n is ultimately bounded.

21.11.6   Results and Special Cases

Result 21.11.3.   1. $a_n = o(b_n)$ if and only if $a_n = |b_n|o(1)$.
2. $a_n = O(b_n)$ if and only if $a_n = |b_n|O(1)$.
3. $a_n = o(b_n)$ implies $ca_n = o(b_n)$.
4. $a_n = O(b_n)$ implies $ca_n = O(b_n)$.
5. $b_n = O(b_n)$.
6. $O(b_n{}^1)O(b_n{}^2) = O(b_n{}^1 b_n{}^2)$.

7. $o(b_n{}^1)o(b_n{}^2) = o(b_n{}^1 b_n{}^2)$.
8. $o(b_n{}^1) + o(b_n{}^2) = o(\max(b_n{}^1, b_n{}^2))$.
9. $O(b_n{}^1) + O(b_n{}^2) = O(\max(b_n{}^1, b_n{}^2))$.
10. In general the order of magnitude of a sum of o and O terms is equal to the largest order of magnitude of the terms in the sum provided that the number of terms does not depend on n.

21.11.7   Extension to Functions

Definition 21.11.13. Let f : $D \mapsto R$ and let g : $D \mapsto R$ where $D \subset R$. If $\ell \in D$ then

(i) $f(x) = o(g(x))$ as $x \to \ell$ means that $f(x_n) = o(g(x_n))$ for every sequence x_n such that $x_n \to \ell$ as $n \to \infty$.
(ii) $f(x) = O(g(x))$ as $x \to \ell$ means that $f(x_n) = O(g(x_n))$ for every sequence x_n such that $x_n \to \ell$ as $n \to \infty$.

Example. 1. If f : $R \mapsto R$ and f is continuous at x_0 then

$$f(x) = f(x_0) + o(1)$$

2. If f : $R \mapsto R$ and f is differentiable at x_0 with derivative $f'(x_0)$ then

$$f(x) = f(x_0) + f'(x_0)(x - x_0) + o(|\, x - x_0\, |)$$

3. (Taylor's Formula) If f : $R \mapsto R$ and f is m times differentiable at x_0 then

$$f(x) = \sum_{i=0}^{m} \frac{f^{(r)}(x_0)(x - x_0)^r}{r!} + o(|\, x - x_0\, |^m)$$

where $f^{(r)}(x_0)$ denotes the rth derivative of f evaluated at x_0.

21.11.8   Extension to Vectors

The notion of o and O extend easily to vectors.

1. $\{\mathbf{a}_n : n \in N\}$ where $N = \{1, 2, \ldots\}$ is the set of natural numbers will denote a sequence of k-dimensional vectors each coordinate of which is a real number. For brevity we will write $\mathbf{a}_n$ to denote such a sequence.

2. $\parallel \mathbf{a}_n \parallel = (a_{n1}^2 + a_{n2}^2 + \cdots + a_{nk}^2)^{1/2}$ will denote the norm or length of $\mathbf{a}_n$. If k=1 then $\parallel \mathbf{a}_n \parallel = \mid a_n \mid$, the absolute value of a_n.
3. b_n will denote a sequence of real numbers.

Definition 21.11.14. $\mathbf{a}_n = o(b_n)$ if for every $\epsilon > 0$ there exists an integer $N(\epsilon)$ such that

$$n > N(\epsilon) \implies \parallel \mathbf{a}_n \parallel < \epsilon \mid b_n \mid$$

Definition 21.11.15. $\mathbf{a}_n = O(b_n)$ if there exists a number $K > 0$ and an integer N(K) such that

$$n > N(K) \implies \parallel \mathbf{a}_n \parallel > K \mid b_n \mid$$

Result 21.11.4. 1. $\mathbf{a}_n = O(1)$ means that $\mathbf{a}_n$ is bounded.
2. $\mathbf{a}_n = o(1)$ means that $\mathbf{a}_n \to 0$ as $n \to \infty$.
3. $\mathbf{a}_n = O(b_n)$ if and only if $\mathbf{a}_n = b_n O(1)$.
4. $\mathbf{a}_n = o(b_n)$ if and only if $\mathbf{a}_n = b_n o(1)$.
5. $\mathbf{a}_n = O(b_n)$ implies $c\mathbf{a}_n = O(b_n)$.
6. $\mathbf{a}_n = o(b_n)$ implies $c\mathbf{a}_n = o(b_n)$.

21.11.9 Extension to Vector-Valued Functions

Definition 21.11.16. Let $f : D \mapsto \mathbf{R}^k$ and let $g : D \mapsto (0, \infty)$ where $D \subset \mathbf{R}^N$. If $\ell \in D$, then

1. $f(\mathbf{x}) = O(g(\mathbf{x}))$ as $\mathbf{x} \to \ell$ means that $f(\mathbf{x}_n) = O(g(\mathbf{x}_n))$ for every sequence $\mathbf{x}_n$ such that $\mathbf{x}_n \to \ell$ as $n \to \infty$.
2. $f(\mathbf{x}) = o(g(\mathbf{x}))$ as $\mathbf{x} \to \ell$ means that $f(\mathbf{x}_n) = o(g(\mathbf{x}_n))$ for every sequence $\mathbf{x}_n$ such that $\mathbf{x}_n \to \ell$ as $n \to \infty$.

Definition 21.11.17. If $f : R^N \mapsto R$, then f is said to be of class $C^{(m+1)}$ if all $(m+1)$th order partial derivatives exist and are equal.

Result 21.11.5 (Taylor's formula in multidimensions). Let $f : R^N \mapsto R$ and let f be of class $C^{(m+1)}$. Then the rth term of Taylor's formula (multidimensional version) is given by

$$T(r) = \frac{1}{r!} \sum_{i_1=1}^{N} \sum_{i_2=1}^{N} \cdots \sum_{i_r=1}^{N} \left[\frac{\partial^r f(\mathbf{x})}{\partial x_{i_1} \partial x_{i_2} \cdots \partial x_{i_r}} \right]_{\mathbf{x}=\mathbf{x_0}} \prod_{k=1}^{r} (x_{i_k} - x_{0 i_k})$$

and Taylor formula's is

$$f(\mathbf{x}) = \sum_{r=0}^{m} T(r) + o(\| \mathbf{x} - \mathbf{x_0} \|^m)$$

Result 21.11.6. An important special case of the multidimensional Taylor formula occurs when $f : R^N \mapsto R$ has continuous partial derivatives at $\mathbf{x} = \mathbf{x_0}$. In this case

$$f(\mathbf{x}) = f(\mathbf{x_0}) + \sum_{j=1}^{N} f_j(\mathbf{x_0})(x_j - x_{j0}) + o(\| \mathbf{x} - \mathbf{x_0} \|)$$

where $f_j(\mathbf{x_0})$ is the jth partial derivative of f evaluated at $\mathbf{x_0}$ and x_j is the jth coordinate of $\mathbf{x}$, i.e.,

$$f_j(\mathbf{x_0}) = \frac{\partial f(\mathbf{x})}{\partial x_j}\bigg|_{\mathbf{x}=\mathbf{x_0}}$$

References

1. Basu, D.: An essay on the logical foundations of survey sampling, part one*. In: DasGupta, A. (ed.) Selected Works of Debabrata Basu, pp. 167–206. Springer, New York (2011)
2. Bayarri, M., DeGroot, M., Kadane, J.: What is the likelihood function? (with discussion). In: Gupta, S.S., Berger, J.O. (eds.) Statistical Decision Theory and Related Topics IV, vol. 1. Springer, New York (1988)
3. Berger, J.O., Wolpert, R.L., Bayarri, M.J., DeGroot, M.H., Hill, B.M., Lane, D.A., LeCam, L.: The Likelihood Principle. Lecture Notes-Monograph Series, 208 pp. IMS, Hayward (1988)
4. Bickel, D.R.: The strength of statistical evidence for composite hypotheses: inference to the best explanation. Stat. Sin., **22**, 1147–1198 (2012)
5. Boos, D.D., Stefanski, L.A.: P-value precision and reproducibility. Am. Stat. **65**(4), 213–221 (2011)
6. Casella, G., Berger, R.L.: Statistical Inference, vol. 70. Duxbury Press, Belmont (1990)
7. Chernoff, H., Moses, L.E.: Elementary Decision Theory. Dover Publications, New York (1959)
8. Cornfield, J.: Sequential trials, sequential analysis and the likelihood principle. Am. Stat. **20**(2), 18–23 (1966)
9. Cox, D.R.: Some problems connected with statistical inference. Ann. Math. Stat. **29**(2), 357–372 (1958)
10. Cox, R.T., Jaynes, E.T.: The algebra of probable inference. Am. J. Phys. **31**(1), 66–67 (1963)
11. Diggle, P., Heagerty, P., Liang, K.-Y., Zeger, S.: Analysis of Longitudinal Data. Oxford University Press, Oxford (2002)
12. Donahue, R.M.J.: A note on information seldom reported via the p value. Am. Stat. **53**(4), 303–306 (1999)
13. Einbeck, J., Augustin, T.: On design-weighted local fitting and its relation to the Horvitz-Thompson estimator. Stat. Sin. **19**(1), 103 (2009)
14. Evans, M., et al.: What does the proof of birnbaum's theorem prove? Electron. J. Stat. **7**, 2645–2655 (2013)
15. Fink, D.: A compendium of conjugate priors, p. 46. http://www.people.cornell.edu/pages/df36/CONJINTRnew20TEX.pdf (1997)
16. Fisher, R.: Statistical methods and scientific induction. J. Roy. Stat. Soc. Ser. B (Methodological) **17**, 69–78 (1955)
17. Fisher, R.A.: Statistical Methods and Scientific Inference. Hafner Publishing Co., New York (1956)
18. Gandenberger, G.: A new proof of the likelihood principle. Br. J. Philos. Sci. axt039, Br Soc Philosophy Sci (2014)

19. Ghosh, M., Reid, N., Fraser, D.A.S.: Ancillary statistics: a review. Statistica Sinica **20**, 1309–1332 (2010)
20. Good, I.J.: The Estimation of Probabilities: An Essay on Modern Bayesian Methods, vol. 258. MIT Press, Cambridge (1965)
21. Goodman, S.N.: A comment on replication, p-values and evidence. Stat. Med. **11**(7), 875–879 (1992)
22. Horvitz, D.G., Thompson, D.J.: A generalization of sampling without replacement from a finite universe. J. Am. Stat. Assoc. **47**(260), 663–685 (1952)
23. Howson, C., Urbach, P.: Scientific Reasoning: The Bayesian Approach. Open Court Publishing, Illinois (2006)
24. Jeffreys, H.: Theory of Probability. Oxford University Press, Oxford (1998)
25. Kalbfleisch, J.G.: Probability and Statistical Inference II. Springer, New York (1979)
26. Lambert, D., Hall, W.J.: Asymptotic lognormality of p-values. Ann. Stat. **10**, 44–64 (1982)
27. Lehmann, E.L.: Testing Statistical Hypotheses. Wiley, New York (1959)
28. Lehmann, E.L.: Elements of Large-Sample Theory. Springer, New York (1999)
29. Lindley, D.V.: Probability and Statistics from a Bayesian Viewpoint: Parts I and II. Cambridge University Press, Cambridge (1965)
30. Lohr, S.L.: Sampling: Design and Analysis. Thomson, Boston (2009)
31. Marin, J.-M., Robert, C.P.: Bayesian Essentials with R. Springer, New York (2014)
32. Mayo, D.G.: On the birnbaum argument for the strong likelihood principle. arXiv preprint arXiv:1302.7021 (2013)
33. Mayo, D.G., Spanos, A.: Severe testing as a basic concept in a neyman–pearson philosophy of induction. Br. J. Philos. Sci. **57**(2), 323–357 (2006)
34. Neyman, J.: First Course in Probability and Statistics. Henry Holt, New York (1950)
35. Neyman, J.: Foundations of behavioristic statistics. In: Foundations of Statistical Inference (Proc. Sympos., University of Waterloo, Waterloo, 1970), pp. 1–19 (1971)
36. Overton, W.S., Stehman, S.V.: The Horvitz-Thompson theorem as a unifying perspective for probability sampling: with examples from natural resource sampling. Am. Stat. **49**(3), 261–268 (1995)
37. Pitman, E.J.G.: Some remarks on statistical inference. In: Bernoulli, Bayes, and Laplace. Springer, New York (1965)
38. Pratt, J.W.: Review of lehmann's testing statistical hypotheses. J. Am. Stat. Assoc. **56**, 163–166 (1961)
39. Pukelsheim, F.: The three sigma rule. Am. Stat. **48**(2), 88–91 (1994)
40. Renyi, A.: Probability Theory. North-Holland Series in Applied Mathematics and Mechanics. North Holland/Elsevier, Amsterdam/New York (1970)
41. Robbins, H.: Statistical methods related to the law of the iterated logarithm. Ann. Math. Stat. **41**, 1397–1409 (1970)
42. Roy, S.N., Roy, S.M.: Some Aspects of Multivariate Analysis. Wiley, New York (1957)
43. Royall, R.M.: Statistical Evidence: A Likelihood Paradigm, vol. 71. Chapman & Hall/CRC, New York (1997)
44. Royall, R.: On the probability of observing misleading statistical evidence. J. Am. Stat. Assoc. **95**(451), 760–768 (2000)
45. Savage, L.J.: The Foundations of Statistical Inference. Methuen, London (1970)
46. Schervish, M.J.: Theory of Statistics, p. 329. Springer, New York (1995)
47. Shafer, G.: What is probability. In: Perspectives in Contemporary Statistics, pp. 19–39. Mathematical Association of America, New York (1992)
48. Siegfried, T.: Odds are, it's wrong: science fails to face the shortcomings of statistics. Sci. News **177**(7), 26–29 (2010)
49. Sprott, D.A.: Statistical Inference in Science. Springer, New York (2000)
50. Stein, C.: Inadmissibility of the usual estimator for the mean of a multivariate normal distribution. In: Proceedings of the 3rd Berkeley Symposium on Mathematical Statistics and Probability, vol. 1, pp. 197–206 (1956)
51. Tsou, T.-S., Royall, R.M.: Robust likelihoods. J. Am. stat. Assoc. **90**(429), 316–320 (1995)

52. Valliant, R., Dorfman, A.H., Royall, R.M.: Finite Population Sampling and Inference: A Prediction Approach. Wiley, New York (2000)
53. Whittle, P.: Probability via Expectation. Springer, New York (2000)
54. Williams, D.: Weighing the Odds: A Course in Probability and Statistics, vol. 548. Springer, New York (2001)
55. Xie, M., Singh, K.: Confidence distribution, the frequentist distribution estimator of a parameter: a review. Int. Stat. Rev. **81**(1), 3–39 (2013)
56. Yang, R., Berger, J.O.: A Catalog of Noninformative Priors. Institute of Statistics and Decision Sciences, Duke University, Durham (1996)
57. Zhang, Z.: A law of likelihood for composite hypotheses. arXiv preprint arXiv:0901.0463 (2009)

Index

© Springer International Publishing Switzerland 2014
C.A. Rohde, *Introductory Statistical Inference with the Likelihood
Function*, DOI 10.1007/978-3-319-10461-4

Printed in the United States
By Bookmasters